Bacteria and
Human Disease

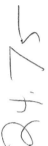

BACTERIA AND HUMAN DISEASE

J. M. Slack, Ph.D.
Professor of Microbiology

and

I. S. Snyder, Ph.D.
Professor and Chairman of Microbiology

West Virginia University Medical Center
Morgantown, West Virginia

YEAR BOOK MEDICAL PUBLISHERS, INC.
CHICAGO • LONDON

1978

Library of Congress Cataloging in Publication Data

Slack, John Madison, 1914–
  Bacteria and human disease.

  Includes index.
  1. Bacteriology, Medical. I. Snyder, Irvin S., joint author. II. Title. [DNLM: 1. Bacteria—Pathogenicity. 2. Disease—Etiology. QZ65 S631b]
QR46.S577   616.01'4   78-55410
ISBN 0-8151-7700-3

To our families who encouraged
and tolerated us and to our
students who helped us learn

Preface

This book provides the student with basic information on the characteristics of pathogenic bacteria, the mechanisms by which these organisms produce disease, and the types of disease they cause. Certain disease states are discussed in depth to give the student a broader insight into the microbiology of these clinical situations. Each chapter on pathogenic organisms ends with a clinical problem and review questions designed to show how microbiology relates to clinical problems. Thereby we hope to enable students at all levels to integrate basic aspects of structure, genetics and mechanisms of pathogenesis, and to understand the prevention and control of infectious disease problems in man.

The book is designed for the student who has little or no background in bacteriology. For this reason chapters have been included on *Bacterial Structures and Their Functions* and on *Host Interactions, Bacterial Pathogenicity and Host Defenses* to give the student a background sufficient for the understanding of the remaining chapters. A chapter entitled *Diagnosis of Bacterial Diseases: Clinical Approach and Laboratory Procedures* is intended to give the student an introduction to methods used for obtaining and handling clinical specimens. The same chapter has a section to orient the student, particularly the medical student, toward use of microbiology in decision-making.

The chapters on pathogenic microbiology are arranged by genus and not by organ systems. There is merit in both approaches but most microbiology courses, including those offered to medical students, are often organized by genus and not by disease or organ system affected.

The authors are indebted to those who permitted us to use figures and photographs from their publications and files.

The following colleagues and friends graciously took the time to read portions of the manuscript and we appreciate their suggestions and criticisms: William Johnson, *University of Iowa College of*

Medicine; S. Kominos, *Mercy Hospital, Pittsburgh, Pennsylvania;* Roger Finch, Herbert Thompson, S. J. Deal, W. K. C. Morgan, Dane Moore, R. G. Burrell, Rama Ganguly, and M. A. Gerencser, *all of the West Virginia University Medical Center.*

J. M. Slack

I. S. Snyder

Contents

Objectives

Perhaps the best way to determine what a textbook is designed to do is to state the objectives or, in other words, what the student should be able to do after completing this textbook. The statements listed below are given as a guide for the teacher and the learner and should be modified to meet one's particular needs.

A. Given the age, sex, environmental conditions, geographic region and symptoms of an infectious disease, the student should be able to do the following:
   1. List the specimens which should be sent to the laboratory
   2. List the organisms which might be found as etiologic agents of disease
   3. Rank order these organisms as to the probability that they are etiologic agents of the disease
   4. Identify the portal of entry and exit for these organisms
   5. Identify the reservoir for the infectious organism and vector
   6. Write a short paragraph on the mechanism by which these organisms are able to establish themselves in the host and cause disease
   7. Write the methods available for prevention and treatment of the disease and give rationale
   8. Write the likelihood of transmission of these organisms to (a) family members; (b) other members of the community

B. Given the age, sex, environmental conditions, geographic region, symptoms, type of specimen collected, and the laboratory report of the organism(s) isolated, the student will be able to interpret the significance of the laboratory findings. The interpretation should include the following aspects:
   1. Whether the laboratory findings are appropriate to the case presented
   2. If the findings are inappropriate, what procedures should be

followed to prevent their recurrence upon the submission of
additional specimens
3. What further tests, if any, should be requested and why these
   tests are necessary

C. Given the type of specimen submitted for isolation and identifica-
    tion of pathogenic microorganisms and a list of suspected micro-
    organisms, the student will be able to indicate the time following
    submission of the specimen to the laboratory at which he might be
    able to obtain the following:
    1. Preliminary information regarding the identification of the
       organism
    2. Final confirmation regarding the identification of the organism

D. Given a list of microorganisms and the specimen from which
    these organisms were isolated, the student should be able to indi-
    cate which organisms are part of the normal flora and indicate
    predominance by rank order.

E. Given a list of infectious diseases, the student should be able to
    indicate the following:
    1. Whether or not antibodies are formed and if antibodies play a
       role in preventing recurrence of the disease
    2. Type of the test used to measure these antibodies
    3. Whether or not immunity is cell mediated
    4. Whether or not hypersensitivity is developed to the etiologic
       agent and methods for measuring this hypersensitivity

1 / Host Interactions, Bacterial Pathogenicity and Host Defenses

OVERVIEW

The human is in constant contact with a wide variety of microorganisms, and the resultant interactions are a dynamic interplay influenced by the attributes of both the host and the microorganism. An appreciation of these interactions is vital, as it is the basis for understanding the initiation of an infectious disease and the subsequent recovery or death of the host. An understanding of these mechanisms of pathogenicity and host defense will help in developing methods for control of disease.

HOST-MICROORGANISM INTERACTIONS

INTERACTIONS.—The interactions between the host and microorganisms are multiple and complex and may be inconsequential, beneficial or harmful. The simple association of host and microorganism is termed symbiosis (living together). Commensalism is that symbiotic relationship in which neither of the participants is benefited or harmed, a situation best exemplified by the normal bacterial flora of the host. However, some of the normal flora produce substances (vitamins K and B) that appear necessary to the host; the host in return offers an abode. This interaction, which is beneficial to both host and microorganism, is a mutualistic form of symbiosis. An interaction which results in harm to the host is termed parasitism, and the organisms are termed pathogens. Some commensals and mutualistic organisms cause disease in an appropriately altered or debilitated host, and under these conditions they are termed opportunists.

The following diagram illustrates the relationships between the host and microbiota:

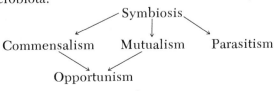

1

BACTERIAL PATHOGENICITY

Pathogens differ from saprophytes in that they are able to: (1) survive in host tissue; (2) multiply; (3) produce substances (such as toxins and extracellular enzymes) that are harmful to the host and (4) survive in transit from one host to the other. These attributes of pathogenicity can be stated as: (1) adaptability, (2) reproducibility (3) toxinogenicity and (4) communicability.

The relative ability of organisms to cause disease (virulence) varies not only between genera but also within species. Organisms that readily survive in transit from one host to the other, are able to multiply in the tissues of the host, or produce large amounts of toxins or more potent toxins are better able to cause disease than those lacking these attributes. Thus, increased survival or production of toxin results in greater virulence. Organisms which cause disease only when present in high concentrations or which generally do not cause serious disease are considered of low virulence. Virulence can be measured in the laboratory by determining the number of organisms which cause a measurable effect in a test system and can be expressed as:

1. number of organisms required to kill 50% of the injected animals = LD_{50}; or
2. number of organisms required to infect 50% of the animals = ID_{50}.

Whether disease will occur after an interaction between the host and a pathogen is determined not only by the virulence of the organism but also by the number of organisms and the resistance of the host as formulated below:

$$D = \frac{nV}{R}$$

D = disease; n = number of organisms; V = virulence of the organism; R = resistance.

In a host with decreased resistance, disease can occur with organisms of low virulence. For example, persons with altered urinary flow or pulmonary function readily become infected by organisms of low virulence such as those which constitute the normal flora, whereas persons with unaltered resistance do not become infected with organisms of low virulence.

Interaction of the host and microorganisms does not always lead to disease (Fig. 1-1). The initial interaction is termed colonization or infection and is defined simply as the presence of microorganisms on tissues of the body. If a clinically manifest injury of the host results

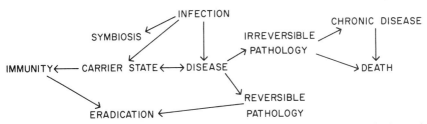

Fig. 1–1.—Results of interaction between a host and a microbe. (Adapted from Simon, H. J.: *Attenuated Infection* [Philadelphia: J. B. Lippincott Co., 1960].)

from this interaction, an infectious disease results which may be reversible or irreversible. Pneumonia caused by *Streptococcus pneumoniae* is usually a reversible disease process, i.e., the architecture and function of pulmonary tissue return to normal after eradication of the organisms. Pneumonia caused by *Klebsiella pneumonia*, however, commonly leads to fibrosis; thus, the architecture and function of the lung tissue remain altered, and such alteration often results in chronic disease, e.g., bronchiectasis. If the damage is extensive, death of the host may ensue. Irrespective of the primary infectious agent, the host usually is susceptible to reinfection with the same organism or may be secondarily infected with a different organism.

In certain diseases the host may continue to harbor the organism after the subsidence of symptoms (carrier state). For example, in a person convalescing from typhoid fever, the gallbladder may become infected and the patient continues to harbor and excrete organisms without evidence of disease. The carrier state may be of short or long duration, and it is significant because this state represents a source of organisms available for transmission to susceptible persons and on occasion for reinfection.

The presence of commensalistic and mutualistic interactions on body surfaces made early studies of the etiology of disease difficult and confusing. Henle in 1840 described the criteria necessary to prove the etiology of an infectious disease. Until Koch applied these criteria, the causal relationship between microorganism and disease was unclear.

The criteria proposed by Henle are known as *Koch's postulates* and state that:

1. The microorganism must regularly be associated with the disease.
2. The observed organism must be grown in pure culture from the lesion.

3. When a pure culture is inoculated into a susceptible animal species, the typical disease must result.
4. The organism must again be demonstrated and grown in pure culture from the experimentally infected animal.

The application of Koch's postulates permitted differentiation of pathogenic organisms from those which constitute the normal flora or indigenous microbiota and also helped differentiate pathogenic species (for example, *Mycobacterium tuberculosis*) from other nonpathogenic bacteria. However, Koch's postulates have not been fulfilled in all diseases of man because of the lack of a susceptible animal or an inability to grow the organism.

EXOTOXINS. — The first description of a specific bacterial product related to disease in humans was the exotoxin of *Corynebacterium diphtheriae* (Roux and Yersin, 1888). In diphtheria, the organism grows on the surface of the oral mucous membranes where it synthesizes and releases a toxin. The toxin first acts locally, causing tissue necrosis; it then spreads to other tissues or organs via the lymphatics and bloodstream where it catalyzes the inactivation of elongation factor II, thereby inhibiting cellular protein synthesis. This interference with the cell metabolism causes local areas of necrosis, and the cumulative effect interferes with organ (particularly kidney, heart and nerves) and body metabolism, which may then result in death from cardiac failure or respiratory paralysis (chap. 10).

The discovery of diphtheria toxin was followed by the demonstration that symptoms of tetanus were also due to an exotoxin (tetanospasmin). *Clostridium tetani,* an anaerobic organism, grows at the site of the infection and releases toxin which travels by retrograde intra-axonal transport to the central nervous system (CNS). In the CNS, it acts on the presynaptic apparatus, disturbing the release of inhibitory transmitters. This results in hyperactivity of motor neurons, causing skeletal muscle spasms and spastic paralysis; paralysis of the respiratory muscles can be fatal (chap. 9). These two discoveries prompted an intensive investigation of almost every pathogen for the production of an exotoxin, and several have now been described (Table 1–1).

ENDOTOXIN AND PEPTIDOGLYCAN. — The endotoxins (Boivin antigens; LPS; pyrogens) were first discovered by Boivin and Mesrobeanu in 1935, and later purified by Westphal and associates. These toxic lipopolysaccharides are complex macromolecules which are part of the cell wall of gram-negative organisms (chap. 13). They differ from exotoxins in many ways (Table 1–2). Their role in causing or

TABLE 1-1.—BACTERIA PRODUCING EXOTOXINS

BACTERIUM	COMMENTS
Bacillus anthracis	Toxin has 3 components which cause edema, hemorrhage and capillary thrombosis.
Clostridium botulinum	Seven antigenic types of the toxin. It is a neurotoxin which prevents release of the transmitter, acetylcholine.
Clostridium perfringens	1. Principal toxin is the enzyme lecithinase which alters membrane structure causing cell lysis. 2. Enterotoxin° which is a heat-labile protein acting in the intestinal tract.
Clostridium tetani	Tetanospasmin acts on the presynaptic apparatus of nerves disturbing release of inhibitory transmitters.
Corynebacterium diphtheriae	Toxin causes inactivation of the elongation factor, thus inhibiting cell protein synthesis.
Escherichia coli	Heat-labile and heat-stabile enterotoxin. Heat-labile toxin has the same action as that of V. cholerae.
Pseudomonas aeruginosa	Heat-labile protein which is cytotoxic and lethal for mice; inactivates elongation factor and thus affects protein synthesis. Its role in human infections is uncertain.
Salmonella enteritidis	Enterotoxin but the mechanism is unknown.
Shigella dysenteriae	Toxin may be cytotoxic for intestinal epithelial cells resulting in diarrhea.
Staphylococcus aureus	1. Enterotoxin which seems to stimulate local neural receptors in the gut with impulses traveling along afferent autonomic fibers to the vomiting center. 2. Exfoliatin which cleaves the epidermis through disruption of the desmosomes. 3. Delta toxin which activates adenyl cyclase.
Streptococcus pyogenes	Erythrotoxin causes an inflammatory reaction and a rash in scarlet fever.
Vibrio cholerae	Heat-labile enterotoxin (choleragen) activates adenyl cyclase resulting in increased cyclic adenosine monophosphate (cAMP). Increased levels of cAMP affect water and electrolyte transport by mucosal cells with resultant diarrhea.

°An enterotoxin is an exotoxin active within the intestinal tract.

mediating the signs and symptoms associated with gram-negative infections is undecided. Suggestions have been made that the LPS may impede host defenses by preventing association of complement with the bacterial cell membrane, and, alternatively, that the host effects are due to activation of complement by endotoxin or through release

TABLE 1-2.—CHARACTERISTICS OF EXOTOXINS
AND ENDOTOXINS

EXOTOXINS	ENDOTOXINS
1. Released from the cell before or after lysis	1. Integral part of cell wall
2. Protein	2. Endotoxin is lipopolysaccharide; lipid is toxic component
3. Heat labile	3. Heat stable
4. Antigenic and immunogenic	4. Antigenic; questionable immunogenicity
5. Toxoids can be produced	5. Toxoids cannot be produced
6. Specific in effect on host	6. Many effects on host
7. Produced by gram-positive and gram-negative organisms	7. Produced by gram-negative organisms

of mediators. Endotoxin is present in the host during infection with certain gram-negative organisms, and studies in man and animals show that endotoxin can cause fever, leukopenia and leukocytosis, changes in hemodynamics and blood clotting mechanism (disseminated intravascular coagulation; DIC). Alterations in blood and liver carbohydrate levels and in synthesis and activity of certain enzymes have also been shown.

The peptidoglycan makes up the basic structure of the bacterial cell wall and is found in all bacteria (gram positive and gram negative) except those which lack cell walls (*Mycoplasma*). It is a disaccharide-peptide polymer (see Figs. 2-2 and 2-3) with biological activities like those of endotoxin. The role of the peptidoglycan in disease is presently under investigation.

SEPTIC SHOCK.—This is a clinical condition described as hemodynamic failure associated with sepsis. Most commonly, septic shock is associated with gram-negative organisms, but it also occurs after infection with gram-positive bacteria, fungi, viruses or rickettsiae. It is characterized by vasospasm of arterioles and venules, microemboli formation and decreased capillary flow. The consequences are poor tissue perfusion, anoxia and cell death. The mechanisms by which shock associated with sepsis occurs are not clear. In animals, endotoxin results in activation of complement and the Hagemann factor, release of lysosomal enzymes and increased adrenergic receptor sensitivity, all of which can contribute to the decrease in tissue perfusion.

DISSEMINATED INTRAVASCULAR COAGULATION (DIC).—This is a condition which occurs in humans with gram-negative sepsis and in animals after injection of endotoxin. Studies in animals suggest that many of the changes occurring after injection of endotoxin (platelet aggregation, thrombocytopenia, endothelial damage, and activation of the Hagemann factor and complement) may account for DIC.

SHWARTZMAN REACTION. — Repeated exposure to endotoxins has been suggested as a means by which microorganisms or their products can cause tissue injury. In rabbits, a subcutaneous injection of endotoxin (preparative injection), followed 18–24 hours later by an intravenous injection (provoking injection) of endotoxin, results in hemorrhage and necrosis at the site of the subcutaneous injection. This reaction occurs within a few hours and is termed a local Shwartzman reaction. Two intravenous injections of endotoxin (preparative and provoking), 24 hours or less apart, result in death of the animal, the primary lesion being bilateral renal cortical necrosis. This type of reaction is called the generalized Shwartzman reaction. Histologically, the vasculature shows the presence of leukocyte-platelet thrombi. Erythrogenic toxin from *Streptococcus pyogenes* can be used in place of endotoxin in production of the Shwartzman reaction. The renal lesions are identical to those obtained with endotoxin and suggest that endotoxin and other bacterial products may act in conjunction to cause tissue injury.

INFLAMMATION. — With very few exceptions (e.g., botulism) a bacterium has to gain entrance into tissue in order to initiate an infection. The entrance is frequently through an injury of the skin or mucous membranes or, in some instances, via a hair follicle or sweat gland. The point of entry may be so small that it is inapparent. Enzymatic reactions have been proposed as a means of entry, but there is no experimental support for this mechanism. After entrance, the bacteria initiate infection through cell injury, which usually begins as inflammation followed by injury and death of cells, migration of leukocytes in response to chemotactic factors and necrosis. Bacteria can initiate inflammation through the activation of complement, which then leads to the formation of vasoactive factors (kinins) causing the release of histamine, which in turn alters the microcirculation. The inflammatory process is discussed further under defense mechanisms.

CELL DEATH AND NECROSIS. — A viable tissue or blood cell must have an intact cell membrane for the bioenergetic systems to function (electron transport, maintenance of ion exchange, regulation of cell volume and substrate transport). In addition, the cell must have an oxygen supply, water, and preferably a slightly alkaline pH. The presence of living bacteria causes injury or death of cells in a variety of ways, such as reducing the amount of available oxygen, producing an acid pH, or utilizing available substrates such as sugars or amino acids. However, a more direct and devastating effect is the alteration or disruption of cell membrane integrity through enzymatic activity, particularly that of lipases. This causes injury and leads to death and lysis of the cell with release of the cell constituents, including cytoplasmic enzymes and lysosomes. Rupture of lysosomal membranes results in release of a wide variety of hydrolytic enzymes which act on proteins, lipids, polysaccharides and nucleic acids. Indirectly, as a result of the presence of bacteria, accumulating granulocytes undergo destruction, releasing lysosomal hydrolases which also contribute to tissue cell injury. Necrosis, or the hydrolytic conversion of dead cells into a mass of debris, results.

Initially, the inflammatory extravascular fluid or exudate is slightly viscous and contains some cellular debris. As the protein, DNA, cell debris and white blood cell content increase, the exudate becomes more viscous and is referred to as pus. Pus accumulates locally and then becomes walled-off by fibroblasts and collagen fibers to form an abscess. At any given site the formation of exudate, pus and necrosis may take place at the same time. It should be noted that the inflammation-to-necrosis sequence can occur in the absence of bacteria (e.g., burns, chemicals), although pus formation is usually not as evident.

ALTERATION OF THE TISSUE ENVIRONMENT. — Bacteria, as well as other invading microorganisms, synthesize their own proteins, carbohydrates and lipids from organic sources of carbon and nitrogen (heterotrophs). Therefore, bacteria in tissue must obtain these necessary nutrients and minerals from plasma, cell constituents, or both. In addition, water, usually oxygen, and a space in which to grow are required by the invading organism. Further, the bacteria have a fast metabolic rate; they synthesize and release extracellular enzymes and are resistant to conditions of low oxygen and pH variation. In addition to producing substances which harm tissue cells, bacteria are more than able to successfully compete with the tissue cells for nutrients, O_2 and H_2O, which results in injury and usually death of the host cells.

ANTIPHAGOCYTIC FACTORS. — During the inflammatory response, the cells migrating through the vessel wall are primarily the polymorphonuclear leukocytes (neutrophils, polys, PMNs). The PMN response is soon supplemented by mononuclear phagocytes or macrophages (derived primarily from blood monocytes). These two cell types, of primary importance in host defense, engulf and promptly kill most invading bacteria. However, certain bacteria are antiphagocytic because of the presence of a capsule *(Streptococcus pneumoniae, Bacillus anthracis)* or other surface components (M protein of *Streptococcus pyogenes*, Vi antigen of *Salmonella typhi*). These structures are the virulence factors for these organisms. In other instances the organism grows and multiplies within the phagocyte *(Mycobacterium tuberculosis, Listeria monocytogenes)*, which is then a protective environment and may even provide a means of spread. The filamentous growth of some organisms *(Actinomyces, Nocardia)* also acts as a mechanical barrier to phagocytosis. In *Actinomyces* the formation of a protein-polysaccharide complex around these filaments contributes to the antiphagocytic ability. The clumping of *Staphylococcus aureus* is also antiphagocytic. In addition, organisms may multiply faster than the rate of phagocytosis, or cytotoxins (hemolysins of *Staphylococcus aureus* and *Streptococcus pyogenes*) may be produced which cause death of the phagocyte. Although bacteria have a variety of antiphagocytic factors, phagocytosis remains an effective means for the host to overcome invading organisms.

ENZYMES. — Bacteria have highly refined mechanisms which respond to the environment by regulating the rate of synthesis and activ-

TABLE 1–3. — BACTERIAL ENZYMES THAT MAY HAVE A ROLE IN PATHOGENICITY

ENZYME	SUBSTRATE	COMMENTS
Coagulase	Fibrinogen	Results in clotting of plasma
Collagenase	Collagen	Results in breakdown of collagen fibers
Deoxyribonuclease	DNA	Cleaves DNA to nucleotides; liquefies pus
Elastase	Elastin	May act on fibrous connective tissue
Glycosidase	Glycoproteins	May release sugars from tissue
Hyaluronidase	Hyaluronic acid	Breaks down the cement between cells
IgA protease	IgA$_1$	Cleaves the proline-threonine bond of IGA$_1$
Lecithinase	Lecithin	Disrupts cell membranes
Lipase	Lipids	Disrupts cell membranes
Neuraminidase	Acetylneuramic acid	Damages cell membranes
Nicotinamide adenine dinucleotidase	NAD	Could interfere with electron transport
Protease	Proteins	Alters cell structure and metabolism
Ribonuclease	RNA	Cleaves RNA to nucleotides
Streptokinase	Plasminogen	Causes hydrolysis of fibrin
Urease	Urea	May be nephrotoxic

ity of a given enzyme. Most of these enzymes are intracellular, but a number of extracellular enzymes—primarily hydrolases—degrade macromolecules such as proteins, lipids, polysaccharides and nucleic acids. These extracellular enzymes could act as pathogenic factors by: (1) directly attacking tissue membranes or blood cells (lipases); (2) interfering with cell function (nucleases); (3) hydrolyzing cell proteins (proteases) and (4) cleaving antibody such as IgA and thereby inactivating the antibody. The cell products released by these enzymatic reactions would then be available for utilization by the invading bacterium. Experimental support for the direct action of such enzymes is lacking except in the case of *Clostridium perfringens*, for which lecithinase is the major pathogenic factor. The bacterial enzymes that have been implicated in pathogenicity are listed in Table 1–3.

HEMOLYSINS AND LEUKOCIDINS.—A hemolytic bacterium causes either complete or partial lysis of red blood cells. This is usually determined by streaking the organisms onto a blood agar plate and, after incubation, observing the change in the erythrocytes around the bacterial colony. This change is referred to as alpha or beta hemolysis or no hemolysis, as follows.

Alpha hemolysis is a green zone around the colony. The green color may be due to: (1) the action of peroxides or hyaluronidase, (2) formation of methemoglobin or (3) formation of an iron-containing derivative of hemoglobin.

Beta hemolysis is a clear zone around the colony due to complete lysis of the erythrocytes.

No hemolysis (gamma hemolysis) means that the bacterium has no visible action on the erythrocytes and there is little or no change around the colony.

With the possible exception of the lytic action of lecithinase in gas gangrene, there is little concrete evidence that beta hemolysins cause sufficient alteration of the red blood cells in human infections to cause anemia, but a number of these hemolysins are cytotoxic. This cytotoxic action causes injury or lysis of neutrophils, macrophages, lysosomes or tissue cells, and in so doing could be: (1) an antiphagocytic factor, (2) the cause of death of phagocytes after ingestion of the organisms, (3) a stimulant to inflammation or (4) the cause of death of tissue cells facilitating the spread of the organism during the infection. Table 1–4 lists some of the beta hemolysins that have been shown to be cytotoxic. In addition, some species or strains of *Haemophilus, Vibrio, Escherichia* and *Pseudomonas* are beta hemolytic, but these have not been adequately studied in relation to cytotoxicity.

TABLE 1-4.—BACTERIA PRODUCING CYTOTOXIC
BETA HEMOLYSINS

HEMOLYSIN	ORGANISM	CYTOTOXIC FOR TYPES OF HUMAN CELLS			
		ERYTHRO-CYTES	NEUTRO-PHILS	MACRO-PHAGES	TISSUE CELLS
Streptolysin O°	*Streptococcus pyogenes*	+	+	±	+
Streptolysin S	''	+	+	+	+
Alpha†	*Staphylococcus aureus*	±	−	+	+
Beta	''	+	±	−	+
Delta	''	+	+	+	+
Alpha‡	*Clostridium perfringens*	+	+	+	+

°Essentially, the same hemolysin is produced by streptococcal groups B, C and G, *Streptococcus pneumoniae, Clostridium tetani, C. perfringens, C. histolyticum, Listeria monocytogenes* and *Bacillus cereus.*
†The terminologies become confusing as these Greek letters are applied to three different hemolysins, but all cause beta hemolysis.
‡This is lecithinase C, which is an enzyme and also designated as the α-toxin. This point emphasizes that the distinction among enzymes, exotoxins and hemolysins is fine, if it exists at all.

All of the hemolysins listed above could be termed leukocidins. In fact, *Streptococcus pyogenes* was considered a classic example of an organism that produced a specific leukocidin, but this product was later demonstrated to be a beta hemolysin and is now termed streptolysin S. However, *Staphylococcus aureus* produces a nonhemolytic leukocidin (Panton-Valentine factor; P-V) which is a complex of two proteins. This complex is specific in that it links only to the surface of leukocytes and not to the surfaces of other cells; the P-V leukocidin is an antiphagocytic factor of *S. aureus* (chap. 5).

HOST FACTORS CONTRIBUTING TO DISEASE OR RESISTANCE

AGE.—In an infant, resistance to disease is a reflection of passive immunity acquired in utero by placental transfer of IgG. This resistance is only partial as, for example, newborns are susceptible to infections with enterics because of the inability of antibody to these organisms (IgM) to be placentally transferred. Also, during the first year the infant is more susceptible to infection because of the lack of active immunological experience with bacterial and viral agents. In later life the immunological responses diminish and the functional ability of the host tissue is impaired, providing increased susceptibility, particularly to respiratory and urinary tract infections.

SEX, HORMONES AND NUTRITION.—The male has a higher incidence of infection than the female (except in the urinary tract); this is probably associated with increased exposure at work or while traveling. Hormonal imbalances are associated with an increased susceptibility to infections, as in Addison's disease (hypoadrenalism), Cushing's disease (hyperadrenalism) and diabetes; in the last there is an increased susceptibility to pyelonephritis, tuberculosis, and staphylococcal and fungal infections. Malnutrition increases the occurrence and severity of infections such as tuberculosis, whooping cough and measles, and there is evidence that antibody synthesis is reduced in persons with protein deficiencies. Although not directly applicable to humans, animal experiments show that deficiencies in vitamins A, C and riboflavin, a reduced protein diet, or a limited food intake results in decreased resistance to bacterial, rickettsial and helminthic infections.

OPPORTUNISM.—Infections are encountered in hosts with an alteration in the inflammatory process, phagocytosis, immune response, tissue metabolism or tissue integrity. The responsible microorganisms (termed opportunists) are frequently part of the normal flora or those commonly found in the environment, including *Escherichia, Pseudomonas, Klebsiella, Serratia, Bacteroides, Listeria, Nocardia, Candida, Aspergillus, Cryptococcus, Pneumocystis*, cytomegalovirus or herpesvirus. Such infections may be severe, difficult to treat, and even life-threatening. Certain opportunities for invasion have always been present, but they have increased with the more complex surgical, medical and chemotherapeutic techniques. The principal conditions which promote infection by opportunistic organisms are as follows: (1) burns which destroy tissue and alter skin flora; (2) corticosteroid therapy which depresses inflammation and antibody formation; (3) immunosuppressive or irradiation therapy which can cause neutropenia, depress antibody formation or cause cell injury; (4) malignancies such as leukemia, lymphomas or Hodgkin's disease which interfere with cell function; (5) diabetes or renal or hepatic failure which deranges metabolic balances; (6) antimetabolite or alkylating drugs which suppress immune responses; (7) obstruction of fluid or blood flow in such organ systems as urinary, intestinal, respiratory tracts or bile ducts, which then interferes with blood supply and cell metabolism; (8) prolonged antibiotic therapy which alters normal flora or selects resistant bacterial strains and (9) catheters or prostheses which damage tissue and interfere with blood flow.

NOSOCOMIAL INFECTIONS (infections of hospital origin).—The advent of antibiotic therapy in the 1940s resulted in a relaxation of attention to aseptic and hygienic techniques in hospitals. Outbreaks of infections with *Staphylococcus aureus*, phage type 80/81, (chap. 5), were reported with increasing frequency in nurseries and in postoperative patients. This prompted a drastic revision of patient-care procedures and resulted in the introduction of surveillance techniques and the employment of personnel trained in infection control. These changes, along with improved therapies, including the more careful selection and use of antibiotics, have reduced the incidence of nosocomial infections. However, nosocomial infections, due mostly to gram-negative bacteria, continue to be a serious problem. These infections cause an increase in morbidity and mortality and extend hospital occupancy, adding millions of dollars annually to patient-care costs. This problem will remain because nosocomial infections are basically dependent on an altered host-parasite relationship. The host is a patient who has entered the hospital because of some alteration in metabolism, tissue function or architecture. In the hospital the resistance of the patient is altered as a result of being subjected to complex diagnostic and therapeutic procedures. Under these conditions the parasite (bacterium, virus or fungus) encounters a host with lowered resistance and is thus able to more easily invade and multiply in the host. The parasite may be from (1) the normal flora of the host, (2) contact or droplets from attending personnel or other patients, (3) hospital equipment such as respirators or (4) uncooked foods such as lettuce or other vegetables. In addition, the hospital environment harbors an increased number of parasites, and some of these may have an increased virulence for the host and be resistant to chemotherapy.

HYPERSENSITIVITY.—The concept of immune injury as a cause of disease is well accepted. Immunological reactions to infectious agents must be considered when one studies the pathogenesis of infectious diseases even though such reactions may also favor host defenses. The currently recognized four major types of immune injury are illustrated in Figure 1–2.

Type I reactions are dependent on antibodies of the IgE class. These reaginic antibodies fix to mast cells or basophils in such a manner that when the antibodies react with their specific antigen the cell membrane is stressed and the cells secrete pharmacologically active substances. This leads to the symptoms of immediate hypersensitivity as seen in allergic reactions.

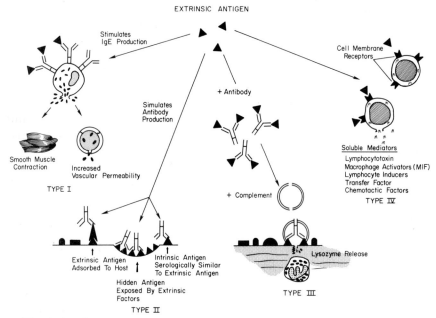

Fig. 1–2.—Summation of the four types of immunologic injury. (From diagram by Burrell, R. G., Morgan, W. K. C., and Seaton, A. (eds): in *Occupational Lung Diseases* [Philadelphia: W. B. Saunders Co., 1975]. Used by permission.)

Type II reactions are due to antibodies reacting directly with antigens on host cells. Such antigens may be extrinsic (not a component of the host), which nonspecifically adsorb to the host cells, or intrinsic.

In rheumatic fever there is considerable evidence that the cytoplasmic membranes of *Streptococcus pyogenes* share antigens with myocardial tissue. The antibodies formed in response to these antigens react with the cardiac tissue, causing tissue cytotoxicity.

Type III reactions are due to circulating antigen complexing with antibodies. This soluble complex deposits at certain anatomic sites, fixes complement and stimulates neutrophils to release proteolytic enzymes which causes tissue damage. Such reactions are involved in the nephritis of systemic lupus erythematosus, poststreptococcal glomerulonephritis and in the Arthus phenomenon.

The *Arthus* reaction is a localized reaction occurring when the antigen-antibody reaction aggregates in tissue and activates complement. Chemotactic factors, formed by activation of complement, attract neutrophils which release lysosomal enzymes resulting in a destructive inflammation of small blood vessels and then edema and hemorrhage. The reaction develops slowly (4–8 hours) but usually subsides in 24 hours with destruction of the antigen; serum can passively transfer the reaction to other animals. Mild and severe Arthus reactions have been reported following repeated injections of antisera, certain vaccines and globulins.

Type IV reactions are due to cell-mediated immune reactions and not to humoral antibodies. Specifically sensitized T-lymphocytes, arising in response to the foreign antigen, react with that antigen, become metabolically active and secrete macromolecular mediators which possess a variety of biological activities, including (1) chemotaxis, (2) inhibition of the migration of macrophages, (3) enhancement of cell transformation and (4) cytotoxicity for tissue cells. Macrophages and lymphocytes accumulate at the reaction site, resulting in swelling of tissue (edema and induration). The tissue damage is due primarily to lysosomal enzyme release from the macrophages with some participation by cytotoxic factors from the lymphocytes.

The classic example of a delayed hypersensitivity reaction is that caused by *Mycobacterium tuberculosis*, in which there is vascular damage, necrosis and tubercle formation. This is harmful to the host, causing death and necrosis of cells, but at the same time it is beneficial by walling-off the area of infection to prevent spread. Localized hypersensitivity reactions occur in infections due to *Staphylococcus aureus, Streptococcus pyogenes, Brucella,* many fungi and certain viruses. These reactions may contribute to the inflammatory responses, but to what extent this aids the pathogenicity of the organism is difficult to evaluate.

STRUCTURAL BARRIERS.—The human body is a closed system covered with skin and lined with mucous membranes which together provide an efficient barrier to bacteria. The skin with its epidermal and dermal layers is normally impervious to bacteria, and reports of penetration by *Yersinia pestis* and *Treponema pallidum* through the intact skin have not been substantiated. In addition to presenting a physical barrier, the skin continually sheds keratinized cells, thereby reducing associated microbial cells. Also, the skin is bathed with an acidic oily emulsion containing unsaturated fatty acids and lysozyme which may be bactericidal to some organisms. The only breaks in the surface barriers are the sweat glands, hair follicles and sebaceous glands, all of which offer possible points of penetration through the intact skin.

The conjunctiva, nose, oropharynx, stomach, intestinal tract and genitourinary tract are covered with a relatively thin mucous membrane. This protective covering in the various areas is supplemented by (1) the adhesive quality of the mucus which traps organisms; (2) the flowing action and lysozyme content of the tears; (3) the ciliary action in the respiratory tract which keeps the mucus stream, with enmeshed bacteria, flowing towards the trachea; (4) the cough reflex; (5) the epiglottal reflex preventing aspiration of large particles; (6) the acidity and enzyme content of the gastric juices; (7) the peristaltic action of the intestinal tract; (8) the flushing action of the urine, along with its acidity and osmolarity and (9) the acidity of the vaginal tract. Any alteration in the mechanism for removal of bacteria, such as the absence of lacrimation, reduced peristaltic action or interference with the cough reflex, may permit excessive bacterial multiplication and can result in a serious infection.

The alveoli are normally free of bacteria and are kept that way by a combination of processes including filtration, mucus flow, cough reflex, and phagocytosis and by humoral and cellular immune mechanisms. The respiratory tract and lungs are continually exposed to particles of dust, carbon, microorganisms or droplets which are normally

Fig. 1–3.—Cilia of a human bronchiole. Scanning electron micrograph. (Courtesy of R. V. Ebert, Department of Medicine, University of Minnesota.)

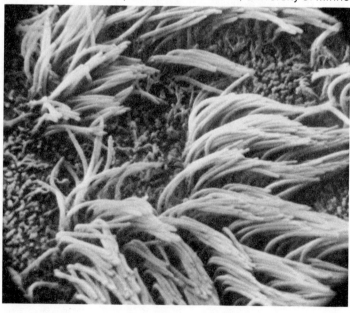

removed prior to reaching the alveoli. This removal process begins with the filtering action of the mucus-covered hairs and cilia, whereby the particles become enmeshed in the mucus, either by direct impaction or by gravitation, and eventually are eliminated by swallowing or expectoration. Particles 10 μm or larger are usually removed in the nasal cavity, nasopharynx or bronchi. Particles 2–10 μm are removed in the bronchi and bronchioles, and those 0.2–2.0 μm are removed in the bronchioles. The smaller particles remain suspended in air and are most likely to reach the alveoli. From the trachea to the terminal bronchioles, the mucociliary system is most active.

The cilia (Fig. 1–3) keep the mucus stream moving toward the trachea at a rate of 10–20 mm/hr resulting in removal, within an hour, of 90% of the particles reaching the area. The filtration system is then aided, as necessary, by (1) the cough reflex, (2) phagocytosis by alveolar macrophages and (3) secretory IgA and other immune mechanisms.

PHAGOCYTOSIS. — When bacteria bypass the structural barriers of the host, inflammation begins. Chemotactic factors are released, which then attract motile leukocytes to the site, and phagocytosis begins. The neutrophil (polymorphonuclear leukocyte, PMN) is the most active phagocytic cell (Fig. 1–4). Phagocytosis consists of three activities: attachment of the microorganism to the surface of the phagocytic cell, ingestion and digestion. This process is facilitated by an alteration of the surface of the microorganism by opsonin, which may be either specific antibodies that react with the particular organisms or nonspecific serum constituents. However, opsonization is not mandatory for phagocytosis to occur.

The exact nature of the chemotactic factors is not known, but when they, along with complement (primarily C5a), reach a critical concentration at the surface of the PMN, there is increased metabolic activity, including increased consumption of O_2, influx of calcium, activation of the hexose monophosphate (HMP) shunt and production of H_2O_2. Microfilaments and microtubules assemble and provide for motility of the PMN towards the bacterium. When the PMN makes contact with the bacterium, C3b fixed to the bacterial surface attaches or binds to receptors on the PMN membrane initiating an invagination of the cell membrane to form a vacuole, the phagosome. The bacterium is then engulfed through a combination of the physical forces of surface tension and the contraction of microfilaments and microtubules. The phagosome then migrates toward the interior of the cell. The membranes of the cytoplasmic granules fuse with the phagosome membrane and discharge hydrolytic enzymes into the vacuole or phagoly-

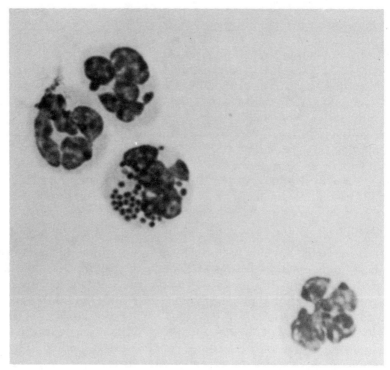

Fig. 1–4.—Phagocytosis of *Staphylococcus aureus* by a polymorphonuclear leukocyte. Wright stain of peritoneal exudate from a mouse injected with *S. aureus.* (Courtesy of M. A. Melly, Division of Infectious Diseases, Vanderbilt University.)

sosome. This process is termed degranulation. There are at least three types of granules: the primary or azurophils, the secondary or specific granules and the tertiary granules. The tertiary granules are small and apparently without an antimicrobial role. The secondary granules seem to degranulate first, releasing lactoferrin and lysozyme followed by the primary granules, releasing myeloperoxidase (MPO), lysozyme, cationic proteins and hydrolytic enzymes.

The ingested bacterium is usually killed within 5–30 minutes (some, such as *Mycobacterium tuberculosis*, survive) as the result of mechanisms either independent of or dependent on H_2O_2. Microbicidal systems independent of H_2O_2 include the action of cationic proteins, elastase, lactoferrin or lysozyme (and probably additional substances), which are liberated by the granules and concentrate in the phagolysosome. The cationic proteins alter the bacterial cytoplasmic membrane; lysozyme acts on the peptidoglycan of the cell wall. The microbicidal action of lactoferrin may be due to its binding of iron. Hydrogen peroxide-dependent systems include the direct action of H_2O_2 and, particularly, the H_2O_2-myeloperoxidase-halide system. The mechanism of action of the latter is not established but H_2O_2 + MPO + Cl$^-$ can cleave peptides from the cell wall and oxidatively decarboxylate amino acids to form aldehydes which may be microbicidal. However, as both mycoplasmae and viruses are susceptible to this system, a cell wall is not always necessary for its action. Neutrophils can also generate superoxide ($O_2{}^-$) which can be bactericidal, although certain bacteria synthesize the inactivating enzyme superoxide dismutase. Thus, the intracellular killing of bacteria is a complex, multifaceted process which is still to be entirely elucidated.

The monocytes of the blood (8–10% of white cells) have limited phagocytic power, but they migrate into the connective tissue during inflammation and are precursors of the tissue mononuclear phagocytes (macrophages), which include the alveolar macrophages of the lung and fixed macrophages in the liver (Kupffer cell), spleen, bone marrow and lymph nodes. These cells are large (25–50 μm) active phagocytes which can divide. They remove and destroy bacteria, damaged tissue, blood cells, neoplastic cells, antigens, colloidal material and macromolecules. These are the scavenger cells of the body. They can also transform into epithelioid cells or giant cells. The process of phagocytosis by macrophages is essentially the same as that described for the neutrophil, although the method of bacterial killing is more dependent on alteration of the bacterial surface and enzymatic digestion (particularly by lysosomal hydrolases). Macrophages do not contain cationic protein or the bactericidal H_2O_2-myeloperoxidase system. They are active against both gram-positive and gram-negative bacteria, although certain organisms can survive and even multiply within the nonsensitized macrophage including *Mycobacterium tuberculosis, Listeria monocytogenes, Brucella abortus, Salmonella typhi* and *Francisella tularensis*. Some workers propose that the macrophage processes antigens in some way so that information is transmitted to immunologically competent cells to stimulate antibody synthesis, but this process needs further clarification and substantiation.

INFLAMMATION. — This reaction in the host is usually precipitated by some type of injury (microorganism, cut, bruise, burn). The inflammatory response is due to a disruption of the microcirculation (capillaries and venules), resulting in vasodilation, transudation of plasma proteins and cellular emigration. The mechanisms of vascular injury are not entirely established, but mediators—primarily histamine—are involved. These cause the endothelial cells to contract, resulting in widening of intercellular junctions and escape of plasma proteins. First, plasma cells and leukocytes stick to the injured endothelium. This is then followed by migration (diapedesis) of neutrophils and monocytes between the endothelial cells into the surrounding tissue. These reactions account for the signs of inflammation: namely, redness, swelling, heat and pain. This process is a host response, resulting in the accumulation of phagocytic cells, antimicrobial factors and tissue responses which combine in an attempt to contain the invading bacteria.

ANTIBODIES. — These are globulins formed in response to an antigen and which react specifically with that antigen. The antigen stimulates either plasma cells or lymphocytes to synthesize any one of the five classes of immunoglobulins (Ig). These classes are distinguishable on the basis of molecular weight, sedimentation constant ($S_{20, w}$), chemical structure and biological activity.

IgM (MW 890,000 – 1,000,000; 19S) is the first antibody to be detected (7 days) after the injection of an antigen. It readily agglutinates particulate antigens such as bacteria and erythrocytes, fixes complement, does not cross the placenta and has a half-life of 5 days.

IgG (MW 150,000; 7S) begins to appear 10–14 days after the initial antigen injection. If a second injection (booster) is given, there is a marked increase in the amount and reactivity of the antibody. It is the principal antibody responsible for immunity to bacterial, viral, fungal and parasitic diseases. IgG crosses the placenta, thus affording passive immunity to an infant. It has a half-life of 23 days and is also able to fix complement.

IgA (MW 170,000; 7, 11, 15S) is referred to as secretory IgA because it is the principal antibody in exocrine secretions including respiratory, intestinal and genitourinary mucin, saliva, tears and milk. When antigens enter the body via inhalation, ingestion, or contact with the conjunctivas, they stimulate cells to produce IgA. This antibody is active in preventing invasion through mucosal surfaces. For example, oral live polio vaccine stimulates IgA, which then prevents virus invasion through the nasopharynx or intestinal tract. IgA can fix complement but only by the alternative pathway; it does not pass the placenta and has a 6-day half-life.

IgE (MW 200,000; 8S) is an antibody termed reagin and is responsible for activating allergic (immediate hypersensitivity) reactions such as hay fever, asthma and anaphylaxis. It is found only in minute amounts in normal serum, fixes complement by the alternative pathway, does not pass the placenta and has a 2.5-day half-life.

IgD (MW 180,000; 7S) does not fix complement; it has a 3-day half-life. Little is known about the activity of this antibody.

The immunoglobulins (particularly IgG, IgM and IgA) serve the host by providing humoral immunity. This is brought about by the specific reactions of agglutination, precipitation, neutralization or opsonization of the invading organism, toxin or foreign antigen. Aggregation and opsonization are particularly important in facilitating phagocytosis by neutrophils and macrophages. The exception to these benefits is IgE, which activates the local and systemic allergic reactions, although this antibody may play a role in recovery from intestinal helminth infections.

COMPLEMENT. — This is a complex constituent of normal serum consisting of eleven plasma proteins (C1q, C1r, C1s, C2, C3, C4, C5, C6, C7, C8 and C9); complement levels do not increase with immunization. Complement is involved in a number of biological activities including cell lysis (erythrocyte, bacteria, tissue), chemotaxis, adherence of particles to leukocytes (opsonization), alteration of blood vessel permeability and enhancement of phagocytosis. The fixation or "cascading" of complement can be initiated through the classic pathway. There is first an antigen-antibody (IgG or IgM) reaction, and then the C1q binds to the antibody, followed by C4-C2-C3-C5 through C9. Certain substances such as immune complexes of IgA and inulin do not fix complement by the classic sequence but initiate a bypass or alternative pathway (C3 shunt), beginning with activation with the C3 component. Complement activation usually benefits the host by increasing the susceptibility of bacteria, viruses and other particles to phagocytosis and by causing lysis of gram-negative bacteria, but under certain conditions it can be detrimental through initiating localized inflammatory reactions and tissue necrosis.

FEVER. — The elevation of body temperature is a common manifestation of disease and is related to inflammation. Neutrophils, or macrophages, are stimulated by bacteria, viruses, fungi, protozoa, endotoxins or other factors in exudate to produce an endogenous pyrogen. This pyrogen is a protein which acts on the thermoregulating centers of the hypothalamus to initiate the physiologic responses resulting in fever. This reaction is diagrammed·as follows:

Neutrophil or Macrophage	+	Exogenous pyrogen (e.g., endotoxin)	→	Endogenous pyrogen (host protein)
Endogenous pyrogen	+	Hypothalamus	→	Fever

It is stated that fever is beneficial in overcoming an infection, but experimental proof is lacking.

SUPPLEMENTARY READING

Bernheimer, A. W.: Interactions between membranes and cytolytic bacterial toxins, Biochim. Biophys. Acta 344:27–50, 1974.

Brachman, P. S., and Eickoff, T. C. (eds.): *Proceedings of the International Conference on Nosocomial Infections* (Chicago: American Hospital Association, 1971).

Ellen, R. P., and Gibbons, R. J.: Parameters affecting the adherence and tissue tropisms of *Streptococcus pyogenes*, Infect. Immun. 9:85-91, 1974.

Green, G. M.: Pulmonary clearance of infectious agents, Annu. Rev. Med. 19: 315–336, 1968.

Klainer, A. S., and Beisel, W. R.: Opportunistic infection: A review, Am. J. Med. Sci. 258:431-456, 1969.

Mudd, S.: *Infectious Agents and Host Reactions* (Philadelphia: W. B. Saunders Co., 1970).

Simon, H. J.: *Attenuated Infection* (Philadelphia: J. B. Lippincott Co., 1960).

Smith, H.: *Microbial Pathogenicity in Man and Animals*, Symposium, Society for General Microbiology (Cambridge: Cambridge University Press, 1972).

Taylor, C. E., and De Sweemer, C.: Nutrition and infection, World Rev. Nutr. Diet 16:203–225, 1973.

Zweifach, B. W., Grant, L., and McCluskey, R. T. (eds): *The Inflammatory Process*, Vols. 1, 2 and 3 (New York: Academic Press, 1973).

2 / Bacterial Structures and Their Functions: Nomenclature

OVERVIEW

Bacteria are unicellular organisms which are morphologically and biochemically quite complex. With few exceptions they are encased in a rigid cell wall which maintains the shape of the organism, i.e., coccus, rod, or spiral. The structure of the cell wall is important because interaction with the host's defense mechanism occurs at the cell wall. Also, many antibiotics have their effect on cell wall synthesis. In addition, the cell wall contains biologically active components, for example, endotoxin and peptidoglycan, which participate in production of disease. The cytoplasmic membrane is an active transport site and protects against variation in osmotic pressure. The cell membrane, in addition to its role in the physiology of the organism, is the site of damage in certain immunological reactions and by certain antibiotics. There may also be various structures adherent to the cell wall (capsule) or penetrating through the cell wall (flagella, pili) which may aid the organism in resisting phagocytosis or in adhering to cell surfaces, or which serve as organs of motility. Certain bacteria produce spores, a bacterial form that is resistant to physical and chemical agents and enables the organism to survive adverse conditions. As with all living organisms, bacterial cells have ribosomes and nuclear material. Alterations in the DNA, or in the acquisition of DNA, result in a change in the properties of the organism, reflected by resistance to chemotherapeutic agents, the ability to produce a toxin, or a change in the bacterial surface which enables the organism to resist phagocytosis. Figure 2–1 is a diagrammatic representation of most of these structures.

CELL WALL

All bacteria, except *Mycoplasma* and *Halobacterium*, are surrounded by a rigid cell wall which (1) maintains the shape of the cell, (2)

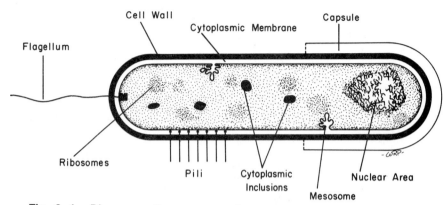

Fig. 2–1.—Diagrammatic representation of microscopic and submicroscopic structures found on or in both gram-positive and gram-negative bacteria. Most of these structures are demonstrable only by special staining techniques or by electron microscopy and are not visible in gram-stained preparations or by the usual laboratory methods of observing bacteria.

determines the gram reaction, (3) contributes to the antigenicity of the cell, (4) provides phage receptor sites and (5) serves as the site of action for certain antibiotics. All bacterial cell walls have as a common structural unit the peptidoglycan, a large macromolecule which forms a meshwork around the entire cell, and which is responsible for the tensile strength and shape of the cell. Linked to or closely associated with the peptidoglycan are a number of proteins, lipoproteins and carbohydrates. These latter compounds supplement cell wall function by adding specificity to the antigens, contributing to pathogenic-

Fig. 2–2.—Amino sugars of the peptidoglycan.

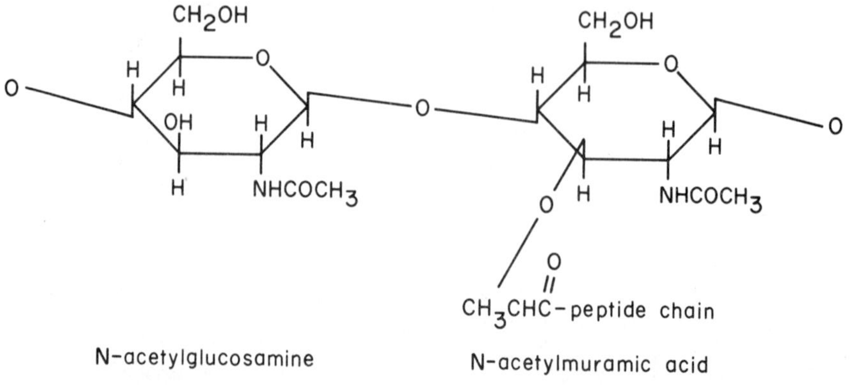

N-acetylglucosamine   N-acetylmuramic acid

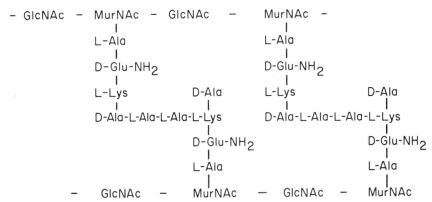

Fig. 2–3.—Diagrammatic representation of the peptidoglycan of *Strep-tococcus pyogenes.*

ity by an antiphagocytic effect and providing receptor sites for phages and antibodies.

Peptidoglycan (murein, mucopeptide) is a heteropolymer composed of glycan strands linked by short peptides. The glycan (Figs. 2–2, 2–3) consists of equimolar concentrations of alternating N-acetylglucosamine and N-acetylmuramic acid residues (N-glycolylmuramic acid in *Mycobacterium*) which are β-1, 4 linked; the chain length varies from 10 to 65 disaccharide units. A peptide chain (Figs. 2–2, 2–4) is bound to the carboxyl group of N-acetylmuramic acid and is composed of alternating L- and D-amino acids, which are usually L-alanine, D-glutamic acid, L-lysine and a terminal D-alanine. Substitutions for these amino acids can occur as listed in Table 2–1. The peptide chains are cross-linked (Figs. 2–3, 2–4) with peptide subunits or bridges extending from the ε-amino group of L-lysine on one chain to the carboxyl group of D-alanine on another chain. In gram-positive bacteria there is extensive cross-linking by peptide subunits, but in gram-negative organisms there is only intermittent linkage between the peptide chains themselves (Fig. 2–4). The structure of the peptidoglycan for any particular organism is constant, but changes may occur under abnormal growth conditions. The synthesis of the peptidoglycan requires a complex sequence of enzymatic steps involving at least 20 different enzymes. There is a partial assembly in the cytoplasm with this complex being transported through the membrane, and then a final assembly of the glycan with cross-linking by transpeptidation occurring outside the membrane.

GRAM-POSITIVE BACTERIA.—The cell wall of these organisms is a

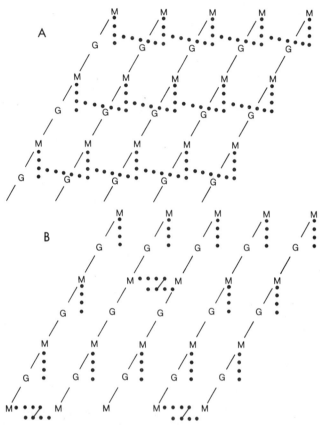

Fig. 2–4.—Diagrammatic representation of the cross-linkages between the peptide chains of the peptidoglycan. **A,** extensive cross-linking found in gram-positive bacteria. The vertical dots indicate the peptide chains and the horizontal dots the cross-linking chain. **B,** intermittent cross-linking through the bonding of two peptide chains (no cross-linking bridges) as found in gram-negative bacteria.

rather dense, uniform layer varying from 200 to 800 Å in thickness (Fig 2–5). It is composed primarily of the peptidoglycan (Figs. 2–3, 2–4), which may be linked to polysaccharides, teichoic acids, teichuronic acid, mycolic acids and proteins. A chemical analysis of hydrolysates of such cell walls may show monosaccharides such as arabinose, galactose, glucose or mannose which may act as specific antigenic determinants and be used to determine either species or serotypes within a species. The source of these sugars is cell wall-associated polysaccharides or glycans.

TABLE 2-1.—VARIATIONS IN THE PEPTIDE CHAIN AND THE CROSS-LINK WITHIN THE PEPTIDOGLYCAN*

COMMON SEQUENCE†	VARIATION†	CROSS-LINK VARIATIONS‡
L-Ala	Gly, L-Ser	None§
D-Glu	Glu-NH$_2$, Gly	(L-Ala)$_{2; 3; 4}$; (L-Ala)$_4$-L-Thr
L-Lys	Dap, Dab, L-Orn	D-Asp-L-Ala
	L-Ala, L-Glu	D-Asp-NH$_2$
D-Ala	(always terminal)	(Gly)$_{2; 5; 6}$
		(Gly)$_3$-(L-Ser)$_2$
		L-Ser-L-Ala

Abbreviations: Ala = alanine; Asp = aspartic acid; Dap = diaminopimelic acid; Dab = diaminobutyric acid; Glu = glutamic acid; Gly = glycine; Orn = ornithine; Ser = serine; Thr = threonine.

*This is not a complete listing but includes the majority of variations. These occur primarily in gram-positive bacteria.
†The usual sequence is L-Ala-D-Glu-L-Lys-D-Ala. Most, but not all, the variations are listed opposite each amino acid; the D-Ala is quite stable, and if there is no cross-linkage there is a terminal dipeptide, D-alanyl-D-alanine.
‡These are linkages between the L-lysine of one chain and the D-alanine of another chain; most variations in the peptidoglycan occur in this linkage.
§There is a direct bonding of the NH$_2$ of L-lysine to the COOH of D-alanine.

GRAM-NEGATIVE BACTERIA.—The cell wall of these organisms is considerably more complex than the gram-positive cell wall. The wall contains at least two layers: the inner layer is the rigid peptidoglycan layer (15–30 Å thick), and the "outer membrane" is a trilaminar structure (75 Å thick) which contains protein, phospholipids, lipoproteins and lipopolysaccharide (endotoxin) (Fig. 2–6).

In *Escherichia coli*, the peptide chains (bound to muramic acid) are cross-linked by a peptide bond between meso-diaminopimelic acid and D-alanine of the adjacent peptide side chains (Figs. 2–4, 2–8). The degree of cross-linking is variable and in *E. coli* ranges from 15 to 30%. Lipoprotein molecules are covalently linked to every 10–12 disaccharide unit of peptidoglycan through meso-diaminopimelic acid. These lipoproteins serve to anchor the peptidoglycan to the outer membrane.

The LPS found in the outer membrane is a complex macromolecule containing three regions: a specific polysaccharide (region I) which determines serological specificity, a core polysaccharide (region II), and a lipid component termed lipid A (region III) (Fig. 2–7). The fatty acid composition of lipid A varies among groups of bacteria and is responsible for endotoxin activity. The LPS is oriented so that the lipid A end is in the lipid bilayer (Fig. 2–6).

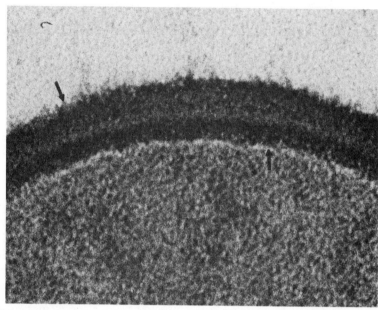

Fig. 2–5.—Electron micrograph of an ultra-thin section of *Staphylococcus aureus* showing the trilaminar cell wall typical of gram-positive bacteria *(upper arrow).* The wall has an outer, middle and inner layer. Because the cytoplasmic membrane is electron transparent, it appears as a space beneath the cell wall rather than a solid membrane *(lower arrow).* (From Cole, R. M., Chatterjee, A. N., Gilpin, R. W., and Young, F. E.: Ann. N. Y. Acad. Sci. 236:22, 1974. By permission of the author and journal.)

Fig. 2–6.—Section through the *Escherichia coli* cell envelope, which consists of outer membrane, the cell wall (peptidoglycan), and the cytoplasmic membrane. For the wall, hypothetical subunits are drawn to represent the major building blocks. (From Braun, V.: J. Infect. Dis. 128s:9–16, 1973. By permission of the author and publisher.)

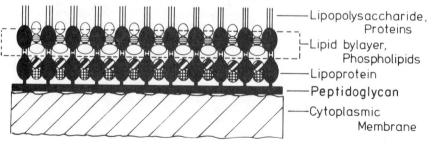

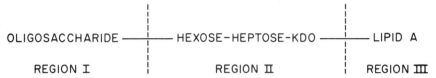

OLIGOSACCHARIDE ————— HEXOSE-HEPTOSE-KDO ————— LIPID A

REGION I   REGION Ⅱ   REGION Ⅲ

Fig. 2–7.—Schematic diagram of the lipopolysaccharide of gram-negative bacteria. R-mutants may lack part or all of region I (oiigosaccharide) or region I and the heptose in region II. All R-mutants contain lipid A and are as toxic as the S-organism. KDO = 2 keto-3 deoxyoctonate.

CYTOPLASMIC MEMBRANE

The cytoplasm is separated from the cell wall by a complex membrane approximately 75 Å thick and composed of lipid and protein in the ratio of 1:5 (Figs. 2–1, 2–5). Electron micrographs show a triple-layered structure which results from two protein layers being separated by a central lipid layer. The major lipids are phospholipids, including phosphatidylglycerol, phosphatidylethanolamine and phosphatidylserine. Glycolipids, diglycerides and polyisoprenoids are present in small amounts. Sterols are not found (except in certain mycoplasmae and fungi); thus certain antibiotics such as amphotericin B are ineffective against bacteria. In and on the membrane are enzymes and components associated with energy production and solute transport.

Fig. 2–8.—Cross-linking of adjacent peptidoglycan chains through diaminopimelic acid and alanine. Abbreviations: MurNAc = N-acetylmuramic acid; GlcNAc = N-acetylglucosamine; Ala = alanine; Glu = glutamic acid; Dap = diaminopimelic acid; Lys = lysine; Arg = arginine.

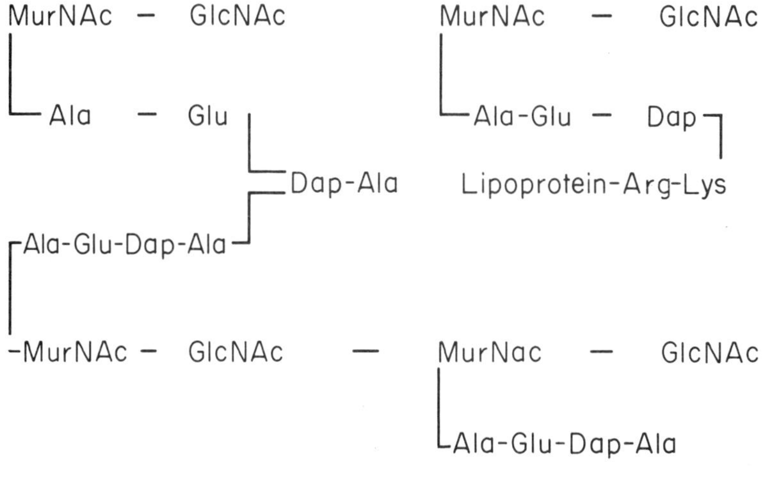

MurNAc   —   GlcNAc   MurNAc   —   GlcNAc

└ Ala   —   Glu   └ Ala-Glu   —   Dap ┐

                    └ Dap-Ala   Lipoprotein-Arg-Lys

┌ Ala-Glu-Dap-Ala ┘

-MurNAc — GlcNAc   —   MurNac   —   GlcNAc

                                                   └ Ala-Glu-Dap-Ala

Although many nutrients pass through the membrane by a non-energy-requiring diffusion process, most solutes are transported by an energy-requiring active transport system. This transport system requires stereospecific protein components at the membrane and a carrier system. The basic membrane structure and the transport system are common to all bacteria. The cytoplasmic membrane forms invaginations called mesosomes, the structure and function of which are not yet established (see Fig. 2–1).

NUCLEUS

The bacterial nucleus or nuclear area (Fig. 2–1) is not enclosed in a membrane as is the nucleus of eukaryotic cells, and in electron micrographs it appears as a region less dense than the ribosome-containing cytoplasm. The nucleus contains a chromosome composed of a circular molecule of DNA about 1 mm in length; no histones are present. The DNA molecule is a double helix consisting of a complementary pair of polynucleotide chains in which adenine is always paired with thymine and guanine paired with cytosine. As in all other organisms, the sequential order of these pairs makes up its genetic code. During cell division these complementary strands separate, and each strand serves as a template for the assembly of a new complementary strand. This mode of replication of DNA insures that two new double helices will be identical to the original helix and that each daughter cell will have the essential properties of the parent cell. Mistakes during replication may be lethal or may result in mutant progeny.

Many species of bacteria contain extrachromosomal, self-replicating, circular DNA molecules. These may carry genetic determinants for resistance to antibiotics and metallic ions, as well as for the biosynthesis of bacteriocins, toxins, some catabolic enzymes and F pili. These DNA molecules carry only a few genes and are called plasmids. The term episome is used if they can integrate with the chromosome. In certain instances, particularly within the enterics, the R (Resistance) plasmid is made up of two parts: (1) a resistance factor (RTF) responsible for conjugation and (2) a determinant for antibiotic resistance which can replicate independently of the RTF. These two factors must fuse together in order for the genes for antibiotic resistance to be transferred from one cell to another. A plasmid consisting of an RTF and the genes for antibiotic resistance is called an R factor.

CAPSULE

Under appropriate environmental conditions, most bacteria produce an extracellular polysaccharide which may contain one or more

TABLE 2-2.—CHEMICAL COMPOSITION OF CERTAIN
BACTERIAL CAPSULES

ORGANISM	COMPOUND	COMPOSITION
Bacillus anthracis	Polypeptide	D-glutamic acid
Haemophilus influenzae	Polysaccharide	Polyribose phosphate in type b
Klebsiella pneumoniae	Polysaccharide	Fucose, glucose, glucuronic acid
Neisseria meningitidis		
Group A	Polysaccharide	N-acetyl, O-acetyl-mannosamine phosphate
Group B	Polysaccharide	N-acetylneuraminic acid
Group C	Polysaccharide	N-acetyl; O-acetyl-neuraminic acid
Streptococcus pneumoniae		
Type 2	Polysaccharide	Glucose, glucuronic acid, rhamnose
Type 3	Polysaccharide	Glucose, glucuronic acid
Type 14	Polysaccharide	Galactose, glucose, N-acetylglucosamine
Type 18	Polysaccharide	Glucose, rhamnose
Streptococcus pyogenes	Hyaluronic acid	Glucuronic acid, N-acetylglucosamine

kinds of sugars. The polysaccharide may be linear or branched and may contain different linkages (Table 2-2). If the polysaccharide accumulates on the surface of the cell wall, it is called a capsule and can be stained (Alcian blue stain) or observed as a clear zone around the organism as in an India ink wet preparation (Figs. 2-1, 2-9). If the polysaccharide is soluble it diffuses throughout the medium, forming a slime, and may make the growth medium quite viscous. Many organ-

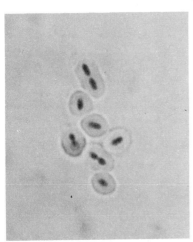

Fig. 2–9.—Capsule of *Streptococcus pneumoniae*. The capsule is polysaccharide and determines the type specificity of the pneumococcus. Note the clear area with a distinct border around the cell. This preparation is a quellung reaction.

isms, particularly the enterics, have an increased concentration of polysaccharide at the cell surface which can be detected immunologically but cannot be visualized in a wet mount; this is referred to as an envelope (microcapsule). On solid media, encapsulated or slime-producing bacteria form smooth (S) or mucoid colonies. Most capsular material is antigenic (some only haptenic), and for certain genera it provides the antigenic specificity necessary for serotype determinations (*Streptococcus pneumoniae;* chap. 6). In some instances the antigenic determinant is shared with other organisms or substances and results in serologic cross reactions. For example, the type 14 pneumococcus reacts with antibodies to blood group A substance because galactose is a common antigenic determinant. The capsular material may increase resistance to desiccation, and in certain organisms (*Streptococcus pneumoniae, S. pyogenes, Bacillus anthracis*) the capsule is antiphagocytic and thereby plays a role in pathogenicity.

FLAGELLA

Flagella are organelles of motility. In general, they are not found on cocci but are present on about half of the bacilli and most of the curved bacteria. The flagellum originates in the cytoplasm in a portion

Fig. 2–10.—Peritrichous flagella of *Proteus vulgaris.* Young agar slant culture stained by the Leifson method.

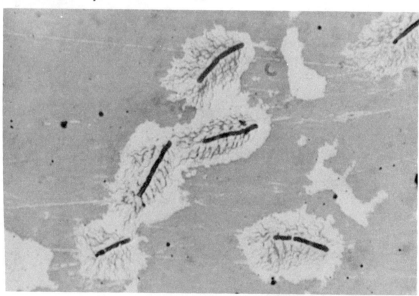

of the cytoplasmic membrane (basal body) and penetrates through the peptidoglycan of the cell wall (Fig. 2-1). It is composed of an antigenic protein (H antigen) termed flagellin. The flagellum is helical in shape with the wavelength and amplitude being quite constant for a given species. The flagellum rotates about its longitudinal axis and moves the organism forward or backward at speeds up to 50 μm/sec. The source of energy for the motion is not yet established, although it apparently is not ATP.

Morphologically, a flagellum consists of (1) a basal structure associated with the cytoplasmic membrane, which is the probable site of flagellin synthesis; (2) a bent region or "hook" extending beyond the cell wall and (3) the spiral filament. Growth of the flagellum is rapid and seems to occur at the apex. The mature flagellum is about 0.02 μm wide and 10 μm or more long. Even with this length it is below the limit of resolution of the light microscope, so special staining procedures are used which precipitate stain onto the flagellum to increase the size and make it visible. The number of flagella on a bacterium is constant for a given species; the organelles are found singly (monotrichous), as a polar tuft (lophotrichous) or distributed over the entire cell (peritrichous) (Fig. 2-10).

PILI

Pili (fimbriae) are filiform strands of protein which are helically coiled; some have a hollow core. The pili (Fig. 2-11) originate in a cytoplasmic, membrane-associated site and extend through the cell wall. They are shorter, straighter and thinner than flagella (0.003-0.014 μm wide and 0.5-20 μm long) and are observable only by the electron microscope. Six morphological types of pili, designated types I-V and F, have been described. Pili have been found on many gram-negative bacteria—particularly the enterics—but rarely on gram-positive organisms; the numbers per cell are variable but may exceed 200. The F pilus or sex pilus is longer than the other pili and there may be 1 to 10 per cell. The production of the sex pilus is determined by an extrachromosomal gene, the F factor; such cells are referred to as "F+". The pilus provides a means for chromosomal transfer from F+ to F− cells; F− cells receive but cannot transfer DNA. The F pilus also acts as a specific receptor for certain bacteriophages. Pili may cause other effects, including (1) adherence to mucosal cells, soil particles, rocks or other particulate matter; (2) nonspecific clumping of erythrocytes and (3) aggregation and pellicle formation of some bacteria. Adherence of bacterial cells to tissue via pili is important in producing disease.

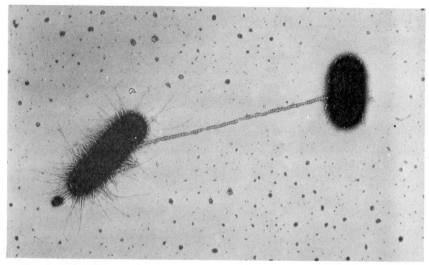

Fig. 2–11.—Bacterial cells connected by an F pilus (conjugation). The F pilus is labeled by phage which infect the cell through the F pilus. Smaller hair-like structures are type I pili which enable the cell to attach to tissue. (Courtesy of Dr. Charles C. Brinton, Jr., Dept. of Life Sciences, University of Pittsburgh, Pittsburgh, Pa.)

SPORES

Species of the genera *Bacillus* and *Clostridium* form endospores (Fig. 2 – 12), which are the most resistant biological structures known. When a vegetative cell with the potential to produce spores reaches the stationary growth phase, depletion of a nutrient turns on the genes determining spore structure and the cell then differentiates into an endospore. Differentiation begins with the chromosome being surrounded by a portion of the cell membrane. Within this septum, a spore which contains a multilayered wall (spore wall, cortex) is synthesized. This differentiation into a spore occurs over 8 – 10 hours. Lytic enzymes then digest the remaining bacterial structure (vegetative structure), liberating the spore. The mature spore has little metabolic activity and is markedly resistant to heat, ultraviolet light, x-irradiation, chemicals and desiccation. Some may be viable after 30 years in dry sand. The spore provides the bacterium with a means of survival in adverse conditions. When the environment favors growth, the spore is activated and germination occurs by outgrowth of a single vegetative cell having all the characteristics of the parent cell.

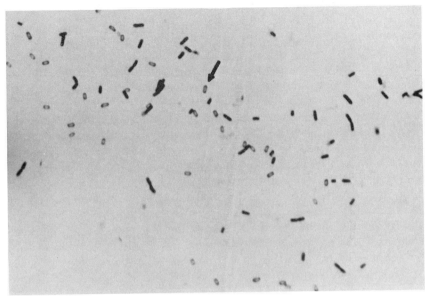

Fig. 2–12.—Stain of a 4-day-old culture of *Bacillus megaterium*. Note the solid staining rods and the spores. The spore appears as an unstained area within the cell with a small portion of stained cytoplasm at either end *(arrow)*.

L-FORMS, PROTOPLASTS AND SPHEROPLASTS

Certain bacteria, either spontaneously or in the presence of inducing agents (enzymes, antibiotics), form fragile, filterable, reproducing structures which lack the peptidoglycan moiety of the cell wall; these are called L-forms. They are usually spherical but may vary in shape and even be filamentous. They will reproduce in liquid media indefinitely and produce small granular colonies on suitable solid media; reversion to the parent cell can occur under appropriate conditions. L-forms synthesize extracellular enzymes, including toxins, and if the parent is motile, the flagella remain attached to the membrane. Some workers suggest that treatment of patients with penicillin or certain other antibiotics can induce conversion of the pathogen into the antibiotic-resistant L-forms. These L-forms may persist until the antibiotic is no longer present and then revert to the pathogen, thus being a source of relapse of the infection. L-forms are produced by many organisms, including *Bacillus, Clostridium, Escherichia, Neisseria, Proteus, Salmonella, Staphylococcus, Streptococcus* and *Streptobacillus*.

Confusion continues in use of the terms L-form and PPLO (pleuropneumonia-like organisms). Early, they were both considered to be virus-like because they were filterable. The PPLO were finally cultured and identified with greater certainty and are now called *Mycoplasma* (chap. 22). The mycoplasmal cell is membrane bound and usually divides by binary fission. The L-forms, as indicated above, arise from bacteria and continue to reproduce as such, but unlike the mycoplasma they can revert to the parent bacterial cell with all the characteristics of the parent cell.

Structures similar to L-forms can be produced experimentally by treating bacteria with lysozyme (other enzymes or antibiotics can be used) in a hypertonic solution which prevents lysis. Lysozyme causes the complete loss of the peptidoglycan from gram-positive bacteria and transforms the cells into osmotically fragile spheres or protoplasts that can metabolize and increase in size but do not divide. Such treatment of most gram-negative bacteria also results in loss of the peptidoglycan but not other cell wall constituents such as the lipopolysaccharide; these forms are called spheroplasts. Removal of the lysozyme (or other inducing agent) from the medium allows some protoplasts or spheroplasts to regain the morphology of their parent cell and resume normal growth. These wall-defective forms have been used primarily in studying the structure and function of the bacterial cytoplasmic membrane.

NOMENCLATURE

Each bacterium, after being adequately described, must have a name so that it can be identified by anyone in the world. Specific names are also necessary for communication among microbiologists, physicians and other allied health personnel. The clinical laboratory reports the results of cultures to the physician by giving the name of the organism(s) isolated. The physician must know the proper nomenclature to interpret these reports and subsequently to determine treatment and to make verbal or written reports about the disease. As in all biological classifications, each distinct bacterium is given a species name, and similar species are placed in a genus, such as *Streptococcus pyogenes*. Then genera are grouped into families and families into orders. Higher ranks of class, division and kingdom then follow.

For years, bacteria were considered to be part of the plant kingdom, but now a separate kingdom, *Procaryotae*, has been established. The essential reason for separating bacteria from plants is that bacterial DNA is not enclosed in a membrane as it is in plants and animals. The classification of bacteria, as presented in the eighth edition of *Bergey's Manual of Determinative Bacteriology*, is given in Table 2-3.

TABLE 2-3.—CLASSIFICATION OF BACTERIA (BERGEY'S MANUAL OF DETERMINATIVE BACTERIOLOGY—8TH ED)

DESCRIPTION	KINGDOM-PROCARYOTAE ORDER	DIVISION—BACTERIA FAMILY	GENUS	
Spirochetes	Spirochaetales	Spirochaetaceae	*Treponema* *Borrelia*	*Leptospira*
Gram-negative aerobic rods and cocci	—	Pseudomonadaceae	*Pseudomonas*	
		Uncertain affiliation	*Alcaligenes* *Brucella*	*Bordetella* *Francisella*
Gram-negative facultatively anaerobic rods	—	Enterobacteriaceae	*Escherichia* *Edwardsiella* *Citrobacter* *Salmonella* *Shigella* *Klebsiella*	*Enterobacter* *Hafnia* *Serratia* *Proteus* *Yersinia* *Erwinia*
	—	Vibrionaceae	*Vibrio* *Aeromonas*	
		Uncertain affiliation	*Flavobacterium* *Haemophilus* *Pasteurella*	*Actinobacillus* *Streptobacillus* *Calymmato-bacterium*
Gram-negative anaerobic bacteria	—	Bacteroidaceae	*Bacteroides* *Fusobacterium*	*Leptotrichia*
Gram-negative cocci, coccobacilli	—	Neisseriaceae	*Neisseria* *Branhamella*	*Moraxella* *Acinetobacter*
Gram-negative anaerobic cocci	—	Veillonellaceae	*Veillonella*	
Gram-positive cocci aerobic-facultative	—	Micrococcaceae	*Micrococcus*	*Staphylococcus*
	—	Streptococcaceae	*Streptococcus*	
Anaerobic	—	Peptococcaceae	*Peptococcus*	*Peptostrepto-coccus*
Endospore-forming rods	—	Bacillaceae	*Bacillus*	*Clostridium*
Gram-positive, asporogenous rod-shaped bacteria	—	Lactobacillaceae	*Lactobacillus*	
		Uncertain affiliation	*Listeria*	*Erysipelothrix*
Actinomycetes and related organisms	—	Coryneform group	*Corynebacterium*	*Arthrobacter*
	—	Propionibacteriaceae	*Propionibacterium*	*Eubacterium*
	Actinomycetales	Actinomycetaceae	*Actinomyces* *Arachnia* *Bifidobacterium*	*Bacterionema* *Rothia*
	"	Mycobacteriaceae	*Mycobacterium*	
	"	Dermatophilaceae	*Dermatophilus*	
	"	Nocardiaceae	*Nocardia*	
	"	Streptomycetaceae	*Streptomyces*	
	"	Micromonosporaceae	*Thermoactinomyces*	
Rickettsias	Rickettsiales	Rickettsiaceae	*Rickettsia* *Rochalimaea*	*Coxiella*
	"	Bartonellaceae	*Bartonella*	
	Chlamydiales	Chlamydiaceae	*Chlamydia*	
Mycoplasmas	Mycoplasmatales	Mycoplasmataceae	*Mycoplasma*	

38   BACTERIAL STRUCTURES AND THEIR FUNCTIONS

SUPPLEMENTARY READING

Braun, V.: Molecular organization of the rigid layer and the cell wall of *Escherichia coli*, J. Infect. Dis. 128S:9–16, 1973.

Braun, V., and Hantke, K.: Biochemistry of bacterial cell envelopes, Annu. Rev. Biochem. 43:89–121, 1974.

Buchanan, R. E., and Gibbons, N. E. (eds.) *Bergey's Manual of Determinative Bacteriology* (8th ed.; Baltimore: Williams & Wilkins Co., 1974).

Guze, L. B.: *Microbial Protoplasts, Spheroplasts and L-Forms.* (Baltimore: Williams & Wilkins Co., 1968).

Keynan, A.: The Transformation of Bacterial Endospores into Vegetative Cells, in Ashworth, J. M., and Smith, J. E. (eds.): *Microbial Differentiation* (Cambridge: Cambridge University Press, 1973).

Luderitz, D., Galanos, C., Lehmann, V., Nurminen, M., Rietschel, E. T., Rosenfelder, G., Simon, M., and Westphal, O.: Lipid A: Chemical structure and biological activity, J. Infect. Dis. 128S:17–29, 1973.

Ottow, J. C. G.: Ecology, physiology and genetics of fimbriae and pili, Annu. Rev. Microbiol. 29:80–108, 1975.

Schleifer, K. H., and Kandler, O.: Peptidoglycan types of bacterial cell walls and their taxonomic implications, Bacteriol. Rev. 36:407–477, 1972.

Smith, R. W., and Koffler, H.: Bacteria flagella, Adv. Microb. Physiol. 6:219–339, 1971.

Szulmajster, J.: Initiation of Bacterial Sporogenesis, in Ashworth, J. M., and Smith, J. E. (eds.): *Microbial Differentiation* (Cambridge: Cambridge University Press, 1973).

3 / Normal Flora

The human fetus in utero is free from bacteria. Within hours after birth it begins to acquire a bacterial flora which then stabilizes within the first week or two. From then on, enormous numbers of bacteria are harbored on the skin and on the mucous membranes of the oral cavity, nasopharynx and intestinal tract, although the internal organs, cavities and muscles remain free from bacteria. The human lives in symbiosis with these billions of metabolizing microorganisms, and evidence suggests that these bacteria may aid the digestive processes and even be a source of some vitamins or micronutrients. However, these bacteria may interfere with absorption and they remain an ever-present source of infection. The various areas of the body are briefly discussed primarily from the standpoint of the kinds of bacteria present. Information on the number of organisms found is minimal because meaningful data are technically difficult to obtain. Table 3–1 attempts to relate the various genera of bacteria with their presence or absence on different body sites.

SKIN

The skin (area approximates 2 sq m) is often considered a dry, nonnutritive surface, but actually the combined secretions of the sweat and sebaceous glands provide an acidic, oily surface film which contains water, amino acids, urea, salts and fatty acids; these ingredients are a source of nutrients for the bacterial inhabitants. The numbers of bacteria range from as few as 100 to as many as 2×10^6 organisms per square centimeter with the greatest numbers being on the head, axilla, groin, perineum, hands and feet. Each person tends to maintain a relatively stable low, intermediate or high level of numbers of bacteria on the skin. This stable resident flora includes primarily *Staphylococcus epidermidis, Corynebacterium xerosis, C. pseudodiphtheriticum* and *Propionibacterium acnes* (the last, particularly

TABLE 3-1.–HUMAN INDIGENOUS BACTERIAL FLORA

BACTERIA	SKIN	EYES	EXTERNAL EAR	TONGUE	PLAQUE	GINGIVAL SULCUS	ORO-PHARYNX	NASO-PHARYNX	URETHRA	VAGINA	UTERUS	SMALL INTESTINE	LARGE INTESTINE
				UPPER RESPIRATORY TRACT					GENITOURINARY TRACT			INTESTINAL TRACT	
Acinetobacter	1°	0	–	–	–	–	1	1	1	1	–	0	0
Actinomyces	0	0	0	–	3	3	0	0	0	0	0	0	0
Bacillus	1	1	1	1	0	0•	1	1	1	1	1	1	1
Bacteroides	0	0	–	1	1	3	1	0	1	1	1	3	3
Bifidobacterium	0	0	–	1	1	2	1	1	1	1	1	2	2
Bordetella	0	0	0	1	0	0	1	1	0	0	0	0	0
Borrelia	0	0	0	1	0	2	0	0	–	–	–	–	–
Chlamydia	–	1	–	–	–	–	–	–	1	1	–	–	–
Clostridium†	–	0	0	0	–	–	–	0	0	–	1	2	2
Corynebacterium	3	2	3	1	1	1	1	1	1	2	1	1	1
C. diphtheriae	1	0	0	–	0	0	1	1	0	0	0	0	0
Enterobacter	1	0	1	1	1	1	1	1	1	1	1	2	2
Escherichia	1	0	1	1	1	1	1	1	1	1	1	2	3
Eubacterium	–	–	–	–	–	1	–	–	–	–	–	2	2
Fusobacterium	0	0	0	1	1	2	1	1	–	–	–	1	1
Haemophilus	–	1	–	–	2	1	1	1	1	1	1	0	0
Klebsiella	1	–	1	1	1	1	1	1	1	1	1	2	2
Lactobacillus	1	0	–	1	2	2	1	1	1	3	2	1	1
Leptotrichia	–	–	–	–	2	2	1	–	0	0	0	0	0
Listeria	–	–	–	–	–	–	–	–	–	1	–	1	1
Micrococcus	1	1	2	1	0	0	1	1	1	1	1	1	1
Moraxella	–	1	–	–	–	–	1	1	1	1	–	–	–
Mycoplasma	–	–	–	1	–	2	1	1	1	1	1	–	1
Neisseria	1	–	1	1	1	1	2	1	0	1	0	0	0
N. gonorrhoeae	1	0	0	0	0	0	1	0	1	1	1	0	0
N. meningitidis	1	0	0	0	0	0	1	1	0	0	0	0	0
Nocardia	1	0	0	0	0	0	0	0	0	0	0	0	0
Peptococcus	–	–	–	1	1	1	–	–	–	1	1	1	1
Peptostreptococcus	–	–	–	1	1	2	1	1	1	1	1	1	1
Propionibacterium	3	1	1	–	1	2	1	1	1	1	1	1	1
Proteus	1	0	1	1	1	1	1	1	1	1	1	2	2
Pseudomonas	1	0	1	1	1	0	1	1	1	1	1	1	1
Salmonella	–	0	0	0	0	0	0	0	0	0	0	1	1
Shigella	–	0	0	0	0	0	0	0	0	0	0	1	1
Staphylococcus													
S. aureus	2	1	1	1	1	1	1	2	1	1	1	1	1
S. epidermidis	3	2	3	2	1	1	1	3	1	1	1	1	1
Streptococcus													
Alpha	1	0	1	3	3	3	3	2	2	2	1	2	2
Beta‡													
S. pneumoniae	1	1	–	1	0	0	3	2	0	0	0	0	0
Treponema§	–	–	–	1	–	3	–	–	–	–	–	–	–
Veillonella	0	0	–	3	2	3	1	1	0	1	1	1	1
Vibrio	0	0	0	1	1	1	1	–	–	–	–	1	1
V. cholerae	–	0	0	0	0	0	0	0	0	0	0	1	1

°3 = present; 2 = usually present; 1 = occasionally present; 0 = not reported; – = insufficient information.

†Primarily C. perfringens and other species; C. botulinum and C. tetani are not indigenous flora.
‡Includes groups A, B, C and G.
§Treponema pallidum is found only in the infected person.

in the follicular canals). These organisms persist throughout life along with highly variable and transient flora, including S. *aureus, Streptococcus, Escherichia, Enterobacter, Klebsiella, Pseudomonas, Acinetobacter, Bacillus, Candida, Pityrosporum* and many others (see Table 3–1).

EYE

The eyes harbor bacteria from birth throughout life, and even immediate post-birth treatment with silver nitrate or penicillin does not free them from bacteria. The consistent bacterial flora at all ages has *Staphylococcus epidermidis* as the predominant organism, followed by *S. aureus*, species of *Corynebacterium*, (diphtheroids) and *Streptococcus pneumoniae*. In 0.1–8% of cultures from either eyelids or conjunctivas, a number of additional organisms are isolated, including *Escherichia, Klebsiella, Proteus, Enterobacter, Neisseria, Bacillus* and *Streptococcus*. Few anaerobic organisms are present.

EXTERNAL EAR

The external ear canal is lined with epithelium containing hairs and sebaceous glands. Specialized glands produce cerumen, a wax which contains a high percentage of lipids. Organisms survive in the cerumen, but it is questionable that they multiply. The basic bacterial flora resembles that of the skin with staphylococci and *Corynebacterium* predominating. *Bacillus, Micrococcus* and *Neisseria* are found less frequently. Gram-negative rods such as *Escherichia, Proteus* and *Pseudomonas* are occasionally found and increase in the summer; studies on the anaerobic flora are lacking. Mycological studies have been done in conjunction with otomycosis, and a wide variety of fungi (which rarely cause infections) have been isolated from healthy subjects. These include *Aspergillus, Alternaria, Hormodendrum, Fusarium, Penicillium, Candida* and *Saccharomyces*.

NOSE

The nares with their mucus-covered hairs are the initial filtering mechanism of the respiratory tract where most particles 10 μm or larger are removed. Thus contact is made with a large variety of bacteria, but the predominant inhabitants are *Staphylococcus epidermidis* and *S. aureus*. Much less frequently, *Streptococcus pneumoniae*, other alpha streptococci and *Haemophilus influenzae* are found. *Neisseria* and *Peptostreptococcus* are occasionally isolated as are many of the gram-negative rods, such as *Escherichia, Proteus* and *Pseudomonas.* Anaerobes are seldom isolated. The sinuses are normally free from bacteria.

NASOPHARYNX

This area at the back of the nasal cavity is separated from the oropharynx by the soft palate. As the nasopharynx is in direct continuity with the oropharynx, which extends down to the epiglottis, the flora of both areas is essentially the same. *Streptococcus pneumoniae* and other alpha-hemolytic streptococci are dominant organisms; beta-hemolytic streptococci are less numerous and *S. pyogenes* is occasionally present. Other inhabitants include *Staphylococcus, Corynebacterium, Neisseria, Haemophilus* and *Micrococcus;* the gram-negative rods such as *Escherichia, Enterobacter, Proteus* and *Pseudomonas* are not common (Table 3-1). The tonsils (palatine and pharyngeal) harbor a similar flora, except that in the crypts there is an increase in the anaerobes, including *Bacteroides, Fusobacterium, Veillonella, Actinomyces* and *Leptotrichia.* The lower respiratory tract (trachea, bronchi, alveoli) does not have a normal flora as the bacteria are removed by the mucus stream or by phagocytosis.

ORAL CAVITY

The oral cavity becomes contaminated with bacteria from the surrounding environment within the first few hours after birth. Initially, the flora consists mostly of lactobacilli, staphylococci, streptococci and coliforms, but the flora rapidly increases in number and variety of bacteria. The same kinds of bacteria (see Table 3-1) seem to be universally present, although there is considerable fluctuation in the number of organisms even from day to day in the same individual. The organisms (predominantly facultatives) are washed from various foci into the saliva, which contains an average of 75×10^7 bacteria per milliliter. The main foci are the dorsum of the tongue, the gingival sulcus and the dental plaque. The plaque-gingival debris has a population approximating 2×10^{11} organisms per gram wet weight made up predominantly of anaerobes, including *Actinomyces, Bacteroides, Fusobacterium, Peptostreptococcus, Veillonella, Treponema* and *Borrelia.*

Because plaque (coronal, supragingival or subgingival) is most important in oral health, its development and composition will be discussed in more detail. First, a pellicle of salivary glycoproteins less than 1 μm thick rapidly absorbs to the tooth surface. Within a matter of minutes bacteria sorb to the pellicle and begin to grow, and visible colonies are formed within 1–2 days. Other organisms then attach, leading to the formation of a confluent microbial layer or plaque. Streptococci are among the first to adhere (*S. mutans* forms a dextran which selectively binds to the tooth surface), followed by cocci, rods, filaments *(Actinomyces, Bacterionema, Rothia)*, vibrios and spirochetes. Ultimately a polymicrobial aggregate of bacteria is found on the tooth surface. This plaque, with its millions of metabolically active organisms, is a precursor to the development of caries, gingivitis and periodontal disease.

INTESTINAL TRACT

The intestinal tract harbors the greatest number of bacteria of any area of the body, totaling in excess of 10^{13} organisms. The numbers in the stomach are low, representing primarily organisms from the oral cavity, pharynx and food. The duodenum and jejunum contain few bacteria (less than 10^3/ml of contents), but there is a significant increase in the ileum reaching a maximum in the large intestine with the formation of feces. Microscopic counts of feces average $10^{11.4}$ organisms per gram wet weight and 10^{11} of these are cultivable. This environment is anaerobic (oxidation-reduction potential of -200 mv or below) with a rich supply of nutrients which favors the growth of anaerobes, including: *Bacteroides, Fusobacterium, Bifidobacterium, Eubacterium, Peptostreptococcus, Clostridium, Veillonella* and *Propionibacterium*. Although these organisms constitute 90% or more of the flora, there are facultative bacteria, yeasts (particularly *Candida*), fungi and protozoa (amebae and flagellates) present. The facultative anaerobes are predominantly gram-negative rods such as *E. coli*, but they also include a variety of other rods and cocci (see Table 3–1). Such enormous numbers of bacteria in the intestinal tract are likely to play some role in the nutrition, physiology and health of the individual, but support for this concept comes only from results obtained in animal experimentation.

Studies in germ-free or antibiotic-treated mice indicate that alterations in the normal flora can (1) increase susceptibility to infections with *Salmonella* and *Shigella;* (2) reduce the rate of peristaltic emptying and decrease the resistance to intestinal infections; (3) alter the structure of the intestinal tract, in that the walls are thinner and the lymphatic system is underdeveloped and (4) result in deficiencies in vitamins, such as thiamine, riboflavin, biotin, B_6 and K.

GENITOURINARY TRACT

The upper (kidneys and ureters) and mid (bladder) urinary tract is normally free from bacteria. Urine, leaving the bladder, is normally sterile. The lower portion of the urethra and the meatus may be colonized with bacteria, although most of the information available is from studies on women. Studies of women with no history of urinary or vaginal infection indicate that the flora of the vaginal vestibule and lower urethra contains primarily *Lactobacillus, Corynebacterium, Staphylococcus epidermidis* and nonhemolytic streptococci. *Haemophilus vaginalis* and yeasts are less common. Interestingly, gram-negative rods such as *Escherichia, Proteus, Klebsiella, Enterobacter* and *Pseudomonas* (which commonly cause urinary tract infections) are infrequently present, but they do increase prior to infection and in individuals having recurrent infections. Numerous organisms have been reported from the vagina and cervix, including (in approximate descending order of frequency): *Lactobacillus, Corynebacterium, S. epidermidis*, beta-hemolytic streptococci (mostly groups C and G, seldom group A), alpha-hemolytic streptococci, *Bacteroides, S. aureus, Escherichia, Proteus, Enterobacter, Haemophilus vaginalis, Trichomonas, Candida, Torulopsis* and *Bacillus*. A similar flora is reported for the uterus, although there are fewer numbers and kinds of bacteria, and approximately 30% of endometrial cultures are sterile; the anaerobic organisms *Clostridium* and *Peptostreptococcus* have been isolated. Bacteria probably enter the uterus during menstruation. There is little information on the normal flora of the male and female genitourinary tracts and a comprehensive study is needed.

POPULATION CONTROL

The flora of many areas of the body, in respect to the kinds of bacteria present, remains rather stable. One good example is the skin where *S. epidermidis, C. xerosis, C. pseudodiphtheriticum* and *P. acnes* predominate, in spite of an almost constant contact with a variety of different organisms. The factors that control such selectivity are not well established but they could include (1) humidity, a factor on the skin; (2) fatty acids which would be antagonistic as on the skin and in the intestinal tract; (3) anaerobiosis as in the gingival sulcus and intestinal tract; (4) production of H_2O_2, which is the antagonistic factor of *Streptococcus sanguis* (chap. 6) and (5) lysozyme, the antibacterial substance in the tears, saliva and milk. In addition, secretory IgA selectively reacts with certain organisms as, for example, in the intestinal tract where adherence by a specific serotype of *E. coli* is inhibited by IgA.

Two bacterial factors that may determine the bacterial population associated with the host are adherence factors, such as pili or polysaccharides, which bind to certain cells or surfaces, and antagonistic factors, such as bacteriocins.

Bacteriocins (colicins). These proteins produced by certain gram-negative and gram-positive bacteria are highly lethal for strains of the same species or closely related bacteria. They attach to specific receptor sites on the cell surface, and then by some mechanism directly or indirectly interfere with protein synthesis; resistant bacteria probably do not have the necessary receptor site. Some bacteriocins resemble defective phage particles or portions of a phage, but there is no concrete evidence that they are derived from a bacteriophage. Although the biologic significance of these highly toxic proteins is not clear, there is some evidence supporting the idea that in the natural environment of the organism they can reduce the numbers of closely related organisms, thus eliminating competition for nutrients and survival.

ADHERENCE

Certain bacteria are capable of adhering selectively to receptors — possibly glycoproteins — on various epithelial surfaces such as buccal mucosa, dorsum of tongue, nasopharyñgeal area, certain portions of the gastrointestinal tract and bladder. Adherence factors are associated with the bacterial cell surface. They include the M antigens and lipoteichoic acids of *Streptococcus pyogenes,* the K-88 antigen of *Escherichia coli,* the pili of *Neisseria gonorrhoeae,* the polysaccharides of *Streptococcus mutans,* and fibrils (composition unknown) extending from the surfaces of *Streptococcus salivarius, S. mitis* and *Actinomyces vicosus.* Certain bacteria are more frequently associated with certain cells and tissues. For example, *S. salivarius* selectively adheres to the dorsal surface of the tongue, *S. mitis* to the buccal mucosa, and *S. mutans* to the teeth. *S. pyogenes* adheres much better to oral mucosa than to the bladder, but the reverse is true of enteropathogenic *E. coli. N. gonorrhoeae* adheres to urethral mucosa and to sperm, the latter property perhaps aiding spread of the organism within the genitourinary tract as well as transmission to the female. Adherence may be prevented by salivary antibodies (IgA and IgG) and by mucinous glycoproteins. It is now obvious that the phenomenon of selective adherence is of biologic importance in determining the indigenous flora of various mucosal surfaces as well as a determinant of pathogenicity by providing the organism with a mechanism for remaining at a given site. Future investigations will more specifically identify the bacterial and tissue factors involved, which may lead to methods of control of certain infectious diseases either through immunization or by the use of adherence inhibitors.

SUPPLEMENTARY READING

Gibbons, R. J., and van Houte, J.: Bacterial adherence in oral microbial ecology, Annu. Rev. Microbiol. 29:19–44, 1975.

Gossling, J., and Slack, J. M.: Predominant gram-positive bacteria in human feces: Numbers, variety and persistence, Infect. Immun. 9:719-729, 1974.

Maibach, H. I., and Hildick-Smith, G.: *The Skin Bacteria and Their Role in Infection* (New York: McGraw-Hill Book Co., 1965).

Marples, M. J.: *The Ecology of the Human Skin* (Springfield, Ill.: Charles C Thomas, Publisher, 1965).

Montagna, W., and Parakkal, P. F.: *The Structure and Function of Skin* (New York: Academic Press, 1974).

Nicolaides, N.: Skin lipids: Their biochemical uniqueness, Science 186: 19–26, 1974.

Reeves, P.: *The Bacteriocins* (New York: Springer-Verlag New York Inc., 1972).

Skinner, F. A., and Carr, J. G.: *The Normal Microbial Flora of Man* (New York: Academic Press, 1974).

Suie, T.: *The Microbiology of the Eye* (Rochester, Minn.: Custom Printing, Inc., 1964).

4 / Diagnosis of Bacterial Diseases: Clinical Approach and Laboratory Procedures

DIAGNOSIS AND CLINICAL APPROACH

Overview

Diagnosis of an infectious disease requires knowledge, not only of clinical signs and symptoms, but also of the epidemiology of infectious diseases. Epidemiology, the study of disease patterns in a population, provides the information necessary for (1) quantitative measurement of disease in a population and (2) development of methods for preventing disease spread. Knowledge of the incidence of disease in a given population group permits the physician to make a judgment as to the probable causative organisms and then to develop procedures necessary to prevent the disease and its transmission. The Center for Disease Control, Atlanta, Georgia, regularly monitors disease and periodically reports the quantitative assessment of disease in the *CDC Morbidity and Mortality Weekly Report.*

Knowledge of the pathogenic capabilities and properties of microorganisms also permits the physician to judge the etiologic agent most likely involved in a disease process. With some exceptions, e.g., staphylococcal food poisoning and botulism, bacteria must multiply in the host to cause disease. Certain organisms, primarily the gram-positive bacteria, are better able by production of enzymes, antiphagocytic factors, toxins, hemolysins and adherence factors to become established and invade the healthy host and thus are primary invaders. Other organisms, particularly the gram-negative bacteria, are not as well equipped with these invasive factors and are more apt to be secondary invaders. These latter organisms are frequently part of the normal flora of the host and are opportunists, i.e., they cause infection in a host with a lowered resistance to disease.

Concepts of infection, epidemiology and laboratory diagnosis must be well understood and appreciated as they are relevant to solving clinical problems associated with bacterial diseases.

47

Epidemiologic Considerations

Several terms are used to express the quantitative measurement of disease in a population. The incidence of disease is expressed as the number of cases reported during a particular time period, usually a year, per 100,000 population. The term *morbidity rate* is synonymous with incidence. Prevalence rate is also used to express the magnitude of a disease. The prevalence rate is that percentage of a particular segment of the population with a given disease. For example, if one were to determine that 10 of every 100 men in a hospitalized population had kidney infections, then the prevalence rate for the male hospitalized population would be 10%. The attack rate is a measure of the number of people in a stated population who acquire a disease during a given period. For example, if 10 cases of food-borne disease occurred in an institution housing 1,000 people, the attack rate would be 10 per 1,000, or 1%. Attack rate refers to cases acquired during a given period. Prevalence rate differs from attack rate in that prevalence rate includes all cases of a disease present in a population, irrespective of when they were acquired.

Mortality rate refers to the number of deaths per 100,000 persons occurring in the population during a specified period of time, usually 1 year. If deaths occurring from a specific disease are used, then the mortality rate is disease-specific and is expressed as number of deaths due to a specific cause per 100,000 persons.

The various measures used to express disease are only reflections of the real magnitude of disease. Many specific diseases may be misdiagnosed or incorrectly reported. Other cases of disease may be insufficiently severe to come to the attention of medical personnel and these are not reported. This phenomenon is referred to as the iceberg effect. As only a small portion of an iceberg is visible with the largest part submerged, similarly, only a small part of the total infectious disease problem may be observed.

Occasionally, diseases which are endemic, i.e., continually present in the population, increase in numbers under certain conditions and an epidemic results. For example, one can expect a certain number of cases of pneumonia to occur in the population at any given time of the year. However, during certain periods, such as when influenza outbreaks occur, the actual number of cases of pneumonia exceeds the number of cases expected. When an epidemic is widespread and affects several countries or continents it is referred to as pandemic.

Source and Transmission of Disease

A logical approach to disease control requires an understanding of the source of disease and its mechanism of transmission. In spite of

TABLE 4-1.—HORIZONTAL AND VERTICAL
TRANSMISSION OF BACTERIAL DISEASES

| DISEASE | TRANSMISSION | |
	MEANS	TYPE
Plague (pneumonic)	Aerosols	Direct—horizontal
Plague (bubonic)	Fleas	Indirect—horizontal
Primary syphilis	Mucous membrane contact	Direct—horizontal
Congenital syphilis	Mother to fetus via placenta	Direct—vertical
Borrelia (relapsing fever)	Ticks to ticks	Direct—vertical
Borrelia (relapsing fever)	Ticks to man	Indirect—horizontal
Typhoid fever, cholera	Ingestion of contaminated food, water	Indirect—horizontal
Tularemia	Contamination of wound	Direct—horizontal
	Ticks to man or animal	Indirect—horizontal

effective chemotherapy, diseases such as bubonic plague, leprosy, tuberculosis and venereal diseases are still important, and control is largely directed at identifying the source and preventing transmission.

An infectious agent may be transmitted from one host to another either by direct contact or by contact with some intermediary such as food or water (horizontal transmission). In some diseases of man (congenital syphilis) the infectious organism may be transmitted in utero from the infected mother to fetus, and in insects certain microbial agents (*Borrelia* and *Rickettsia*) are transmitted from the female to the eggs and thereby perpetuate the organism from generation to generation. This type of transmission of an infectious agent from one generation to another is referred to as vertical transmission (Table 4-1).

The reservoir for an infectious disease is that inanimate (soil, water) or animate (man, animal, insect) source in which the organism normally lives and reproduces. Zoonosis is a disease of animals that can be transmitted to man, and epizootic is an epidemic of a disease that occurs in an animal population. From the reservoir the organism may spread by either direct or indirect means. Direct transmission may result from direct contact with an infected host or from contact with secretions of an infected host.

Indirect transmission requires a vector or intermediate vehicle by which the organism is transmitted from the reservoir to the host. Vectors include insects, food, water or fomites. Fomes (pl. fomites) is an inanimate object, such as clothing or an eating utensil that may harbor infectious agents.

Three general approaches are used to control infectious disease: (1) preventing direct contact with infected persons and infective secretions, (2) preventing transmission via the reservoir, vectors and other methods found to transfer organisms from the source of infection to susceptible persons and (3) increasing host resistance and the general level of immunity in a population (herd immunity).

Specific methods employed to reduce or eliminate direct contact with the source include (1) isolation of infected persons, (2) elimination of the animal reservoir or vector and (3) institution of appropriate therapy to reduce or eliminate the infectivity of the diseased persons. Methods employed to prevent indirect transmission include chlorination of water, milk pasteurization, supervision and inspection of food and food handlers, destruction of insect vectors, detection of carriers and elimination of the carrier state through chemotherapy or surgery.

Methods directed at increasing host resistance and raising the level of herd immunity include active and passive immunization. Under natural conditions herd immunity is increased by infection, either clinical or subclinical, or as a result of colonization. The greater the proportion of immune persons in a population, the greater the probability that an infected individual will come in contact with a nonsusceptible individual, thus preventing further spread of the infection.

Two approaches, prospective and retrospective, are used to study the epidemiology of disease and to determine its etiology, or cause. Prospective studies are designed and implemented before the occurrence of disease. In these studies data such as occupation, geographical area, sex, blood chemistry values, microorganisms present and diet are recorded. The data obtained from those who develop disease are compared with the same data collected on those without disease and analyzed in order to understand the epidemiology and etiology of a disease.

Prospective Studies
Data Collection → Clinical Diagnosis → Etiology

In retrospective studies, one tries to determine the cause and effect after disease has occurred. For example, one might be able to identify the disease but not know why it occurred. Thus one tries to determine by careful questioning, history taking and other data collection the factors that may have contributed to disease production. In a retrospective study on the occurrence of kidney disease, for example, it was noted that skin infections seemed to occur prior to the onset of kidney disease. Retrospectively, then, skin infection with a specific organism was associated with kidney disease. Subsequently, a prospective study was done in which a selected population was observed and the occurrence of skin infection and kidney disease was recorded. These studies revealed that only patients with a preceding skin infection developed kidney disease. This clearly established the relationship between skin infections and kidney disease as suggested by the retrospective study.

Retrospective Studies
Clinical Diagnosis → Data Collection → Presumed Etiology

Most disease diagnosed by the physician is diagnosed retrospectively.

Clinical Diagnosis and Problem Solving

Specific knowledge of the individual bacterium is important in making an accurate clinical diagnosis. Therefore, one must understand certain characteristics of the microorganism and the disease process to establish the data base necessary for making a clinical diagnosis. Some of the information required for this data base is listed below:
1. What are the relative morbidity and mortality rates?
2. Is the bacterium gram positive or gram negative; what are its morphological features?
3. Does it possess invasive factors or is it opportunistic?
4. Is it usually a primary or secondary invader?
5. Does it have physiologic limitations, i.e., aerobic or anaerobic; what is the optimal temperature for growth?
6. Does it infect all organ systems or just specific organ systems?
7. Does it produce any characteristic symptoms and are these symptoms associated with specific toxins, e.g., enterotoxin, neurotoxin?
8. What specimens are sent to the laboratory and how are they collected?
9. How is it identified and differentiated from other bacteria?
10. What are the most appropriate methods for prevention and treatment?
11. How is it transmitted, and how can it be controlled?

The stepwise discussion below represents a logical approach to problem solving in infectious disease (for summary, see Fig. 4–1).

1. History and Physical Examination of Patient

A careful and accurate history must be taken and thorough physical examination performed. Factors such as age, sex, environment, occupation and geographic location of the patient are important in deter-

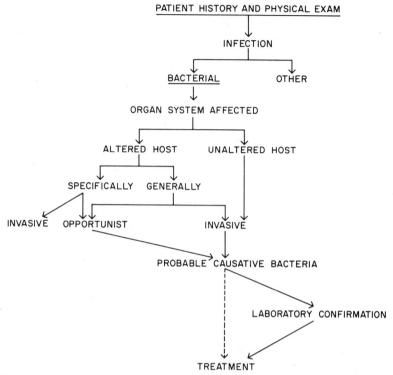

Fig. 4–1.—A step-by-step problem-solving approach to the diagnosis and treatment of a bacterial disease.

mining the cause of a bacterial disease. Other important data include a complete blood cell count with a differential cell count, and the patient's temperature, blood pressure and pulse rate. Such observations influence decisions throughout the remainder of a problem-solving approach.

2. Infection

It must be determined that the patient is actually infected. The characteristics of a bacterial infection are fever, inflammation, pain and a relative leukocytosis.

3. Organ System

The site of infection (the organ system) must be identified. Predictably, symptoms are associated with infection of specific organ systems. The particular organ system and the physiology of the bacteria limit the kinds of bacteria that can be present.

4. Altered Versus Unaltered Host

When the site of infection is known, the physician determines whether the infected organ system or individual is "normal" or if there is a predisposing cause.

    a. If a healthy, unaltered host is infected, invasive bacteria should be considered as the causative agent.

    b. If the alteration is of a specific type (previous tissue damage or infection), opportunistic bacteria should be suspected.

    c. If the host alteration is of a generalized type, both invasive and opportunistic bacteria must be considered.

5. Probable Causative Bacteria (Presumptive Diagnosis)

At the conclusion of step 4, the physician should have sufficient information to consider certain bacteria as the probable cause of the disease.

6. Laboratory Confirmation of Diagnosis

The presumptive diagnosis must be confirmed by collection of specimens and by appropriate laboratory studies (see Laboratory Procedures).

7. Treatment

Treatment involves not only administration of antibiotics but also correction of the host alteration and institution of methods for preventing transmission. Based on the presumptive diagnosis, therapy is sometimes started before laboratory confirmation is obtained. The appropriateness of this therapy must then be confirmed by laboratory studies.

LABORATORY PROCEDURES

The most important step in isolating microorganisms from clinical material is proper collection of the specimen. It is the responsibility of the physician to either collect or insure that proper procedures are used in the collection of specimens and to keep in mind the following criteria: (1) the area of collection must be carefully prepared to prevent contamination of the specimen; (2) adequate material must be collected from the site to insure inclusion of the organisms in the specimen; (3) specimens must be handled or treated properly to prevent death of the organisms; (4) the laboratory must be provided with all the necessary information to insure that the specimen is cultured on appropriate media under appropriate conditions and (5) the specimen must be transported to the laboratory as expeditiously as possible. *The results that the laboratory obtains depends on the care with which the above criteria are fulfilled. Proper treatment of the patient is dependent, in part, on reliable laboratory data.*

The following sections include methods of collection along with culture techniques applicable to different types of specimens, but they do not include methods for identifying the various bacteria or the procedural aspects of laboratory techniques; these can be found in the chapters of this book or in those books listed in the references at the end of this chapter.

Gram Stain

The gram stain is one of the most underutilized but most useful techniques available to the physician and clinical microbiologist. The technique is rapid and, along with clinical judgment, can often provide a basis for a preliminary clinical diagnosis and guide the necessary therapy. It is essential, particularly in patients with meningitis, that gram stain of cerebrospinal fluid be done immediately and the results used to initiate therapy for this life-threatening disease. In persistent infections, in which the patient is not responding to therapy, a gram stain may indicate the type of organism present even when cultures are difficult to obtain. In the laboratory direct gram stains should be made of most clinical specimens because there is a high correlation between the type of organisms seen in direct smears and those obtained in cultures. If stained smears are negative and organisms are isolated on culture, the cultured organism may be a contaminant and not actually involved in the disease process. Gram stains of specimens from patients with a possible infection not only help in determining whether organisms are present, they also indicate the presence or absence of inflammatory cells. Inflammatory cells indicate infection and some bacterial diseases are differentiated by the type of cell response.

Blood Cultures

From the standpoint of the patient's welfare, blood cultures are the most important clinical microbiologic procedure and the one most demanding with respect to techniques of collection, specimen handling and cultivation. Blood cultures are important in any condition in which bacteremia is a possibility. Bacteremia usually indicates the onset of an infectious process or a complication of an existing infection and is manifest by a sudden onset of high fever, chills, increased pulse rate and malaise. Blood cultures are done in patients with endocarditis, meningitis, pneumonia, deep-seated abscesses, urinary tract infections, brucellosis, leptospirosis and enteric fever.

Blood should be collected before administration of antibiotics. If antibiotics are already being administered, cultures should be obtained at the point of lowest antibiotic blood concentration. Opinion varies as to the number of cultures that should be done, but the rationale is to repeat the cultures to be certain that there is a bacteremia and to avoid the question of whether the organism isolated is a contaminant. A minimum of three, and perhaps six, cultures should be taken at 15- to 30-minute intervals. By preference, one should take cultures as the fever is developing. The most important step in taking a blood culture is careful preparation of the venipuncture area to eliminate skin contaminants. A time-tested procedure is (1) cleanse the area with acetone (preferably) or 70% alcohol, (2) apply tincture of iodine and allow it to dry and (3) cleanse with alcohol and then "keep your fingers off." Usually 10 ml (1–2 ml from infants) of blood is collected by venipuncture. The blood is inoculated into two broth culture bottles at the bedside in the ratio of 1:10 (blood:medium), with one bottle for aerobic and the other for anaerobic incubation. The cultures are examined daily for growth for up to 3 weeks, and when growth is evident (usually 24–48 hours), smears and gram stains are done and procedures for isolation and identification of the organism are initiated. The laboratory should immediately report, usually by phone, the results of all blood cultures.

Throat Swabs, Sputum, and Percutaneous Transtracheal Aspiration

Throat swabs are usually done in instances of pharyngitis, tonsillitis, diphtheria and pertussis and for the detection of oropharyngeal carriers. The tongue is depressed with a tongue blade, and then a sterile swab is vigorously rubbed from one side of the uvula, across the uvula and down the other side; repeating with a second swab improves the chances of a meaningful culture. If exudate or membranes are present, these should be collected. Culture media can be directly inoculated or the swabs can be placed in a transport medium for delivery to the laboratory. Smears should be made and gram stained, as the numbers and morphological features of the organisms may reveal their identity. The presence of increased numbers of polymorphonuclear leukocytes also indicates bacterial infection. Culture reports are usually available in 18–24 hours.

Sputum specimens are required for isolation of organisms from patients with tuberculosis, lobar pneumonia and pulmonary fungus infections. The specimen should result from a deep cough and must be promptly taken to the laboratory. A satisfactory specimen is usually mucoid, frequently blood tinged or rusty in color. Saliva does not substitute for sputum. A common problem for both the physician and the laboratory is whether the cultural reports indicate infection or contamination with normal flora of the mouth and pharynx. To determine suitability of the specimen, some laboratories employ the following procedure. Gram-stained smears from sputum are examined under low power (×100). Specimens with fewer than 10 squamous epithelial cells per microscopic field provide results by culture which correlate with those obtained from transtracheal aspirates. Leukocytes indicate infection but are not indicators of a satisfactory specimen. When stained smears are examined for bacteria they often show the predominant organism and are a key to therapy or an indicator for additional direct procedures such as the capsular swelling test or the fluorescent antibody technique.

Specimens obtained directly from the lung are free from normal oral flora. Percutaneous transtracheal aspiration is particularly useful for anaerobic cultures. In brief, the skin site is disinfected and anesthetized; a large-gauge needle is introduced at the cricothyroid ligament into the trachea, and a small-gauge catheter is threaded through the needle and into the trachea. The specimen is aspirated by suction into a syringe or a Lukens trap, stained and then cultured both aerobically and anaerobically. The smear often indicates the etiologic agent and the correlation is high that the same organism will be cultured.

Pus, Exudate and Abscesses

Almost any bacterial infection results in the formation of pus or exudate. If the infection is close to the surface, drainage results, but if not, then an abscess forms (muscle, liver, brain, lung, or other site). If there is drainage, then a swab (preferably moistened) is suitable for collection, subsequent inoculation of media and preparation of smears. For closed abscesses, the skin is disinfected (iodine, alcohol rinse), an incision is made and a specimen is collected by swab or aspiration with a syringe. An alternative method is to aspirate the material directly. If the specimen volume is inadequate, saline can be injected followed by aspiration. Smears and cultures are completed as usual, but if anaerobic cultures are to be done the specimen is placed in an oxygen-free vial or kept in the syringe.

Eye and Ear Specimens

Infections of the eyes may be caused by bacteria, fungi, viruses or protozoa and may involve the lid, conjunctiva, lacrimal glands, or cornea. The frequently encountered bacteria are *Staphylococcus*, *Streptococcus*, *Neisseria*, *Haemophilus* and *Pseudomonas*. Moistened cotton swabs can be used to collect material from the lid, lower palpebral conjunctiva or fornix. For corneal ulcers, a topical anesthetic is applied and then a moistened swab is applied to the edge of the corneal lesion. The swabs are used for direct inoculation of culture media. Smears are made for gram, Giemsa, and fungus stains.

Acute suppurative otitis media is an infection of the middle ear, usually caused by *Streptococcus pneumoniae, Haemophilus influenzae* or *Streptococcus pyogenes*. For specimen collection, the ear wax is removed, the eardrum is cleansed and a disinfectant is applied. A small incision is made in the drum, a Lukens-type tube is inserted and the fluid is aspirated with carefully controlled vacuum. The fluid is streaked onto blood and chocolate agar with incubation in CO_2. Smears are made and gram stained. Chronic infections usually show gram-negative rods.

Cerebrospinal Fluid

Examination of cerebrospinal fluid from patients with meningitis is the only emergency procedure done in the clinical microbiology laboratory. Any delay in the tentative identification of the organisms, and in appropriate treatment based on this identification, may result in death of the patient or, at the least, severe neurologic complications.

The cerebrospinal fluid is collected by lumbar puncture. The skin is disinfected (povidone-iodine) and the CSF is collected into a screw-capped tube. Such aseptic precautions are necessary to prevent contamination. The specimen is immediately taken to the laboratory. If the specimen is collected after the usual working hours, the laboratory personnel must be notified so that they are available to process the specimen immediately. Once in the laboratory, the specimen is centrifuged. A gram stain and an India ink wet mount are made from the pellet, and acid-fast stains are done if requested. The results of the smears are reported immediately and include the types of inflammatory cells observed. Polymorphonuclear leukocytes indicate a bacterial infection, whereas lymphocytes indicate a possible tubercular, leptospiral, fungal, protozoan or viral cause.

The cerebrospinal fluid pellet is immediately cultured in CO_2 and anaerobically at 37 C. A portion of the noncentrifuged CSF is also incubated.

Alternatively, the CSF can be filtered through a 0.45-nm membrane filter and the filter placed on an appropriate medium. If the inflammatory cells in the CSF are predominately lymphocytes, then cultures for mycobacteria and fungi are done. The cultures are observed daily for 3 days before being reported as negative. The organisms most frequently isolated are *Haemophilus influenzae, Streptococcus pneumoniae, Neisseria meningitidis, Listeria monocytogenes* and *Cryptococcus neoformans*.

Urine

All urine submitted for culture should be either (1) mid-stream, clean-voided urine, (2) urine collected by catheterization or (3) urine collected by suprapubic aspiration. Proper collection is necessary because the urethra in men contains a normal flora, and contamination via the glans is possible. The glans is washed with detergent, rinsed with a wet sponge and dried with a dry sterile sponge to minimize contamination. A clean catch specimen is collected after the patient has partially voided (mid-stream specimen). The urethra of women contains a bacterial flora and the urine is therefore contaminated with organisms from both the labia and urethra. To minimize contamination the patient is instructed to spread the labia with one hand and to wash the urethral area with soaped sponges, working from front to back. Then the patient is instructed to urinate, and after some urine has flowed the specimen bottle is inserted into the urine stream for collection of the specimen (mid-stream urine). Collection of specimens via catheterization should be avoided, but specimens can be collected from patients catheterized for other reasons. Suprapubic aspiration is done to obtain specimens from patients on whom reliable specimens cannot be obtained or who present diagnostic problems because of apparent urinary tract disease but from whom only a few bacteria are isolated from urine. The abdominal wall is carefully cleaned with skin disinfectant; a local anesthetic is injected into the skin, and the abdominal wall and bladder are penetrated with a 20-gauge needle. Then 20 ml of urine is withdrawn for culture and other diagnostic tests.

Urine specimens should be gram stained, and the morphological and staining characteristics of the bacteria reported. The observation of inflammatory cells in smears suggests infection. The presence of bacteria in the smear indicates 100,000 or more bacteria per milliliter and is presumptive of bacteriuria.

All urine specimens should be cultured within 1 hour of collection or refrigerated. Quantitative urine cultures should be done by the extinction-dilution method or by using known volumes of urine obtained with a calibrated loop (0.001 ml). Urine should be cultured on blood agar and on an enteric isolation medium such as eosin-methylene blue (EMB) agar. The blood agar plates should be incubated in CO_2. Both the number of organisms per milliliter and the identity are reported to the physician. All plates should be observed for 48 hours. Counts of 100,000 or more bacteria per milliliter are indicative of an infection, whereas counts less than 1,000 usually are not significant. Numbers between 1,000 and 10,000 are of questionable significance.

Feces

Fecal specimens can be either freshly passed stools or rectal swabs. Gram stains are employed when pseudomembranous colitis (S. aureus) is suspected and to determine the presence or absence of pus cells. Specimens that cannot be cultured immediately should be placed in an appropriate transport medium to control pH changes and prevent desiccation and loss of bacterial viability. Stool specimens should be examined and portions of the stool which contain blood or mucus should be placed in the transport medium and sent for culture.

A moderately heavy suspension of feces is made in saline and cultured on appropriate media. Serologic testing might be necessary (e.g., E. coli, Salmonella spp., Shigella spp.) for complete identification. In some laboratories, fluorescent antibody (FA) testing permits rapid identification. Isolation of enteric pathogens may require more than one specimen, and at least three specimens should be obtained from suspected carriers before they are considered negative.

Urethral Cultures

Culturing of the urethra is most frequently done for the diagnosis of gonorrhea. Exudate is obtained by inserting the tip of an inoculating needle into the urethra or by "milking" exudate from the urethra and collecting the exudate directly onto a culture plate or swab. Gram stains are done on all urethral specimens and results reported.

Vaginal, Cervical and Uterine Cultures

A vaginal speculum is used to visualize the culture source and minimize contamination. Swabs of material are inoculated directly onto culture media. Thioglycollate broth is also inoculated. The cultures are incubated at 37 C and examined daily for 3 days. Gram stains can also be done. Smears must be interpreted carefully, particularly in attempting to diagnose gonorrhea, because gram-negative cocci which resemble the gonococcus are present in the normal flora.

Determination of Susceptibility to Antimicrobial Agents

From the standpoint of importance to the physician and to treatment of patients, determination of susceptibility to antimicrobial agents is the most important procedure performed by the microbiology laboratory. The procedure for any such test is to bring a standardized suspension of a pure culture of the bacterium in contact with varying dilutions of the antimicrobial agent, and then to report as soon as possible the degree of susceptibility or resistance of the bacterium to each antimicrobial tested. The two general procedures used are the tube or agar plate dilution method and the disk-agar diffusion technique; the latter is more widely used. These procedures can be modified to monitor the concentration of an antibiotic in the blood or other fluids of the patient during treatment.

DISC-AGAR DIFFUSION METHOD (KIRBY-BAUER TEST).—A standardized inoculum is prepared by transferring 2–5 isolated colonies of the bacterium from the streak-plate to a small quantity of broth which is incubated for 4 hours at 37 C. The turbidity of the inoculum is adjusted to a standard, and a calibrated loop (0.001 ml in diameter) is used to transfer a loopful of the bacterial suspension to a molten tube of agar; the suspension is then mixed and poured over the surface of a prepared Mueller-Hinton agar plate, forming an overlay. After the inoculated-agar-overlay hardens, antibiotic-containing disks are applied to the surface and the plate incubated at 37 C for 16–18 hours. The disks used in both methods are commercially available and have been impregnated with predetermined amounts of the various antimicrobials (for example, penicillin G, 10 units; tetracycline, 30 μg; clindamycin, 2 μg; ampicillin, 10 μg). The drug diffuses out from the disk forming a decreasing concentration gradient around the disk. After incubation, the diameter of the zone of complete inhibition around each disk is measured to the nearest whole millimeter, and depending on the diameter, the results are reported in terms of sensitive (S), intermediate (I) or resistant (R) (Fig. 4–2). The zone sizes for each antimicrobial agent vary depending on the concentration, solubility and rate of diffusion of the drug; these zone sizes have been established and published in tabular form; for penicillin G, R=20 mm; I=21–28 mm and S=29 mm. The zone of inhibition indicates that the drug has either a bactericidal or a bacteriostatic effect. In general, a linear relationship exists between zone diameter and the inhibitory concentration for a given antibiotic, and this fact allows interpretation of the degree of sensitivity or resistance. Obviously, several factors affect the zones of inhibition obtained with a chemotherapeutic agent. These are type of medium, depth of the agar, pH, inoculum size, solubility and molecular size of the antibiotic. The Kirby-Bauer technique establishes a standard method for sensitivity testing which helps control these variables.

The laboratory, in consultation with the various medical services, determines the number and kinds of antimicrobial agents to be used for routine antibiograms. From the laboratory standpoint, this is an exacting procedure, requiring attention to details and inclusion of adequate controls to insure reliable and prompt results.

The same general techniques can be used for testing the antibi-

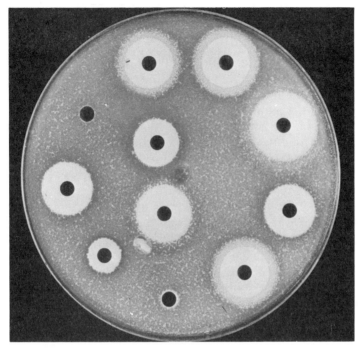

Fig. 4–2. – Kirby-Bauer antibiotic susceptibility test.

otic sensitivities of anaerobes (*Clostridium, Bacteroides, Eubacterium, Peptococcus, Peptostreptococcus, Fusobacterium* and *Veillonella*). The Kirby-Bauer method has not yet been standardized for testing of anaerobes because the inhibitory activity of the antibiotic is altered by changes in CO_2, pH and medium composition occurring in the anaerobic environment; the variability in growth rate of the anaerobes is also a factor (*C. perfringens* grow rapidly, *B. fragilis* slowly).

TUBE-DILUTION METHOD. – Antibiotic sensitivity can also be measured with dilutions of antibiotics in liquid medium. Various concentrations (usually twofold dilutions) of antibiotic are added to broth media, which are then inoculated with a standardized suspension of organisms. After incubation at 37 C for 18–24 hours, the minimal inhibitory concentration is obtained by determining the least amount of antibiotic which does not allow growth. This minimal inhibitory concentration (MIC) represents either a bactericidal or bacteriostatic effect. To differentiate between these effects, one inoculates those dilutions without growth into media without antibiotics. If growth occurs on subculture, then the inhibition was due to a bacteriostatic effect. If growth does not occur, the inhibition was due to a bactericidal effect.

LEVELS OF ANTIMICROBIAL AGENTS IN SERUM (SCHLICHTER TEST). — It is often desirable to determine the concentration of an antibiotic in the patient's serum. This information is useful in regulating the dosage of the antibiotic and in determining whether or not therapeutic concentrations are present in the serum. Usually, the bacterium isolated from the patient is used as the test organism, although an organism of known sensitivity can be used.

Blood is collected from the patient before therapy is begun or just before another injection of antibiotic is given. A second blood sample is taken after an intramuscular injection or an intravenous injection of an antibiotic. Serum is removed from the clotted blood and twofold dilutions are prepared in 0.5-ml volumes using broth as a diluent; the first tube contains 0.5 ml of undiluted patient's serum. A young culture of the isolate from the patient is diluted to contain 2×10^5 viable organisms per milliliter, and 0.5 ml of this suspension is added to each of the serum-dilution tubes. Controls must be included. All tubes are incubated at 37 C overnight and observed for the presence or absence of turbidity (compared to the density of the control). If necessary, each tube can be subcultured to determine viability of the organism and thereby differentiate bacteriostatic from bactericidal effects. Results are reported in terms of the highest dilution of the patient's serum causing an inhibition of the growth of the test organism. In general, the antibiotic dosage is considered adequate if bactericidal activity is demonstrated in the 1:8 or 1:16 dilutions. For staphylococcal infection the minimum dilution is 1:32.

Determination of serum or tissue level of antibiotic is important in managing serious infections such as endocarditis and in treating patients with altered excretion rates or other physiologic alterations. Some antibiotics are toxic at high concentrations, and the level of antibiotic in the body helps the clinician adjust the administration of the antibiotic so as to maintain selective toxicity.

Recently, sophisticated methods for determining levels of aminoglycoside antibiotics and chloramphenicol in fluids have been described. These methods use the plasmid-associated enzymes obtained from resistant organisms which adenylate or acetylate antibiotics. In essence, the techniques use radiolabeled acetyl-CoA or adenosine triphosphate. The radiolabeled acetyl or adenosine group is transferred to the antibiotic in the presence of antibiotic and enzyme.

The inactivated radiolabeled antibiotic readily binds to phosphocellulose paper and can be quantitatively removed from the reaction mixture by filtration and measured by a scintillation counter. The amount of radiolabel is then a measure of the amount of antibiotic present in the sample.

Fluorescent Antibody Technique

The fluorescent antibody technique (FA, immunofluorescence) can be used in identifying bacteria, viruses, fungi or protozoa in culture, in tissue or in their natural environment. Location and identification of tissue antigens are also possible. The principle of the procedure is that a specific antiserum is conjugated with a fluorochrome, and then when the antiserum reacts with the specific antigen, it carries along the fluorochrome. Subsequently, when this antigen-antibody-fluorochrome complex is exposed to UV light, the fluorochrome emits a visible light, making the antigen-antibody complex visible microscopically.

Darkfield Microscopy

For darkfield microscopy, the microscope is fitted with a special condenser in which the central portion of the upper lens is blacked-out. The darkfield condenser permits the rays from the light source to come up around the periphery and then bends them at an angle so they do not enter the objective. Thus, when one looks into the eyepiece, the field is dark. If an object such as a spirochete is in the plane of focus of the objective, the light rays strike the sides of the spirochete and are deflected up into the objective, outlining the bacterium in an observable band of light. The organism seems to be self-luminous in the dark field. Darkfield microscopy can be used to observe any bacterium or any other cell or object that can be prepared as a wet mount for microscopic observation. For the chancre stage of syphilis, the lesion is gently rubbed with gauze and the exuding plasma (blood free) is collected in a capillary pipette. The collected fluid is expelled onto a slide, covered with a coverglass and sealed. The slide, with oil on both top and bottom, is transferred to the microscope and observed for the presence of the actively motile spirochetes.

SUPPLEMENTARY READING

Bauer, A. W., Kirby, W. M. M., Sherris, J. C., and Turck, M.: Antibiotic susceptibility testing by a standarized single disc method, Am. J. Clin. Pathol. 45:493, 1966.
Bodily, H. L., Updyke, E. L., and Mason, J. O. (eds.): *Diagnostic Procedures*

for Bacterial, Mycotic and Parasitic Infections (5th ed.; New York: American Public Health Association, 1970).

Kunin, C. M.: *Detection, Prevention and Management of Urinary Tract Infections* (2d ed.; Philadelphia: Lea & Febiger, 1974).

Lennette, E. H., Spaulding, E. H., and Truant, J. P. (eds.): *Manual of Clinical Microbiology* (2d ed.; Washington, D.C.: American Society for Microbiology, 1974).

Murray, P. R., and Washington, J. A.: Microscopic and bacteriological analysis of expectorate sputum, Mayo Clin. Proc. 50:339–344, 1975.

Rose, N. R., and Friedman, H. (eds.): *Manual of Clinical Immunology* (Washington, D.C.: American Society for Microbiology, 1976).

Slock, J., Snyder, I. S., and Galask, R. P.: Advance organizers in microbiology, ASM News 40:641–644, 1974.

5 / Staphylococcus

OVERVIEW

Staphylococci were observed in pus by Koch in 1878, but it was Ogston in 1881 who experimentally produced abscesses in animals and demonstrated that these organisms caused production of pus. Staphylococci continue to be one of the principal causes of suppurative infections, which may vary from the insignificant infection caused by a splinter to the life-threatening abscesses in various internal organs. When penicillin was introduced, severe staphylococcal infections were among the first infections to be treated and with remarkable success. But shortly thereafter, reports of staphylococcal resistance to penicillin began to appear which focused attention on studies on the mechanism of action of penicillin and on how organisms developed resistance to the antibiotic. The occurrence of resistance has resulted in reintroduction of stricter hygienic and aseptic hospital procedures in order to reduce the incidence of hospital-acquired infections. Obviously, staphylococci will continue to be a health problem, but perhaps a better understanding of the mechanisms of staphylococcal infections will provide a basis for altering host defenses and thus prevent infections with these ubiquitous organisms.

GENERAL CHARACTERISTICS

Staphylococci are gram-positive cocci (0.8–1 μm in diameter), irregularly arranged in clusters (Fig. 5–1). Adjacent cocci in a cluster may be connected by intracellular bridges (Fig. 5-2). Neither spores nor flagella are produced. Capsules are not usually produced but capsulated strains have been isolated. They are facultative anaerobes with an optimum growth temperature of 35–37 C. On solid media they produce entire, hemispherical, soft, glistening colonies 1–2 mm in diameter. Carbohydrates are fermented with the production of acid but gas is not produced; lactic acid is the principal end product from glucose fermentation. They are catalase positive; this characteristic helps differentiate staphylococci from streptococci. The staphylococci

65

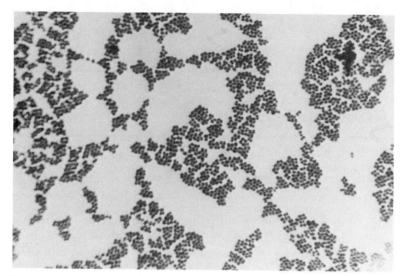

Fig. 5–1.—Gram stain of *Staphylococcus aureus.* Note the arrangement in clusters.

Fig. 5–2.—Scanning electron microscope picture of *Staphylococcus aureus.* Note the cluster arrangement of the cells and the intracellular bridges, which are of unknown composition. (From Klainer, A. S., and Geis, I.: *Agents of Bacterial Disease* [Hagerstown, Md.: Harper & Row, 1973]. By permission of the author and publisher.)

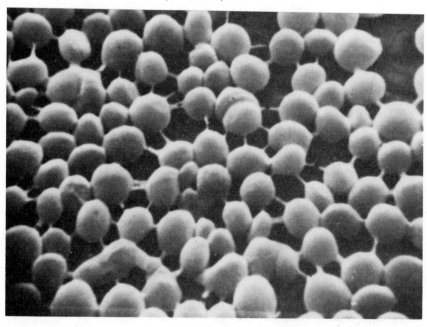

are quite resistant to drying (often cultured from dried pus), and will withstand temperatures up to 60 C. They grow in 10% sodium chloride but are inhibited by 0.001% crystal violet.

SPECIES

STAPHYLOCOCCUS AUREUS forms orange colonies which are usually beta-hemolytic (90% of isolates) (Fig. 5–3). They are coagulase positive and produce acid from mannitol. They produce α toxin and contain cell wall-associated ribitol teichoic acid and protein A. The nucleases are heat resistant, which helps differentiate S. aureus from S. epidermidis. This is the principal pathogenic species causing such infections as boils, osteomyelitis and food poisoning.

STAPHYLOCOCCUS EPIDERMIDIS forms white colonies that are usually not beta-hemolytic (10% are hemolytic). Unlike S. aureus, they are coagulase negative and usually do not ferment mannitol nor do they produce toxin. They have a cell wall-associated glycerol teichoic acid but not protein A. The nucleases are denatured by heat as contrasted with those of S. aureus. This organism is a normal inhabitant of the skin and may occasionally cause abscesses and even endocarditis.

MICROCOCCUS SPP.—These gram-positive cocci resemble staphylo-

Fig. 5–3.—Colonies of *Staphylococcus aureus* on blood agar. Note the large zone of beta hemolysis and the faint zone due to incubation at room temperature.

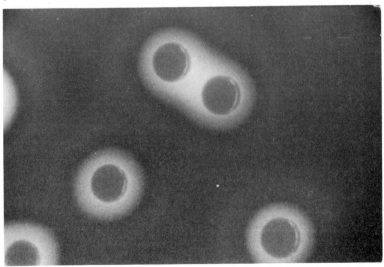

TABLE 5-1.—SCHEME FOR IDENTIFICATION
OF STAPHYLOCOCCI

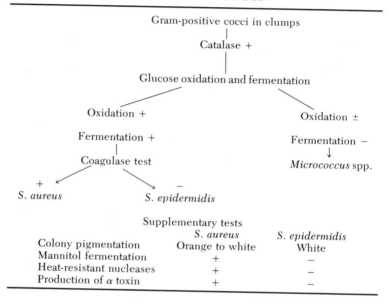

	Supplementary tests	
	S. aureus	S. epidermidis
Colony pigmentation	Orange to white	White
Mannitol fermentation	+	−
Heat-resistant nucleases	+	−
Production of α toxin	+	−

cocci, except the cells are frequently larger. The smooth, nonhemolytic colonies are usually pigmented (yellow or red). They are coagulase negative; glucose may or may not be oxidized but acid is not produced anaerobically. There are three established species. These organisms may be isolated from the skin, nasopharynx, or from clinical material and are confused with staphylococci but are not pathogenic.

A simple scheme for differentiating the *Staphylococcus* and *Micrococcus* is shown in Table 5-1.

ECOLOGY

Staphylococci begin to take up residence on the skin and in the nose during the first day of life and are carried on various mucocutaneous surfaces for the remainder of a person's existence. Nasal carriers are of primary importance as transmitters via aerosols, and although the percentage of such carriers in a given group is variable, it is usually between 30 and 50%. The site of colonization in these individuals is the surface of the squamous epithelium of the vestibule.

Some individuals are persistent carriers and even maintain the same phage types for long periods of time. *S. epidermidis* is a normal inhabitant of the skin surfaces, but *S. aureus* can be isolated from a wide variety of animals, including dogs, cats, cows, horses and pigeons, and certain of these strains are the same phage types as those isolated from humans.

CELL WALL

The structure (Fig. 5–4) of the staphylococcal peptidoglycan is the same as that of other bacteria (chap. 2; Figs. 2–1 and 2–2). *S. aureus* has pentapeptide bridges of glycine residues connecting the free amino group of L-lysine of one chain with the carboxyl group of D-alanine of the adjacent chain. Attached to the N-acetylmuramic acid by phosphodiester bonds are teichoic acids; these are linear polyphosphate polymers. Teichoic acids of *S. aureus* are made of ribitol 5-phosphate with α- or β-N-acetylglucosamine (strain variable) substituted at C-4 of ribitol. N-acetylglucosamine is the determinant of immunologic specificity and acts as a phage receptor site. The teichoic acids of *S. epidermidis* are polymers of glycerol 3-phosphate with α- or

Fig. 5–4.—Electron micrograph of ultrathin section of *Staphylococcus aureus.* Note the trilaminar cell wall, the nuclear material, and the granular cytoplasm composed mostly of ribosomes; the indentations are part of a cross wall which forms prior to cell division. (From Cole, R. M., Chatterjee, A. N., Gilpin, R. W., and Young, F. E.: Ann. N. Y. Acad. Sci. 236:22, 1974. By permission of the author and journal.)

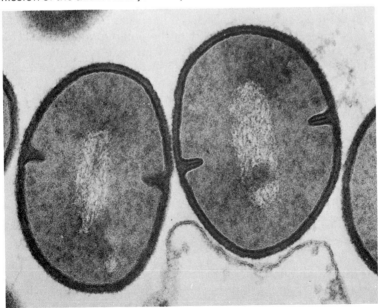

β-linked glucose residues substituted at C-2 of glycerol. The glucose residues are the determinants of immunologic specificity. An additional constituent of the *S. aureus* cell wall is a low molecular weight protein, protein A, which reacts nonspecifically with the Fc portion of IgG. Some work suggests that protein A may also react with IgM and IgA (see Antigens).

ANTIGENS

S. AUREUS.—*S. aureus* is antigenically complex. Approximately 30 antigens are demonstrable and these are designated as antigen a, b, c, etc. With the slide agglutination test and sorbed antisera, *S. aureus* has been divided into 18 serotypes. Of all these antigens, only the cell wall teichoic acids and protein A have been thoroughly studied.

All *S. aureus* contain the species-specific teichoic acid (polysaccharide A). The teichoic acids are antigenic with N-acetylglucosamine being the determinant of specificity; they stimulate antibody production in humans, and titers may increase during staphylococcal infections. Hypersensitivity to teichoic acids has been demonstrated in animals. Protein A (Jensen's antigen A) is a cell wall surface antigen which stimulates antibody production in animals and humans. It also reacts nonspecifically with the Fc fragment of IgG from a variety of mammals. In humans it reacts with IgG subclasses IgG1, 2 and 4 but not 3. This reaction causes staphylococcal cells to agglutinate in normal serum. Protein A can initiate the complement cascade (chap. 1), which is then chemotactic; it can also injure platelets. Because it interferes with opsonization of the cells, it may act as an antiphagocytic factor. Hypersensitivity to protein A including local and systemic anaphylaxis is demonstrable in animals; hypersensitivity reactions could play a role in the inflammatory responses in humans.

S. EPIDERMIDIS.—Little information is available on the antigenicity of *S. epidermidis*, except that the cell walls contain either α- or β-glucosylglycerol teichoic acid (polysaccharide B) with glucose sugar residues as determinants of specificity. Serologically, cross reactions between *S. aureus* and *S. epidermidis* may be due to intracellular glyceroteichoic acids in *S. aureus*.

BACTERIOPHAGE

PHAGE.—Staphylococcal phages contain DNA and have been placed into six serologic groups (A, B, D, F, G, L); each group has similar buoyant densities, morphologies and homologies. Antibodies, particularly to groups A and F, are demonstrable in serums of patients. All the phages have elongated or hexagonal heads with tails of varying lengths (150–300 nm). The specific receptor sites on the staphylococcal cell involve both teichoic acid and peptidoglycan. This host cell is referred to as the phage type, with each being arbitrarily assigned a number. For laboratory convenience staphylococci are placed in phage groups as follows:

Group I—phage types 29, 52, 52A, 79 and 80
Group II—phage types 3A, 3B, 3C, 55 and 71
Group III—phage types 6, 7, 42E, 47, 53, 54, 75, 77 and 83A
Group IV—phage type 42D
Miscellaneous—phage types 81, 187

Lysogenic phages can be determinants for the synthesis of alpha and delta hemolysins, staphylokinase, enterotoxin, lipase, leukocidin and pigment production. Mutants that have lost these properties are no longer lysogenic, but lipase production, hemolysis and fibrinolysis have been shown to be regained by lysogenic conversion.

Phage typing is done by seeding an agar plate heavily with the culture of *S. aureus* to be typed. Single drops of a highly diluted suspension of each numbered phage are placed at designated positions on the agar surface. After incubation, phage susceptibility is indicated as a clear area (bacterial lysis). Since the phage number is known, the type can be designated. If the culture is lysed by phage number 52, then the culture is designated phage type 52. If the culture is lysed by two different phages, for example, 80 and 81, then the designation is phage type 80/81. Certain cultures cannot be phage typed, perhaps because (1) specific receptor sites are not available, (2) the phage is unable to penetrate the cell, (3) penetration occurs but replication does not take place or (4) the cell is lysogenic. Phage typing has been used in epidemiologic studies to correlate phage types with antibiotic resistance and to relate types with a particular infection. There has been a high incidence of phage type 80/81 in hospital-acquired staphylococcal infections.

GENETICS

When penicillin was introduced in the early 1940s, there were dramatic results in the treatment of severe staphylococcal diseases, but by 1946 there were numerous reports of penicillin-resistant strains, particularly from hospital-acquired infections. This resistance was due to the production by the bacteria of β-lactamase (penicillinase).

Antibiotic use resulted in selection of resistant strains already in existence before the use of penicillin; this is also true for resistance to subsequently used antibiotics. Resistance to penicillin is under the genetic control of a large, circular plasmid. Plasmids also carry the genetic determinants for resistance to tetracyclines, chloramphenicol, kanamycin, neomycin, erythromycin, certain metallic ions such as mercury and cadmium, and for bacteriocin synthesis. A single staphylococcal cell may harbor a number of plasmids (or multiple copies of a plasmid) and one plasmid can carry several genetic markers such as production of β-lactamase, resistance to erythromycin and metallic ions. Certain antibiotic resistance markers can also be chromosomal as occurs in resistance to streptomycin, novobiocin and methicillin. Gene transfer has allowed these determinants to be spread among the staphylococci. The primary mechanism is transduction, in which case the mature phage (transducing phage) is released and enters a recipient staphylococcal cell, which then takes on the new phenotypic properties of resistance to an antibiotic. The transduction of antibiotic resistance is readily demonstrable in vitro, and there is experimental evidence that this can occur on the skin and in the oropharynx. Transformation of resistance determinants has also been accomplished in vitro.

S. epidermidis frequently exhibits multiple antibiotic resistance with a plasmid carrying the determinants. Gene transfer is primarily by transduction, but attempts to transduce S. epidermidis plasmids to S. aureus have not been successful.

ENZYMES, HEMOLYSINS AND TOXINS

COAGULASE. — Staphylocoagulase, a protein produced by 90% of S. aureus, reacts with fibrinogen in the following manner:

Staphylocoagulase + Coagulase-Reacting Factor →
   Coagulase − Thrombin.
Coagulase − Thrombin + Fibrinogen → Fibrin.

The coagulase-reacting factor is prothrombin or an active component of the molecule. The reaction requires no calcium and takes place in the presence of anticoagulants. Coagulase is antigenic and there are at least seven serologic types. The presence of coagulase correlates with the pathogenicity of staphylococci, but its role in pathogenicity is probably indirect in that the fibrin produced contributes to the inflammatory process and may protect the organisms from phagocytosis. Coagulase differs from clumping factor, a cell wall-bound protein which causes cells to clump in the presence of fibrinogen.

ENTEROTOXINS. — These are heat-resistant and proteolytic enzyme-resistant proteins synthesized by *S. aureus*. Enterotoxin-producing strains are lysogenic and are found primarily in phage group III. On the basis of antigenic specificity they are separated into toxins A, B, C_1, C_2, D and E. Enterotoxin A is a single polypeptide chain with a molecular weight of approximately 29,000 and glutamic acid as the N-terminal residue. It is produced during the exponential growth period and is the most frequent cause of food poisoning. Enterotoxin B is a single polypeptide chain containing approximately 239 amino acid residues. There is less specific information about the other enterotoxins. The enterotoxins are antigenic in humans. In one study involving 600 persons, antibodies to toxins A, B and C_1 were detectable in 22% of healthy and in 32–67% of infected persons with staphylococcal abscesses, bacteremia or pneumonia, with titers ranging from 1:2 to 1:32. Titers were highest with enterotoxin B. The ingested enterotoxins cause food poisoning in humans, and an experimental enteritis can be produced in cats, dogs and monkeys.

EXFOLIATIN (exfoliative or epidermolytic toxin). — This protein has a molecular weight of approximately 26,000. The toxin is produced by most strains of phage group II staphylococci (3A, 3B, 3C, 55, 71), and its synthesis is probably under plasmid control. When injected into newborn mice (1–6 days) or humans it produces a positive Nikolsky sign, bullae and exfoliation. In humans it causes the scalded skin syndrome (toxic epidermal necrolysis).

HEMOLYSINS (toxins). — Hemolysins will lyse human or animal erythrocytes. Four have been identified from *S. aureus* (α, β, γ, δ). The term *hemolysin* implies disruption and dissolution of red cells, but there may be interference with cell membrane function without lysis. Hemolysins can damage a wide variety of cells, including leukocytes, macrophages, platelets, tissue cells and bacterial protoplasts. The α-hemolysin is a heat-labile protein which lyses rabbit and sheep erythrocytes, but human red cells are more resistant. Production of this hemolysin is phage mediated. It is cytolytic for many types of cells in tissue culture and also acts as a leukocidin, causing damage by altering cell membrane functions. It may contribute to pathogenicity through either disruption of metabolism or its cytolytic effect on tissue cells. The β-hemolysin (sphingomyelinase C) is a heat-labile protein which lyses goat, bovine, human and sheep erythrocytes. Its activity is enhanced by certain metal ions. It is an enzyme hydrolyzing phospholipids with an activity resembling that of phospholipase C. If an inoculated blood plate (sheep or bovine blood) is incubated at 37 C and then refrigerated, the zone of hemolysis is enhanced and enlarged by this hemolysin. The reaction is termed *hot-cold lysis* (Fig. 5 – 3). Leukocidal and cytolytic activities have been associated with the β-hemolysin, but this is questioned by some workers. As a factor of pathogenicity, it may cause cell lysis. The γ-hemolysin is a protein with two components that will lyse human, rabbit and sheep erythrocytes. It is inactivated by pronase, and cell lysis is inhibited by lipids. Antibodies have been demonstrated in humans with osteomyelitis. The δ-hemolysin is a heat-stable polypeptide with surfactant properties. It will lyse erythrocytes from humans and a variety of animals; this action is inhibited by lipoproteins which can also mask antigenicity. In addition, it is cytolytic for leukocytes, platelets, fibroblasts, various tissue culture cells, lysosomes and protoplasts and will produce dermonecrosis in rabbits and guinea pigs. The role of this hemolysin in staphylococcal metabolism is not defined, but it may contribute to pathogenicity through its leukocidin and cytolytic activities. Some work indicates that δ-hemolysin increases the cyclic adenosine monophosphate (cyclic AMP) concentration in the guinea pig ileum, thereby inhibiting water absorption.

Beta-hemolytic strains of *S. epidermidis* produce α-hemolysin and perhaps small amounts of δ-hemolysin.

HYALURONIDASE. — This spreading factor hydrolyzes hyaluronic acid and, in this manner, aids pathogenicity. It differs antigenically from streptococcal hyaluronidase. Three types (I, II, III) have been described on the basis of electrophoretic patterns.

β-LACTAMASE (penicillinase). — This enzyme inactivates both penicillin and cephalosporin by catalyzing the hydrolysis of the amide bond in the β-lactam ring of 6-aminopenicillanic acid and 7-aminocephalosporanic acid to form inactive penicilloic acid and inactive cephalosporanic acid. This enzyme is found in *S. aureus*, *S. epidermidis*, some *Bacillus* and the enterics.

LEUKOCIDIN (Panton-Valentine). — This protein links to the cell membrane surface of polymorphonuclear leukocytes and macrophages causing increased permeability to cations, secretion of proteins and interference with phagocytosis. The protein consists of F and S components; both are necessary for the leukocidin activity with the F component binding to the membrane. It is an antiphagocytic factor. Antileukocidin antibodies are demonstrable in man.

LIPASES. — These enzymes hydrolyze both long- and short-chain triglycerides to fatty acids; they are demonstrable in both *S. aureus* and

S. epidermidis. It has been suggested that the lipolytic activity of staphylococci in the sebaceous duct may contribute to the development of acne.

LYSOZYME. — This glycosidase attacks the β-1, 4-glycosidic bonds of the cell wall peptidoglycan of prokaryotic cells and may result in the formation of protoplasts or in cell lysis. The role it plays in staphylococcal disease, if any, is not evident.

NUCLEASE. — This enzyme is located on or near the cell surface and can cleave DNA or RNA. Purification studies indicate that it is composed of a single polypeptide chain of 149 amino acids.

PHOSPHATASE. — Staphylococci produce both acid and alkaline phosphatases. The acid phosphatase is constitutive and loosely bound to the cell. The exact role of phosphatases in cell function is not known.

PROTEASES. — Both *S. aureus* and *S. epidermidis* produce enzymes that can hydrolyze casein, elastin, gelatin and hemoglobin.

STAPHYLOKINASE. — This enzyme converts plasminogen into the active enzyme, plasmin. Plasmin causes lysis of a fibrin clot.

STAPHYLOCOCCAL INFECTIONS

Staphylococcal infections in man are due primarily to *S. aureus* with the type and severity of infection dependent on the site of invasion and the response of the host to the bacteria. These infections tend to be more severe in the young, the aged and in the individual compromised by immunologic deficiency, diabetes, debilitation, burns or extensive surgery. The infections are suppurative and develop into abscesses due to tissue necrosis and the accumulation of dead and dying leukocytes. The infections may remain localized or drain to the outside, or the staphylococci may metastasize via the lymphatic and vascular system to produce abscesses in other areas of the body. Staphylococci may produce a wide range of infections, including: pustules of hair follicles or sweat glands, sties, boils, carbuncles, meningitis, endocarditis, pericarditis, pyelonephritis, enterocolitis, osteomyelitis and wound infections. A number of these infections are discussed below.

Whenever the skin surface is broken as by a wound, cut, abrasion, incision or suture, either *S. aureus* or *S. epidermidis* may be introduced and result in inflammation and abscess formation with the extent and severity of the infection dependent on the effectiveness of

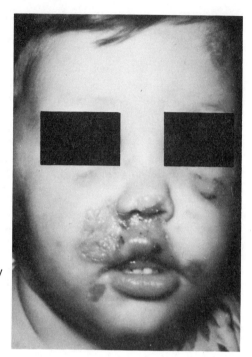

Fig. 5–5.—Impetigo in a young child. *Staphylococcus aureus* was isolated. (Courtesy of W. A. Welton, Division of Dermatology, West Virginia University.)

Fig. 5–6.—Gram stain of a direct smear from a carbuncle. Note the phago-cytized staphylococci and the numerous polymorphonuclear leukocytes. *Staphylococcus aureus* was isolated.

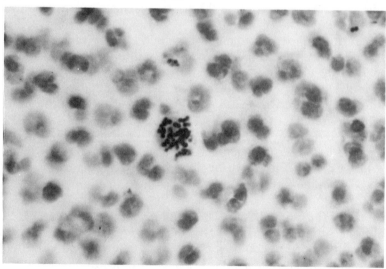

the defense mechanisms of the host. Impetigo occurs primarily in children and may be caused by either S. *aureus* or S. *pyogenes* (Fig. 5–5). It begins as localized areas of inflammation, becomes papular, then forms vesicles that rupture, leaving a crust. Impetigo lesions usually heal without a scar; impetigo may be contagious. The carbuncle (boil) begins with the staphylococci growing in a hair follicle (folliculitis) and penetrating into the subcutaneous tissue to form an abscess and eventually a draining sinus. Carbuncles may be single or multiple and frequently recur (furunculosis) (Fig. 5–6). Bloodstream invasion may result in secondary sites of infection in any organ or tissue but is more likely in the heart valves, kidneys, lungs or meninges. Endocarditis (chap. 6) is not frequently caused by staphylococci, although there is an increasing incidence in narcotic addicts. Meningitis due to staphylococci may be hematogenous or traumatic in origin but is not common. Staphylococcal pneumonia may be lobar, bronchial or interstitial with abscess formation; it can be primary or secondary to viral pneumonia, whooping cough or measles. Staphylococci frequently cause pulmonary infections as a complication of cystic fibrosis.

Osteomyelitis is an infection of the bone (usually the long bones), resulting from hematogenous or traumatic inoculation of the marrow, although in some instances the origin is never established. S. *aureus* is most frequently involved, but a variety of other organisms have been isolated. The organism grows in the bone marrow, invades the bone producing sequestered areas of necrosis, and may then erode to the skin surface, forming a draining sinus. Chronic osteomyelitis may develop in spite of surgery and intensive chemotherapy, and months or years after apparent healing the infection may become active again—often with the same strain of the organism. Some authors postulate that the organisms survive as L-forms.

Enteritis (staphylococcal enteritis, pseudomembranous colitis) may follow oral administration of broad-spectrum antibiotics which markedly reduce the bacterial flora of the intestinal tract. If antibiotic-resistant S. *aureus* are present, they normally are greatly outnumbered and suppressed by the *Escherichia-Bacteroides-Bifidobacterium-Streptococcus* flora. Freed from this competition for nutrients by chemotherapy S. *aureus* will grow rapidly, producing areas of acute suppurative necrosis, pseudomembrane development and bacteremia with a high mortality. Enterotoxin and δ-toxin may be factors in the pathogenesis of these diseases.

The majority of cases of food poisoning are due to S. *aureus, Clostridium perfringens,* or species of *Salmonella.* In cases caused by S. *aureus,* the foods (frequently pastries, but almost any food can be involved) are usually contaminated during preparation, and then the organisms grow and produce their enterotoxins (see above). After the food has been ingested there is an incubation period of 1–6 hours, followed by a sudden onset of nausea, vomiting and diarrhea which persists for 24–48 hours. Mortalities are rare except at the two extremes of life. The mechanism of action of the toxin is controversial, but the oral feeding of enterotoxin B to monkeys indicates that vomiting is due to stimulation of local neural receptors in the gut with impulses traveling along afferent autonomic fibers to the vomiting center. Proof of staphylococcal involvement in cases of food poisoning is dependent on demonstration of enterotoxin production by S. *aureus* isolates or its presence in foods. Through the use of concentration methods and immunodiffusion techniques with specific antisera, as little as 0.001 μg quantities of enterotoxin can be detected. The δ-toxin may be important in production of the symptoms of diarrhea.

Toxic epidermal necrolysis (Ritter's disease, Lyell's syndrome, scalded skin syndrome) is a generalized exfoliative dermatitis occurring primarily in children (newborn to 10 years). It is rare in adults. This syndrome includes three types of dermatologic responses. One form is exfoliative disease in which there is an abrupt onset of diffuse erythema, usually generalized, with the skin being sensitive to touch. A positive Nikolsky sign develops (peeling or wrinkling of skin to light stroking), and large bullae appear followed by a peeling of sheets of skin with healing usually in 7–10 days. The other forms include generalized scarlatiniform rash with desquamation of large flakes of dried skin and localized bullous lesions without exfoliation. The focus of the infection may be at a location distant from the skin. Treatment is with intravenous antibiotics.

S. *epidermidis* is often considered to be nonpathogenic, but it may cause endocarditis after cardiac surgery, infections of cerebrospinal shunts in hydrocephalic patients and urinary tract infections, particularly in children.

HOSPITAL INFECTIONS (nosocomial infections).—Antibiotic-resistant strains of S. *aureus*, particularly of the phage type 52/52A/80/81 complex, have been a major cause of hospital-acquired infections (chap.1). These occur more frequently in surgical patients, burn patients and newborns, with hospital personnel frequently being the source. Transmission from these persons to the patient may be by contact (hands) but more frequently is via droplets from a nasal carrier. Within a hospital the carrier rate is highly variable, but on some services it may include 50–70% of the hospital personnel, and about 25%

of these persons are persistent carriers harboring the same phage type for extended periods. Recently there has been a decrease in staphylococcal hospital infections due, in part, to careful and discriminatory use of antibiotics with more attention given to aseptic and hygienic techniques. Colonization of the umbilical stump of the newborn with a *S. aureus* strain (502 A) of low virulence interferes with colonization by the hospital strains. This may be due to production of bacteriocins. This technique has received only limited acceptance.

MECHANISMS OF PATHOGENICITY

Most microorganisms causing disease must first enter tissue where they use available nutrients for growth and reproduction. As staphylococci are present on most mucocutaneous surfaces, they easily circumvent the skin and/or mucous membrane defenses via cuts, abrasions, traumatic lesions, burns or operative sites. In the absence of obvious lesions, we must assume entrance through sweat glands, hair follicles or microscopic abrasions of the skin or mucous membranes. Once in the injured tissue, the staphylococci use nutrients from plasma or the products of enzymatic degradation of tissue cells. The staphylococci increase in numbers and spread locally by direct continuity. Further extension may then occur via the lymph or bloodstream with the bacteria free or transported by leukocytes resulting in metastatic foci of infection. Phagocytized staphylococci have a prolonged survival rate in PMNs, which favors this distribution and survival in the host.

The mechanisms of pathogenicity of the *Staphylococcus* are extremely complex, and although a number of extracellular products have been shown to be cytolytic, degrading or antiphagocytic, none of these presently identified—with the exception of the enterotoxins, exfoliatin and perhaps δ-toxin—correlate directly with pathogenicity. Thus, there is an interplay of many factors, including competition for tissue nutrients, changes in pH, reduction of oxygen tension, and enzymatic action on tissue cells resulting in tissue cell death and necrosis. In addition, there is interference with phagocytosis through (1) growth in clusters, (2) action of the clumping factor, (3) presence of protein A and (4) neutralization of intracellular hydrogen peroxide production by catalase. Supplementing these processes is the direct action of leukocidin and some hemolysins (particularly α) on the leukocytes. This is most important as phagocytosis is a primary defense mechanism of the body against staphylococcal infections.

Staphylococcal infections are characterized by abscess formation as contrasted with those of streptococci and pneumococci, which usually produce vascular lesions. Experimental evidence indicates that abscess formation may be the result of host reaction to cell wall components. As yet, no specific abscess-forming factor has been isolated, although protein A does fix complement and promotes chemotaxis. Staphylococcal infections tend to recur in a given individual even though humoral antibodies are demonstrable. As such infections tend to be less pustular, more necrotic, and have a greater degree of cellulitis, it is suggested that these represent to some degree a hypersensitivity reaction.

The nausea and vomiting commonly associated with S. aureus food poisoning are due to the enterotoxin. Feeding micrograms of this toxin to humans results in nausea and vomiting, clearly identifying the role of enterotoxins. Some patients with S. aureus food poisoning have diarrhea in addition to nausea and vomiting. The alteration in water absorption mediated by increased cyclic AMP which has been shown to occur in the guinea pig ileum challenged with δ-toxin suggests that this toxin may also be important in human disease.

The exfoliative toxin is clearly associated with the scalded skin syndrome and may also be important in production of bullae. The toxin causes splitting and disruption of the desmosomes at their intercellular contact sites within the granular layer of the epidermis, resulting in intraepidermal separation and exfoliation.

IMMUNITY

Using a variety of serologic procedures, it is possible to demonstrate antibodies in human serum against staphylococcal coagulase, hemolysins, hyaluronidase, leukocidin, protein A, staphylokinase, teichoic acids and even staphylococcal phages. Antibody titers rise during staphylococcal infections, particularly in response to α-hemolysin, γ-hemolysin, leukocidin and the teichoic acids (titers to teichoic acids rise during S. aureus endocarditis). However, there is little correlation between the presence of these antibodies and recovery from staphylococcal disease or prevention of colonization. IgG antibodies reactive with the cell wall and which require complement, are present in normal serum and the opsonin antibody titer increases in staphylococcal infections such as endocarditis. Hypersensitivity to whole cells, lysates and a number of antigens is demonstrable in humans and probably contributes little to immunity but may well add to the disease process through initiating an inflammatory response to the organisms.

A number of vaccines have been used in the treatment or prevention of staphylococcal disease, including toxoids of α-hemolysin and leukocidin, capsular polysaccharide, teichoic acids, whole-cell lysates and killed whole-cell autogenous vaccines. The toxoids, capsular antigens, and teichoic acids are of no value for active or passive immunization. There have been some reports of success in patients with osteomyelitis or furunculosis using the whole-cell vaccines. It appears that if a vaccine is to prevent colonization or promote recovery, it must increase the opsonin titer and aid phagocytosis.

TREATMENT

Staphylococci continue to be a major problem from the standpoint of resistance to antibiotics. Some 85% of S. *aureus* isolated in the clinical laboratory are resistant to benzylpenicillin with varying percentages being resistant to several antibiotics. These may include any combination of the semisynthetic penicillins (ampicillin, methicillin, oxacillin), chloramphenicol, erythromycin, aminoglycosides (gentamicin, kanamycin, neomycin, streptomycin) or any other antibiotic in use.

In the absence of antibiotics, resistant strains tend to be replaced by sensitive strains, which may be due to the loss of a genetic marker or dilution by susceptible strains in a population; this supports the concept that the use of antibiotics for treatment of staphylococcal infections should be limited. The antibiotics most frequently in use are methicillin, cloxacillin, gentamicin, and in refractory infections, rifampicin and erythromycin. The resistance pattern of a given staphylococcal isolate is determined by antibiotic sensitivity testing (chap. 4), and the results are used to guide antibiotic therapy.

In addition to chemotherapy, the infection must be drained to decrease the bacterial load and to facilitate penetration of antibiotics.

LABORATORY PROCEDURES

Materials collected from suspected staphylococcal infections usually include pus, exudate, or both, but also may be blood, cerebrospinal fluid, urine or stool. The procedures outlined here refer only to specimens of pus or exudate, which may be collected by aspiration or with sterile swabs. A smear should be made directly from the specimen and gram stained. If gram-positive organisms are observed, a preliminary report is made indicating that a gram-positive coccus was observed in the smear. Blood agar plates and a tube of thioglycollate broth should be inoculated and incubated 18–24 hours at 37 C for isolation. Stool cultures should also be plated on a selective medium such as mannitol-salt agar. Flat, soft, orange or white colonies with a zone of beta-hemolysis (pigmentation and hemolysis are variable) indicate staphylococci. These should be gram stained, and catalase, coagulase and other tests should be done as required.

Antibiotic sensitivity tests (antibiograms) are done and results are reported in terms of sensitive, intermediate or resistant for each antibiotic tested (chap. 4); the results guide the antibiotic therapy of the patient.

PROBLEM SOLVING AND REVIEW

No. 1. GIVEN: — A 55-year-old man was hospitalized because of pain below the knee. Two months previously he had injured his left leg; the roentgenograms revealed no abnormal findings, pain subsided, a swelling occurred in 2 weeks but disappeared. The present pain had started 2 weeks earlier. No chills or fever were reported and the patient appeared in good health. Three years previously he had been hospitalized for pemphigus vulgaris and treated with prednisone, which he was still taking. He developed a S. aureus septicemia but became asymptomatic after 4 weeks of treatment with oxacillin. Roentgenographic examination of the left leg revealed an osteolytic lesion in the proximal shaft of the tibia and an area of rarifaction in the distal shaft of the right femur. A skeletal survey, laboratory findings and blood cultures revealed no abnormalities. Surgery revealed a cavity in the left tibia. The cavity was drained; smears showed gram-positive cocci. Intravenous cephalothin was administered for 6 weeks and then oral cephalexin for a prolonged period. The tibia lesion healed and the femur lesion decreased in size.

PROBLEMS: — 1. What is the probable diagnosis? 2. What is the most likely organism? 3. What is the most likely way that this infection started? 4. What procedures would you use to cultivate the organism from such a case? 5. How would you identify the organism and differentiate it from *Micrococcus*? 6. Would an antibiogram be necessary? If so, how would this be done? 7. Would a vaccine be of any value in this case? (Ans. p. 84.)

No. 2. GIVEN: — A Boeing 747 jet with 344 passengers left Anchorage on an 8-hour flight to Copenhagen. Snacks including tuna salad and pastries were served shortly after takeoff. A ham and omelet breakfast was served approximately 2 hours before arrival. As the plane arrived in Copenhagen about 30 passengers experienced nausea, vomiting and abdominal cramps. The flight out of Denmark was canceled, and within 5 hours 142 passengers and 1 crew member were hospitalized and 53 others had milder symptoms. This total of 196 sick persons comprised over half of the passengers. The flight crew was not affected as they had a different menu. All patients except 2 had recovered within 48 hours, and these 2 were back to normal in a week.

PROBLEMS: — 1. What would you suspect as being the cause of the food poisoning? 2. What procedures would you initiate to try to determine the source of the organisms? 3. How would you explain that only slightly more than half of the passengers became ill? 4. How would you determine the cause of the outbreak? (Ans. p. 84.)

SUPPLEMENTARY READING

Baird-Parker, A. C.: A classification of micrococci and staphylococci based on physiological and biochemical tests, J. Gen. Microbiol. 30:409–427, 1963.

Cohen, J. O.: The Staphylococci (New York: Wiley-Interscience, 1972).

Coyette, J., and Ghuysen, J. M.: Structure of the cell wall of Staphylococcus aureus, Biochemistry 7:2385–2389, 1968.

Dillon, H. C.: Impetigo contagiosa: Suppurative and non-suppurative complications, Am. J. Dis. Child. 115:530–541, 1968.

Elwell, M. R., Liu, C. T., Spertzel, R. O., and Beisel, W. R.: Mechanisms of oral staphylococcal enterotoxin B-induced emesis in the monkey, Proc. Soc. Exp. Biol. Med. 148:424–427, 1975.

Greenberg, L.: Staphylococcal vaccines, Bull. N.Y. Acad. Med. 44: 1222–1226, 1968.

Grov, A., Oeding, P., Myklestad, B., and Aasen, J.: Reactions of staphylococcal antigens with normal sera, gamma G-globulins, and gamma G-globulin fragments of various species origin,. Acta Pathol. Microbiol. Scand. [B]78: 106–111, 1970.

Hughes, J. M., Merson, M. H., and Pollard, R. A.: Foodborne disease outbreaks in the United States, 1973, J. Infect. Dis. 132:224–228, 1975.

Kamme, C.: Antibodies against staphylococcal bacteriophages in human sera, Acta Pathol. Microbiol. Scand. [B]81:741-748, 1973.

Lacey, R. W.: Antibiotic resistance plasmids of Staphylococcus aureus and their clinical importance, Bacteriol. Rev. 39:1-32, 1975.

Melish, M. E., Glasgow, L. A., Turner, M. D., and Lillibridge, C. B.: The staphylococcal epidermolytic toxin: Its isolation, characterization and site of action, Ann. N.Y. Acad. Sci. 236:317–342, 1974.

Montie, T. C., Kadis, S., and Ajl, S. J. (eds.): Microbial Toxins, vol. III: Bacterial Protein Toxins (New York: Academic Press, 1970).

Musher, D. M., and McKenzie, S. O.: Infections due to Staphylococcus aureus, Medicine (Baltimore) 56:383–409, 1977.

O'Brien, A. D., and Kapral, F. A.: Increased cyclic adenosine 3',5'-monophosphate content in guinea pig ileum after exposure to Staphylococcus aureus delta-toxin, Infect. Immun. 13:152–162, 1976.

Rosendorf, L. L., and Kayser, F. H.: Transduction and plasmid deoxyribonucleic acid analysis in a multiple antibiotic resistant strain of *Staphylococcus epidermidis*, J. Bacteriol. 120:679–686, 1974.

Waldvogel, F. A., Medoff, G., and Swartz, M. N.: Osteomyelitis: A review of clinical features, therapeutic considerations and unusual aspects, N. Engl. J. Med. 282:198–206; 260–266; 316–322, 1970.

Wiseman, G. M.: The hemolysins of *Staphylococcus aureus*, Bacteriol. Rev. 39:317–344, 1975.

Yotis, W. W. (ed.): Recent advances in staphylococcal research, Ann. N.Y. Acad. Sci. 236:5–520, 1974.

ANALYSIS

No. 1.—1. Staphylococcal osteomyelitis of the tibia and femur. 2. *Staphylococcus aureus*. 3. This cannot be definitely established, but it is likely that the previous staphylococcal septicemia was inadequately treated, and viable organisms lodged in the bone marrow slowly metabolized to produce the abscesses; the trauma may have aggravated the process and prednisone may have lowered resistance. 4. Blood cultures should be done (chap. 4) and the exudate cultured using blood agar and thioglycollate broth. 5. Gram-positive coccus in clusters, beta hemolytic, coagulase positive, positive α-toxin and heat-resistant nucleases; *Micrococcus* is nonhemolytic, coagulase negative and oxidative. 6. Antibiograms should be done to determine antibiotic sensitivities; the disk-agar diffusion method is used (chap. 4). 7. Vaccine therapy for staphylococcal infections has been controversial and now is rarely used; autogenous vaccines have been reported beneficial in osteomyelitis.

No. 2.—Rather than answering the questions directly, we will relate the procedures and results. A listing of all the foods and beverages was prepared and each passenger filled out a questionnaire. The attack rate was 86% for the passengers eating ham prepared by one cook and 0% for ham prepared by another cook; for those eating the omelet there was some correlation with the cases, but none with other foods or beverages.

The short incubation period suggested that the disease was caused by a pre-formed toxin. Nausea and vomiting are typical in food-associated disease caused by *S. aureus* enterotoxin. Diarrhea is a common feature of infections associated with *Salmonella*- and *Shigella*-contaminated food.

An investigation of the food handlers and processing of the food showed that one cook had open lesions on his hand. After preparation the ham was kept at room temperature for 20 hours before serving.

Cultures from the lesions of the cook, the ham and vomitus of patients were positive for *Staphylococcus aureus*, phage type 53. This culture produced enterotoxin and enterotoxin was demonstrable in extracts of ham and some omelet. Stained smears from the surface of the ham revealed heavy contamination with gram-positive cocci.

6 / Streptococcus

OVERVIEW

In 1883 Fehleisen inoculated human subjects and showed that S. *pyogenes* (pus producing) was the cause of erysipelas. Since then the streptococci have become recognized as a diverse group of organisms causing a variety of suppurative and nonsuppurative diseases in humans. These infections range from pharyngitis with an acute onset, which must be differentiated from viral infection, to the more insidious postinfection sequelae such as rheumatic fever, all of which present diagnostic problems.

Even though streptococci have been recognized for decades, the exact mechanisms of disease production are still elusive but do include the antiphagocytic action of both the M protein and capsule, one or more enzymes, hemolysins and the erythrogenic toxin. The major problem in establishing such mechanisms is that neither the symptoms nor the pathologic features of the various streptococcal diseases can be duplicated in experimental animals, although in both man and animals, the streptococci do survive and metabolize in tissue or organs, causing inflammation and necrosis or granulomatous reactions. The species most frequently involved in human disease are the beta-hemolytic S. *pyogenes* and the alpha-hemolytic S. *pneumoniae* and S. *faecalis*.

GENERAL CHARACTERISTICS

Streptococci are gram-positive cocci which occur in pairs or chains (Fig. 6–1). The cells within the chain are attached by intracellular bridges, at which point cell wall synthesis occurs. Spores and flagella are not produced but motile strains have been described. Some species produce capsules. They are facultative anaerobes with an optimum growth temperature of 37 C. Enriched medium is required for growth. On blood agar, hemolysis may be alpha, beta, or gamma (nonhemolytic). Streptococci are catalase negative, which differen-

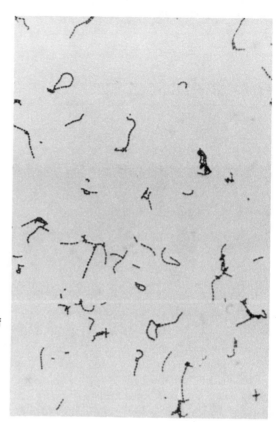

Fig. 6-1.—Gram stain of *Streptococcus pyogenes*. Note the chains and that some appear to be diplococci.

tiates them from *S. aureus*. Glucose is fermented by the hexose diphosphate pathway with lactic acid as the principal end product.

SPECIES

The principal species causing infections in humans and their differential characteristics are listed in Tables 6-1 and 6-2. This large and complex group can be divided into three groups based on type of hemolysis on blood agar or absence of hemolysis: the alpha-hemolytic, the beta-hemolytic and the non-hemolytic (gamma) streptococci. The beta-hemolytic streptococci are subdivided into serogroups (A through U) based on cell wall antigens (C carbohydrate) and then into serotypes based on a protein (M protein). Further differentiation is accomplished by determining physiologic characteristics. The differential characteristics of the streptococci are briefly summarized

TABLE 6-1.—DIFFERENTIAL CHARACTERISTICS OF SPECIES OF *STREPTOCOCCUS**

| SPECIES | GROUP† | GROUP ANTIGEN‖ | TYPE | | HEMOL-YSIS‡ | BAC. SEN.§ | FA‖ | GROWTH | | | HYDROLYSIS | |
			NO.	ANT.				45C	6.5% NaCl	40% BILE	HIPP.	ESCUL.
S. pyogenes	A	Rha-GlcNAc, P	63	Prot.	β	+	+	–	–	–	–	+
S. agalactiae	B	Rha-Gal-GlcNAc, P	5	Poly.	β	–	+	–	±	+	+	–
S. equisimilis	C	Rha-GalNAc, P	8	Prot.	β	±	+	–	–	–	–	±
S. faecalis	D	Glycerol T.A.	11	Poly.	α, γ	–	+	+	+	+	±	+
S. infrequens	E	Rha-Glu-GlcNAc, P	5	Poly.	β	±	+	±	–	–	–	+
S. anginosus	F	Rha-Glu-GlcNAc, P	5	Poly.	β	–	+	–	–	±	–	+
S. sp.	G	Rha-Gal-GlcNAc, P	3		β	±	+	±	–	–	–	+
S. sanguis	H	Glycerol T.A.?	5		α	–		±	–	–	–	+
S. salivarius	K	Rha, P	2		γ	–		–	–	+	–	–
S. mitis	–	–	2		α	–		±	–	–	–	–
S. mutans	–	–	7	Poly.?	γ	±		±	–	±	±	–
S. pneumoniae	–	Ribitol T.A.	82	Poly.	α	±		–	–	–	±	–

*Abbreviations: Ant. = antigen; Bac. Sen. = bacitracin sensitivity; Escul. = esculin; FA = fluorescent antibody technique; GalNAc = N-acetylgalactosamine; GlcNAc = N-acetylglucosamine; Hipp. = hippurate; Let. = letter; No. = number; P or Poly. = polysaccharide; Prot. = protein; Rha = rhamnose; T.A. = teichoic acid.

†The Lancefield Group as determined by the precipitin test. There are additional species in groups C, D and E. Groups L through U are not listed as they rarely cause infections in humans.

‡Hemolysis as determined on animal blood agar.

§Sensitivity to bacitracin is sometimes strain variable; 1–4% of S. pyogenes are resistant.

‖The fluorescent antibody technique is used to identify the species indicated; results with the other species not yet reported.

¶Either polysaccharide or teichoic acid.

TABLE 6-2.—DIFFERENTIAL CHARACTERISTICS OF ALPHA-HEMOLYTIC STREPTOCOCCI°

SPECIES	LANCEFIELD GROUP	HEMOLYSIS	HIPPURATE HYDROLYSIS	ESCULIN HYDROLYSIS	ARGININE HYDROLYSIS	ACID ARABINOSE	LACTOSE	MANNITOL	RAFFINOSE	SORBITOL	SUCROSE	TELLURITE	GROWTH 45 C	6.5% NaCl	40% BILE
S. faecalis†‡	D	α, γ, β§	−	+	+	−	+	+	−	+	+	+	+	+	+
S. faecium‡	D	α	−	+	+	+	+	+	−	−	−	−	+	+	+
S. durans‡	D	α	−	+	+	−	+	−	−	−	−	−	+	+	+
S. bovis	D	α, γ	−	+	−	±	+	±	+	−	−	−	−	−	+
S. equinus	D	α	−	+	−	−	−	−	−	−	−	−	−	−	+
S. sanguis	H	α	−	+	+	−	+	−	−	−	+	−	±	−	+
S. salivarius‖	K	γ, α	−	+	−	−	+	−	+	−	+	+	+	−	−
S. mitis	−	α	−	−	±	−	+	−	±	−	+	+	−	−	−
S. mutans	−	γ, α, β	−	+	−	−	+	+	±	+	+	−	−	−	±
S. pneumoniae	−	α	±	−	−	±	+	−	+	−	+	−	−	−	−

°Note that although called "alpha" some may be non- or beta-hemolytic. The term *viridans streptococci* is sometimes used; the name *S. viridans* should not be used as it is not a valid species name.

†*S. faecalis* may be separated into *S. faecalis* var. *liquefaciens*, which liquifies gelatin, and *S. faecalis* var. *zymogenes* which is beta-hemolytic; otherwise, they have the same reactions as above.

‡The term *enterococcus* includes *S. faecalis, S. faecium* and *S. durans*, all of which hydrolyze arginine and grow both at 10 C and in 6.5% NaCl.

§The usual reaction is listed first but the others given may occur.

‖Produces large mucoid colonies on 5% sucrose agar.

in Tables 6-1 and 6-2. For convenience of discussion, this chapter is divided into several sections covering the major groups of streptococci.

ECOLOGY

The streptococci are found primarily in the human upper respiratory and intestinal tracts and can also be present on the skin, around the anus, and in the vagina and cervix. All groups have been isolated from a variety of infectious processes in domestic animals. *S. pyogenes* is present in the upper respiratory tract of 2-10% of individuals. In one survey with over 22,000 throat cultures taken over an extended period of time from school children, 18% of the cultures were positive for beta-hemolytic streptococci, and of these 60% were group A with the remainder being groups B, C or G. *S. agalactiae* has been reported as the most frequently isolated beta-hemolytic streptococcus from the cervix. The alpha-hemolytic streptococci, particularly *S. salivarius*, *S. sanguis*, *S. mitis* and *S. mutans*, are universally present on the surfaces of the teeth, tongue, cheeks and in saliva. Dental plaque may contain 10^{11} streptococci per gram wet weight. The enterococci, *S. faecalis*, *S. faecium* and *S. durans*, are found in the oral cavity and genitourinary tract, but the greatest numbers are in the intestinal tract where counts of 10^8 per gram of feces are reported. Studies on the carrier rate of *S. pneumoniae* in the upper respiratory tract indicate a variation from 20 to 60% with the highest rates during the winter months (chap. 3).

ANTIGENS

The streptococcal cell contains a variety of intracellular and cell wall protein and carbohydrate antigens. The cytoplasm has over 20 antigenic components. The cell wall antigenic components are used for identification, and because they are related to pathogenicity, they are discussed below with particular emphasis on the antigens associated with *S. pyogenes*.

C CARBOHYDRATE OR GROUP ANTIGEN.—Lancefield in 1933 divided beta-hemolytic streptococci into three groups A, B and C on the basis of specific polysaccharide antigens extractable with hot acid and identifiable serologically. Subsequently, numerous other serogroups were determined. In group A, the antigen (termed C carbohydrate) is composed of N-acetylglucosamine and rhamnose in the ratio of 1:2, which is linked to the peptidoglycan. The terminal N-acetylglucosamine is the antigenic determinant and is the source of cross-reactivity among antigens from other organisms of mammalian tissue, including valvular heart tissue. When injected intravenously into rabbits, the purified C antigen does not produce heart lesions, but when coupled with protein or other complexes and injected, it provokes valvular and myocardial lesions. After a streptococcal infection in humans, antibodies to this antigen are demonstrable and they persist for months or years. Group antigens of Lancefield groups A through U are either polysaccharides with differing determinant groups or teichoic acids (see Table 6–1).

M, T AND R PROTEINS.—The M (term derived from "Matt" used to describe colony morphology) protein antigen of *S. pyogenes* is a surface component of the cell wall which extends outward and is associated with hair-like fimbriae. The protein is antigenic and is the basis for dividing *S. pyogenes* into 63 serotypes. Some strains contain two different M antigens. This antigen is extractable from the cell by hot hydrochloric acid and identifiable by serologic means such as precipitation, immunodiffusion, hemagglutination, complement fixation or fluorescent antibody procedure. Functionally, the M protein is antiphagocytic and aids in adherence to mucosal cells which promotes colonization in the oral cavity. Both of these activities are absent in M⁻ mutants. Adherence and resistance to phagocytosis can be inhibited by specific antiserum. Anti-M antibodies are formed in response to an infection and persist for extended periods of time. They provide the host with a type-specific immunity but may not eliminate the carrier state; hypersensitivity (delayed and immediate) may develop. The M antigen may play a role in the development of poststreptococcal rheumatic fever and glomerulonephritis, but this etiologic relationship has not been established.

The term *M antigen* has been applied to protein antigens in other streptococcal groups and in *S. pneumoniae*, but these are neither biologically nor serologically related to the M antigen of *S. pyogenes*.

The *T antigen* is a cell wall-associated protein which is resistant to proteolytic enzymes but is denatured by hot acid. It is antigenic, but antibodies are not demonstrable following streptococcal infections; it is not a virulence factor. A T antigen-agglutination test can be done using a trypsinized suspension of cells if M typing is negative. However, the usefulness of this agglutination test is limited by the presence of multiple T antigens in the same cell and because of cross-reacting antigens in groups C and G. The R antigen is found in a limited number of strains and in groups B, C and G. It is not a virulence factor, and there are no reports of antibodies being formed in response to streptococcal infections.

TEICHOIC ACIDS. — The group D streptococcal antigen is a membrane glycerol phosphate teichoic acid with glucopyranosyl residues being the antigenic determinant. A glycerol teichoic acid is probably the group H antigen of *S. sanguis*. The glycerol or ribitol cell wall teichoic acids are covalently linked to the peptidoglycan; the membrane glycerol phosphate teichoic acid is covalently linked to a glycolipid (lipoteichoic acid), but the long glycerol phosphate chains can extend to the outer surface of the cell wall. On the outer surface of the cell wall they act as a surface antigen and as a factor in adherence.

GENETICS

TRANSFORMATION. — Griffith in 1928 reported that when mice were injected intraperitoneally, first with a rough (R), avirulent, noncapsulated pneumococcus (derived from his type 2R), and then with a heat-killed suspension of a smooth (S) virulent strain (type 3S), a living virulent capsulated pneumococcus (type 3S) could be recovered from the mice. This observation was extended in 1944 when Avery, MacLeod and McCarty demonstrated that DNA donated by the heat-killed virulent strain was the factor responsible for the R to S transformation. It is now established that fragments of the bacterial chromosome can enter the living cell and replace, in part, a homologous segment of the bacterial genome of the recipient by recombination. In the case of the pneumococcus, the new genetic determinant regulates and codes for the synthesis of capsular polysaccharide. Transformation has been demonstrated in streptococcal groups A, F, H and O, as well as in species of *Escherichia, Haemophilus, Neisseria, Bacillus, Moraxella* and *Acinetobacter*. Any genetic characteristic, whether located on the bacterial chromosome or on a plasmid, can be transformed.

TRANSDUCTION.—Bacteriophages have been isolated from streptococcal groups A, C, G and H and from *S. pneumoniae;* they are DNA phages of similar structure. Transduction of the genetic determinants for resistance to streptomycin, erythromycin and lincomycin has been demonstrated. Lysogeny is common in group A streptococci and is necessary for erythrotoxin synthesis (lysogenic conversion). There is evidence that DNase and streptokinase synthesis is phage mediated.

PLASMIDS.—Plasmids have been demonstrated in streptococcal groups D and N and in *S. mutans*. In group D they can carry the genes for beta-hemolysis, bacteriocin activity (chap. 3) and antibiotic resistance.

BETA-HEMOLYTIC STREPTOCOCCI

Of the streptococci, *Streptococcus pyogenes,* Lancefield group A, is the most important human pathogen and is characterized by producing pinpoint, convex, beta-hemolytic colonies (Fig. 6–2) on the surface of blood agar, being sensitive to bacitracin (1–4% resistant) and containing the group A carbohydrate. The group antigen provokes an antibody response in infected individuals, but so far has not been demonstrated to play a direct role in pathogenicity. The M protein serotyping antigen (63 types) is a virulence factor, and the nonantigenic hyaluronic acid capsule supplements the antiphagocytic property of the M antigen (see Antigens and Pathogenicity for further discussion). *S. pyogenes* produces a number of enzymes, including streptokinase, hyaluronidase, proteases, nucleases and diphosphopyridine nucleotidase, which enhance pathogenicity and aid the organism in the fulfill-

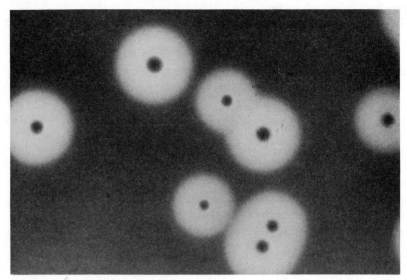

Fig. 6–2. — Beta-hemolytic colonies of *Streptococcus pyogenes* growing on blood agar. Note the small "pinpoint" colony with a proportionately large zone of complete hemolysis.

ment of its nutritional requirements when causing infections in man and animals. *S. pyogenes* and group D streptococci produce L-forms (chap. 2), which are fragile, filterable, reproducible structures that lack a cell wall but are able to synthesize certain enzymes and the M protein. They may occur spontaneously or in the presence of penicillin. L-forms have been implicated in rheumatic fever and endocarditis but proof is lacking. They can persist in tissue for long periods and conceivably may be the source for relapse.

Streptococcus equisimilis, group C, is similar to *S. pyogenes* in cell and colonial appearance. It is beta-hemolytic and produces streptokinase. Infections in humans are usually mild, involving the skin or pharynx, but puerperal sepsis, bacteremia and fatal endocarditis have been reported. The other species in this group are animal pathogens, causing mastitis in cattle and strangles (a lymphadenitis) in horses, but they rarely infect humans.

S. infrequens, group E, is beta-hemolytic, with both group and type antigen being polysaccharides. It is a common cause of lymphadenitis in swine (sometimes called *S. suis*). *S. uberus* is related since some strains have E antigen, but others have P or U group antigens. It causes bovine mastitis. Group E streptococci are not frequently encountered in man but have been reported from bacteremia and genitourinary infections.

Streptococcus anginosus, group F, forms small β-hemolytic colonies and has five polysaccharide type antigens which are responsible for cross reactions with groups A, C, G, L and T. *S. MG* is an encapsulated, nonhemolytic organism containing the F antigen. Originally it was isolated from two fatal cases of primary atypical pneumonia whose sera agglutinated this organism. However, this infection was due to *Mycoplasma pneumoniae,* which has an antigen in common with *S. MG* and the I antigen of human erythrocytes. This antigen is responsible for the increased agglutinin titer to *S. MG* and erythrocytes in patients. Group F organisms are present in the oral cavity and produce abscesses and bacteremia.

Streptococcus sp., group G, is beta-hemolytic and produces rather large colonies. In the clinical laboratory, group G is next to group A in frequency of isolation and causes a diversity of infections, including pharyngitis, empyema, endocarditis, wound infections, genitourinary tract infections and bacteremia. Some strains contain the type M-12 antigen and have been implicated as a cause of glomerulonephritis.

STREPTOCOCCUS PYOGENES (GROUP A)

Capsule and Cell Wall

CAPSULE.—Group A streptococci have a hyaluronic acid capsule, composed of equimolar quantities of N-acetylglucosamine and glucuronic acid. The capsule supplements the antiphagocytic activity of the M antigen. Similar capsules are found in group C, particularly the animal pathogens. Groups B and C also have capsules of a different chemical composition.

CELL WALL.—The complex cell wall of *S. pyogenes* is composed of a peptidoglycan which is linked directly or indirectly to a variety of proteins, carbohydrates and lipids (chap. 2; Figs. 6-1, 6-2, 6-3). The peptidoglycan structure of other streptococcal species is similar except the cross-linking chains may have an additional alanine, lysine, threonine, glycine or aspartic acid. The M, T and R proteins, teichoic acids and the C carbohydrate are linked to the cell wall (see Antigens for a discussion).

ANTIGENIC MIMICRY.—It is established that the group A cell wall and cytoplasmic membrane components share a number of common antigenic determinants with mammalian tissue. This is referred to as antigenic mimicry. The cytoplasmic membrane of these streptococci

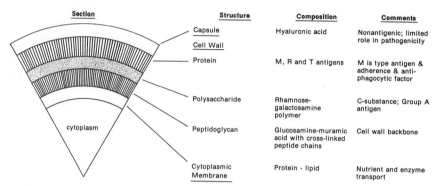

Section	Structure	Composition	Comments
	Capsule	Hyaluronic acid	Nonantigenic; limited role in pathogenicity
	Cell Wall		
	Protein	M, R and T antigens	M is type antigen & adherence & anti-phagocytic factor
	Polysaccharide	Rhamnose-galactosamine polymer	C-substance; Group A antigen
cytoplasm	Peptidoglycan	Glucosamine-muramic acid with cross-linked peptide chains	Cell wall backbone
	Cytoplasmic Membrane	Protein - lipid	Nutrient and enzyme transport

Fig. 6–3.—Diagrammatic section through the cell wall of *Streptococcus pyogenes*.

shares antigens with muscle sarcolemma, renal basement membranes and perhaps with histocompatibility antigens. The group A carbohydrate shares antigens with heart valve tissue, whereas M protein shares antigens with myocardial tissue. There is considerable supporting evidence that antibodies formed in response to these streptococcal cell fractions combine with these tissue antigens causing a localized reaction resulting in myocardial, valvular or glomerular lesions. It is also possible that they have a role in graft rejection.

Hemolysins, Toxins and Enzymes

S. pyogenes produce two hemolysins: streptolysins O and S. Streptolysin O is inactivated by oxygen and cholesterol. It links to bound cholesterol in the cell membrane, causing holes to form in the red blood cell resulting in lysis. It is cytotoxic for a variety of cells including cardiac tissue and leukocytes. Antistreptolysin O (ASO) antibody production indicates a streptococcal infection. Streptolysin O can be demonstrated by streaking the organism on blood agar, incubating anaerobically and observing the zone of beta-hemolysis around the colony. Streptolysin S is not inactivated by oxygen or cholesterol and is closely associated with a carrier such as serum albumin or RNA. It binds to phospholipids and alters cell wall permeability thereby allowing an increase in water and salts in the cell and subsequent lysis. It is cytotoxic for tissue cells, particularly leukocytes. It previously has been referred to as a leukocidin and is a small nonantigenic molecule responsible for aerobic blood agar plate hemolysis. A similar hemolysin is produced by groups B, C, E and F.

Lysogenic strains of *S. pyogenes* produce an erythrogenic (scarlatinal) exotoxin which is composed of: (1) a sensitizing heat-stable protein; (2) three immunologically distinct toxins, A, B and C, which are produced separately by different strains and (3) a hyaluronic acid carrier. In a nonhypersensitive host, the toxins alone can cause the rash of scarlet fever. If the individual is hypersensitive, then the rash can be a delayed hypersensitivity reaction to the nontoxic protein; this latter reaction can be enhanced by the non-immunologic activity of the toxin. The presence or absence of circulating antitoxin can be determined by the Dick test, in which erythrogenic toxin is injected intradermally. If antitoxins are present, they neutralize the toxin and no localized erythema develops, thus the Dick test is negative. If no antitoxin is present, erythema is produced, resulting in a positive test. These erythrotoxins have additional biological activities, including pyrogenicity, cytotoxicity and the ability to transform lymphocytes and alter membrane permeability. These alterations in the defense mechanisms of the host may be an important adjunct to the pathogenicity of group A streptococci.

Deoxyribonucleases (DNase, streptodornase, dornase) degrade DNA. Four serological types — A, B, C and D — can be specifically neutralized by their respective antibodies. S. pyogenes produce all four but predominantly B. Anti-DNase B antibodies are demonstrable in patients who have had or who are recovering from a streptococcal infection. The deoxyribonucleases are not cytotoxic. DNase can depolymerize the DNA in exudates and promote liquefaction, which may enhance the spread of the streptococci; otherwise, a role in pathogenicity has not been demonstrated. The enzymes have been used alone (streptodornase) or in conjunction with streptokinase (varidase) in the enzymatic debridement of wounds or for the liquefaction of purulent exudates.

Five serologically distinct extracellular esterases are produced by S. pyogenes. Neutralizing antibodies are demonstrable in humans following streptococcal infections.

Beta-glucuronidase is produced by groups A, B, C, G and L but has not been reported for groups D or H. Additional glycoside hydrolases are produced by various streptococci, and these may release sugars from tissue glycoproteins, making them available as a source of energy to the bacteria.

Nicotinamide adenine dinucleotidase (NADase) hydrolyzes the respiratory enzyme cofactor, NAD. It has been reported particularly from nephritogenic strains, such as type 12. A role in nephritis has not been demonstrated, although it is a leukocidin and antibodies are formed in humans.

Protease activity is demonstrable in culture filtrates of S. pyogenes and will hydrolyze a variety of proteins including M antigen, streptokinase, fibrin and others. Injected into animals it causes extensive focal necrosis in muscle, including the myocardium, but whether it is active in human infections is not known.

Streptokinase, an antigenic, single-chain protein with MW of 47,000, is produced by groups A and C streptococci. It reacts with plasminogen (a plasma globulin) cleaving an arginyl-valine bond to form plasmin. Plasmin, a trypsin-like enzyme, hydrolyzes fibrin to form a number of soluble peptide fragments. Streptokinase is used in the treatment of early (3-day or less) occlusive vascular diseases, such as pulmonary emboli, arterial occlusions, deep vein thrombi and myocardial infarcts. The plasmin liquefies the fibrin deposits, and the soluble peptide fragments are removed by the circulation. Once a vessel is occluded, the kinase has little effect as it cannot penetrate the clot to complex with the intrinsic plasminogen. Also, as most individuals have circulating antistreptokinase, an initial antibody neutralizing dose must precede the therapeutic dosage.

Infections

The streptococci cause a great variety of infections, with the majority being suppurative (pus producing). These include pharyngitis, adenitis, peritonsillar abscesses, otitis media, meningitis, brain abscess, peritonitis, puerperal sepsis and pneumonia. The principal nonsuppurative infections are rheumatic fever and acute glomerulonephritis. The majority of these infections are discussed below.

SKIN. – In man, the two most common areas of infection are the upper respiratory tract and the skin. The two types of skin infections are erysipelas and pyoderma. Pyoderma, including impetigo, begins as a vesicle and becomes a thick, crusted nonscarring lesion. Staphylococci are often present in the lesion. Adenopathy and bacteremia may occur with nephritis being a serious complication in 10–15% of the cases. The infection usually responds to local treatment, so antibiotics (primarily penicillin) are not necessary unless the lesions are extensive. Pyoderma is more common in young children and may involve groups or families. It is spread by direct contact or fomites, and entrance into the skin is facilitated by trauma, cuts or insect bites. Group A streptococci types 2, 25, 49, 55, 57 and 60 are more frequently involved. The ASO titer response is minimal; anti-DNase B or anti-hyaluronidase antibody responses are more reliable indicators of this infection.

Erysipelas (red skin) (Fig. 6–4) is an acute lymphangitis of the skin, often beginning around the nose as a painful spreading area of inflam-

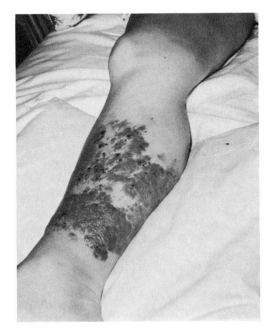

Fig. 6–4.—Erysipelas of the leg in a young patient. *Streptococcus pyogenes* isolated. (Courtesy of W. A. Welton, Division of Dermatology, West Virginia University.)

mation with an advancing bright red margin. Bacteremia or metastatic infections may occur. Omphalitis is an infection of the umbilical stump which may spread to adjacent areas of the skin. Perianal cellulitis may occur in children or adults.

PHARYNGITIS (tonsillitis).—The majority of episodes of acute pharyngitis are due to viruses. When bacteria cause the infection, *S. pyogenes*, (95%) and group C or G (5%) are most frequently isolated, with a few cases due to *H. influenzae, C. diphtheriae, S. pneumoniae,* and *Mycoplasma pneumoniae.* The source of the infection is usually nasal carriers. Within 48–72 hours after invasion of the streptococci, the manifestations are sore throat, fever, headache, malaise, aching, and often nausea and vomiting. The pharynx is edematous, inflamed and sore (Fig. 6–5), adenitis develops, and a yellowish exudate may appear, which in a smear shows numerous polymorphonuclear leukocytes (viral exudate shows monocytes). The majority of patients recover in 4–10 days with an elevated ASO titer. Suppurative complications such as sinusitis, otitis media, mastoiditis, meningitis, brain abscess, pneumonia or endocarditis may develop. The most serious nonsuppurative complications are rheumatic fever and acute glomerulonephritis. Both may occur in the same patient.

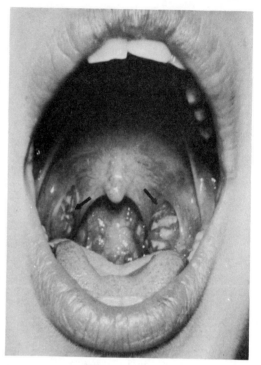

Fig. 6–5.—Acute suppurative tonsillitis in a young child. *Streptococcus pyogenes* was isolated. Arrows indicate tonsillar abscesses. (Courtesy of P. M. Sprinkle, Division of Otolaryngology, West Virginia University.)

SCARLET FEVER.—Although its incidence and severity have decreased in the past several years, scarlet fever can still be a severe disease in children 2–10 years old. The incubation period and early symptoms are those described above for pharyngitis with the development of a rash in 24–48 hours which begins on the neck and spreads over the chest and abdomen to the extremities. The exanthum consists of a diffuse erythema with punctate red spots. As described in the discussion of erythrogenic toxin, this eruption may be due to the toxin, hypersensitivity to a protein, or a combination of both. The complications may be any of those listed with pharyngitis, including rheumatic fever and glomerulonephritis. Penicillin, the antibiotic of choice for treatment, causes the acute symptoms to subside and prevents complications but does not alter the characteristics, duration or the ultimate desquamation. In the untreated patient one can usually demonstrate the development of or increase in ASO, anti-DNase B, anti-hyaluronidase and anti-NADase titers within 7 to 10 days. Early antibiotic treatment negates an antibody response (see Erythrogenic Toxin).

PUERPERAL SEPSIS (childbirth fever). — In 1847 Semmelweis demonstrated this acute endometritis to be transmitted primarily by the hands of those attending women in labor. The infection starts 24–48 hours post partum when *S. pyogenes* (on occasion, group B, C, D or G) from the vagina infects the denuded uterine surface causing fever, leukocytosis and pelvic tenderness. The infection may spread through the cervical wall or via the fallopian tubes, causing bacteremia or peritonitis. Death occurs unless antibiotic therapy (usually penicillin) is promptly instituted. Presently, puerperal sepsis is comparatively rare in this country except in instances of uterine trauma during an attempted abortion, which may then result in anaerobic myositis due to *Clostridium*, an anaerobic organism. Streptococcal vaginitis can occur, particularly in young girls.

RHEUMATIC FEVER. — This poststreptococcal disease has the classic symptoms of fever, acute migratory polyarthritis and carditis; the first manifestation of carditis is the development of mitral or aortic regurgitation. Other symptoms or signs can include chorea, erythema marginatum, epistaxis, subcutaneous nodules over joints and abdominal or pleuritic pain. Most attacks subside in 6 weeks but some persist for 6 months or more. The arthritis usually subsides without joint damage. The valvular lesions may either heal, remain unchanged or undergo progressive sclerosis and calcification, resulting in rheumatic heart disease. Rheumatic fever is more common in children 5–15 years old, but no age group is exempt. Patients usually give a history of a recent (1–3 weeks) streptococcal upper respiratory tract infection which is frequently exudative. In 10 to 50% of persons recovering from the initial attack of rheumatic fever, the disease recurs after subsequent streptococcal infections. Such recurrences are prevented by keeping the individual on continual penicillin prophalaxis. Early antibiotic therapy eradicates the streptococci but does not appreciably alter the course of the disease. Rheumatic fever is worldwide with an increased attack rate (normally 1–3%) prompted by overcrowded living conditions. Any of the 62 group A streptococcal types can cause rheumatic fever, and patients may have increased ASO, anti-NADase, anti-DNase B, anti-C carbohydrate, C-reactive protein and anti-heart tissue antigen titers. Rheumatic fever is an immunologic complication which follows infection. Consequently, blood cultures are negative and organisms are not demonstrable in the joint or valvular lesions.

ACUTE GLOMERULONEPHRITIS (nephritis; Bright's disease). —

Streptococcal infections of the throat or skin may result in the development of acute poststreptococcal glomerulonephritis which is immunologically (chap. 1) mediated and involves complement. The patient may exhibit some or all of the symptoms of proteinuria, hematuria, edema of the face and legs, hypertension and renal function impairment. The nephritis develops on the average about 10 days after pharyngitis or 18 days after pyoderma. Classically, it is short and self-limited, particularly in children, but it can become chronic or even fatal. The development of hematuria, hypertension and decreased renal function indicates a poor prognosis. Epidemiological studies have identified streptococcal types 1, 4, 12, 49, 55, 56 and 57 as nephritogenic. Chronic renal disease may follow the development of streptococcal glomerulonephritis. A large number of patients, after several years of no apparent disease, develop progressive glomerular sclerosis and sometimes acute renal failure.

Mechanisms of Pathogenicity

Probably no single organism can cause as many different kinds of infections in humans as S. pyogenes. Yet the mechanisms involved are unknown, a subject of theoretical consideration, or only partially understood. This problem is compounded by the fact that there is no good animal model in which all the symptoms or pathological features of the human infections can be duplicated. In animals it can be shown that certain enzymes, hemolysins or cell wall components of the streptococci can cause a variety of cell or tissue changes, and these no doubt contribute to the pathologic features of the human infections.

The M protein is antiphagocytic and is a major factor in pathogenicity. This antiphagocytic property is enhanced by the hyaluronic acid capsule, as demonstrated by the fact that capsulated strains have twice the survival time of noncapsulated strains in the presence of phagocytes. The M protein (as well as the lipoteichoic acid) aids in adherence to mucosal cells which is a factor in colonization of the oral cavity. In addition to these factors, the erythrogenic toxin can cause an erythematous reaction, but this may also be due to a hypersensitivity to the carrier protein. Streptolysin O is cytotoxic and a leukocidin; streptolysin S is a major leukocidin and is capable of disrupting lysosomes and altering cell membrane permeability. Streptokinase, hyaluronidase and protease degrade the connective tissue matrix and thus facilitate the spread of the streptococci through tissue. Other antigenic components, such as the C carbohydrate, M protein, cytoplasmic membrane proteins or carbohydrates, can initiate immunopathologic changes through Arthus reactions, delayed hypersensitivity, antigenic mimicry reactions or possibly from antigen-antibody complexes. Coupled with all of these is the ability of the organism to grow and multiply in tissue. Intracellular and extracellular enzymes degrade tissue components which supply nutrients for growth and also cause areas of necrosis and inflammation.

Nonsuppurative Streptococcal Diseases

There is now essentially universal agreement that S. *pyogenes* is the etiologic agent of rheumatic fever based on: (1) clinical observations, (2) the fact that antibiotic prophylaxis prevents attacks and (3) demonstration of elevated antistreptococcal antibodies. However, proof of the pathogenesis is still lacking because the disease has not been reproduced experimentally. Numerous theories have been advanced to explain the mechanisms of pathogenesis, with three being most accepted. (1) The toxin or toxin-antibody theory involves the cardiotoxin streptolysin O and proposes that a toxin-antibody complex is formed which initially prevents the action of the toxin. However, it is proposed that this complex slowly dissociates allowing the streptolysin O to exhibit its cardiotoxicity. (2) The autoimmune theory proposes that a streptococcal product such as an enzyme acts on the cardiac tissue, releasing antigens. The resulting antibodies then react with the cardiac tissue, initiating an inflammatory reaction. (3) According to the cross-reactive antigen theory, determinant groups are shared between streptococcal components and cardiac tissue (antigenic mimicry). There are at least two antigenic possibilities: *(a)* the C carbohydrate cross-reacting with cardiac glycoprotein has been reported but not entirely confirmed, and *(b)* the well-documented cross-reactivity between proteins of the cytoplasmic membrane and sarcolemma of cardiac and skeletal muscle. It is suggested that these microbial antigens stimulate formation of antibodies which react with cardiac tissue. The manner in which this latter antigen-antibody reaction initiates the valvular and myocardial lesions is not clear, but indirect evidence of this occurrence is the demonstration of γ-globulin in the Aschoff bodies by the fluorescent antibody technique. The Aschoff body is usually found in the myocardium and is pathognomonic of rheumatic fever. Histologically, it is a focus of fibrinoid degeneration, surrounded by a granulomatous response. It is now thought to be a reaction to injury of the terminal branches of nerves and derived from Schwann cell proliferation. This third concept, cross-reactive antigens, has the support of many workers in this research area.

The streptococcal product(s) responsible for production of acute glomerulonephritis have not been clearly defined but could be the M protein, membrane antigens or a toxic product. Of these, there is experimental evidence for M protein and for membrane antigens. In brief, an immune complex or an antibody-fibrinogen-M protein complex would be deposited in the mesangial area of the glomerulus and then become fixed to the glomerular membrane. Here, there is an accumulation of IgG, and complement (C3) is fixed, resulting in the liberation of chemotactic factors (serum complement is reduced). Leukocytes migrate into the area, release hydrolytic enzymes and initiate injury to the glomerular membrane. This leads to the coagulation process, fibrin organization and obliteration of the glomerulus. Type 12 apparently shares an antigen with the glomerular basement membranes, which supports the proposal that antibodies, formed against the bacterial antigen, could react directly with the basement membrane, fix complement and cause nephritis. An increase in ASO, anti-DNase B and anti-NADase titers is demonstrable with an increased anti-DNase B titer being the best indicator. Acute glomerulonephritis can also develop following infective endocarditis, staphylococcal bacteremia, pneumonia, quartan malaria or certain virus infections.

Immunity

The M protein of S. pyogenes stimulates antibody (opsonin) response in the infected individual. These antibodies persist for months or years and neutralize the antiphagocytic effect of the M antigen and protect the individual from reinfection with the particular serotype. Opsonic antibodies can be demonstrated by the in vitro bactericidal test. However, these antibodies are type specific, and suppurative streptococcal infections can recur with other serotypes to which the host has not developed an immunity. In glomerulonephritis, in which a limited number of types of streptococcal infections are involved, such an immunity can reduce the chance of repeated attacks. The erythrotoxin stimulates antibodies which neutralizes the toxin and the erythematous reaction resulting from this toxin. However, this does not alter the pharyngitis. Antibodies are produced against a number of streptococcal antigens, including streptolysin O, NAD, DNA, hyaluronidase, streptokinase and the C carbohydrate, but their role in immunity, if any, has not been demonstrated. As pointed out, the antibodies or antigen-antibody complexes may be factors in the pathogenesis of nonsuppurative disease. Hypersensitivity develops in response to the erythrogenic toxin (protein carrier), the M protein and perhaps other antigens. During an infection such reactions could initiate an inflammatory response, fix complement, produce an Arthus reaction or interfere with macrophage migration.

Vaccines

M protein vaccines administered to humans provoke type-specific antibodies which neutralize the antiphagocytic action of the M protein. Some of the vaccines used in early studies caused severe local and systemic reactions, but highly purified M proteins of types 2, 12, 42 and 52 can be injected subcutaneously without causing a reaction. The antibody response is variable. Recently a purified soluble M-1 antigen was prepared and administered as an aerosol; it was nonirritating and stimulated secretory IgA antibody formation. The protective response to this vaccine was determined by swabbing the throats of vaccinees with a virulent M-1 culture, and in comparison to controls there was a 75% reduction in pharyngitis. Of equal importance, there was a greater reduction in colonization of the throats by the M-1 strain. This may lead the way to an effective S. pyogenes vaccine.

Treatment and Prophylaxis

S. pyogenes and groups B, C and G streptococci respond to penicillin, which is the antibiotic of choice for suppurative and nonsuppurative infections. If the patient is allergic to penicillin, erythromycin is effective. Treatment of suppurative pharyngitis should be maintained a full 10 days. This may inhibit antibody response, in which case the patient remains susceptible to infection with the same serologic type of S. pyogenes. In the treatment of rheumatic fever penicillin therapy is maintained until the subsidence of fever, arthritis and cardiac symptoms. Treatment may be supplemented with glucosteroids or salicylates to suppress the cardiac inflammatory reaction. After recovery, the patient is maintained on prophylactic monthly injections of penicillin for an extended period of time. Children with positive throat cultures, particularly in overcrowded conditions, should be maintained on penicillin for at least 10 days as a prophylactic control measure to reduce the incidence of rheumatic fever.

STREPTOCOCCUS AGALACTIAE (GROUP B)

Characteristics

Streptococcus agalactiae, group B, forms convex colonies that may be larger than those of S. pyogenes and are sometimes pigmented.

They are beta-hemolytic but some strains are nonhemolytic. Hippurase is produced and *S. agalactiae* is one of the few beta-hemolytic streptococci to synthesize this enzyme. Hippurase hydrolyzes hippuric acid to benzoic acid and glycine, a reaction used for the identification of group B streptococci.

The group B streptococci also produce a unique reaction termed the *CAMP reaction*, which is useful in identifying this group. If one inoculates *S. agalactiae* in a line perpendicular to a line inoculum of *S. aureus*, an enhanced area of hemolysis resembling an arrow point appears where the cultures of the two organisms meet. This reaction apparently represents synergy between products of the two organisms. This test has been modified and employs a soluble product from *S. aureus* cultures.

Ecology

S. agalactiae is a pathogen for humans and bovines and has been isolated from a number of other animal sources. Animal isolates differ serologically and physiologically from human strains and are apparently not a source of human infections. In humans, the bacteria are constituents of normal flora of the vaginal-cervical area and the intestines. The intestinal tract is the primary reservoir. Colonization rates vary but approximate 25% for both the genital and intestinal tracts. The organism can also be isolated from the throat (approximately 10%). Type II and type III serotypes are most prevalent.

Antigens, Hemolysins and Toxins

The group antigen (Lancefield group B) is a rhamnose-glucosamine polysaccharide. Unlike group A streptococci in which typing is based on a protein antigen (M antigen), the group B streptococci are separated into types based on carbohydrate antigens in the envelope. There are three types, designated I, II, III. Type I can be further subdivided into types Ia, Ib and Ic. Passive protection with antisera against the type antigens can be demonstrated in animals. A microcapsule composed of sialic acid has been demonstrated in type III strains.

A protein antigen, shared among all types except type Ia, is antigenic and protects against infection.

A hemolysin, distinct from streptolysins O and S, as well as the enzyme hyaluronidase, has been demonstrated.

Infections

In neonates, two types of diseases are produced by *S. agalactiae*. "Early onset" disease, characterized by septicemia and respiratory distress, usually occurs within the first 5 days of life and frequently during the first 24 hours. The source of the infection is the mother with the infection acquired either in utero or during birth. The portal of entry may be either oral or through the respiratory tract via aspiration or swallowing of contaminated amniotic fluid. Early onset disease has features similar to the respiratory distress syndrome of the newborn (hyaline membrane disease) and may in fact be confused with hyaline membrane disease clinically, radiologically and by pathology. Hyaline membranes in the alveoli, probably resulting from exudate with a fibrin matrix containing necrotic epithelial cells and red cells, are seen in many patients with group B infection. Both type I and type III organisms are associated with early onset disease, with type I being the most frequent isolate. Mortality in early onset disease may be 40–80%.

The second disease pattern, "delayed onset" disease, is a meningitis that occurs about 10 days after birth. Sepsis may or may not accompany this form of the disease. The disease is primarily a nosocomial infection with the organisms acquired from the mother, other neonates or nursery personnel. The disease is a diffuse purulent leptomeningitis. Some studies report only type III S. agalactiae from infants with delayed onset disease.

The group B streptococci can cause other diseases in young children, among which are impetigo, otitis media, septic arthritis, osteomyelitis, ethmoiditis, pulmonary infection, urinary tract infection, postpartum infection and pharyngitis. In adults, the infections are more frequently seen in patients with underlying diseases such as diabetes and genitourinary disorders.

Mechanisms of Pathogenicity

Little is known about the virulence of S. agalactiae. Hyaluronidase is produced and may play a role in spread of the organism in tissue. A hemolysin is produced but its role in disease is unknown. Some work suggests that type III organisms may have a predilection for the meninges, which may be related to a sialic acid capsule, but further studies evaluating this role must be done.

Immunity

Antibody is obtained from the mother by transplacental transfer, and the presence of these antibodies correlates with neonatal protection. A thermolabile opsonin, which crosses the placenta, has been described. Present knowledge of immunity in this disease suggests that neonatal disease may be due to lack of maternal immunity, an immature immune system and a defect in phagocytic and bactericidal capacity of leukocytes.

Prevention and Treatment

In an attempt to minimize early onset disease, some physicians have recommended vaginal culturing late in pregnancy with treatment of carriers with penicillin G. Oral and skin cultures of neonates may be taken to detect colonization and as a guide for prophylactic treatment of the neonate with penicillin. Delayed onset disease is a nosocomial disease and the regimen described above would not be effective.

Penicillin is the antibiotic of choice for treatment of both neonatal and adult disease. The organisms are also sensitive to ampicillin, cephalothin, erythromycin, clindamycin and chloramphenicol. A majority of isolates are resistant to tetracycline.

GROUP D STREPTOCOCCI

Characteristics

Streptococcus faecalis is one of five species in the alpha-hemolytic (some strains may be beta- or nonhemolytic) group D. The term *enterococcus,* implying presence in the intestinal tract, is applied to three species of group D streptococci—S. *faecalis,* S. *faecium* and S. *durans*—but not to S. *bovis* or S. *equinus.* All grow at 45 C and in 40% bile, but only the enterococci grow at 10 C and in 6.5% NaCl. These species share the group D antigen, a glycerol teichoic acid associated with the cytoplasmic membrane.

Infections

The group D streptococci are found on the skin and in the oral cavity and intestinal tract. Under appropriate conditions these organisms can leave their normal ecological niche and cause several different types of infections. Any of the species can cause otitis media, genitourinary tract infection, meningitis or endocarditis, but S. *faecalis* is most frequently isolated.

Infective endocarditis (subacute or acute bacterial endocarditis, SBE) is a consequence of bacteremia and may be caused by any organism. In a survey of 450 cases, 60% were due to streptococci and the rest to staphylococci, gram-negative enterics, diphtheroids, *Pseudomonas Haemophilus* or fungi (particularly *Candida albicans*). Of the streptococci, 90% were alpha- or gamma-hemolytic and the rest were S. *pyogenes* or *Peptostreptococcus.* Endocarditis may occur at any age. Antibiotics are now used to successfully treat what used to be a uniformly fatal disease. If death occurs, it is usually due to congestive heart failure from a valvular perforation. In endocarditis any infected site can be the source of the bacteremia, but the oral cavity, genitouri-

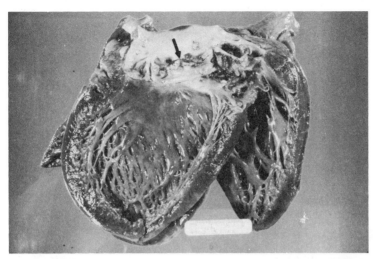

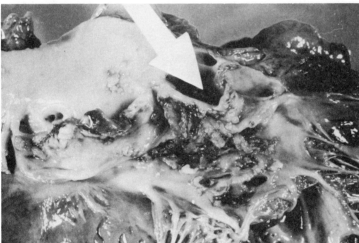

Fig. 6–6.—Infective endocarditis in a young adult male. **Top,** gross specimen of the heart showing involvement of all cups of the aortic valve and posterior aspect of anterior leaflet of the mitral valve *(arrow)*. **Bottom,** enlargement of the involved area showing perforation and vegetations on the leaflets. (Courtesy of W. S. Albrink, Department of Pathology, West Virginia University.)

nary and intestinal tracts predominate. A normal cardiac valve can become infected (particularly with S. *aureus*), but in the majority of cases some type of cardiac disorder (rheumatic fever, prosthesis, congenital defect, atheromas) or predisposing factor (such as cardiac catheterization, hemodialysis, drug addiction or infection at some other site) results in a bacteremia. For the valvular infection to occur, the evidence is that a sterile platelet-fibrin thrombus develops on the endocardium of these valves and the bacteria become implanted in the thrombus during a transient bacteremia. The organisms grow and colonize the thrombus and are then shed from the vegetation at an almost constant rate (Fig. 6–6). The avascularity of the thrombus inhibits phagocytosis and reduces the effectiveness of antibiotics. The principal symptoms of infective endocarditis include fever, cardiac murmur, petechiae and splenomegaly. Blood cultures should be taken as soon as possible (prior to antibiotic therapy) to aid in the diagnosis. Diagnosis includes identification of the etiologic agent and determination of antibiotic sensitivities, which dictate the therapeutic regimen.

Treatment

The enterococci are frequently resistant to the penicillins. Infective endocarditis is one of the few diseases in which combinations of antibiotics, such as penicillin and streptomycin, are used. The non-enterococci (S. *bovis* and S. *equinus*) are more sensitive to antibiotics than the enterococci. The choice of antimicrobial therapy in infective endocarditis depends on the blood culture information, indicating the organism involved and the antibiogram. Except in the acutely ill, therapy can be withheld until the identity of the organism is tentatively established. Patients with a history of endocarditis or rheumatic fever should be given prophylactic penicillin when undergoing operative dentistry or open heart surgery.

STREPTOCOCCUS PNEUMONIAE

Characteristics

Streptococcus pneumoniae is a lancet-shaped diplococcus (Fig. 6–7) that forms chains in broth cultures. It does not contain a Lancefield group antigen but has a species-specific, cell wall-associated ribitol teichoic acid. The polysaccharide capsule is the basis for differentiation into 82 serotypes. The colonies on blood agar are glistening, smooth, sometimes mucoid, with the center becoming depressed as the colony ages. It is alpha-hemolytic, but grown anaerobically produces beta hemolysis due to pneumolysin O. Its cell and colonial

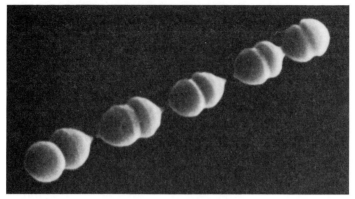

Fig. 6–7.—Scanning electron micrograph of *Streptococcus pneumoniae.* Note the indented central portion of the cell, giving it a diplococcus shape. (From Klainer, A. S., and Geis, I.: *Agents of Bacterial Disease* [Hagerstown, Md.: Harper & Row, 1973]. By permission of the authors and publisher.)

morphological features resemble those of the other alpha-hemolytic streptococci, but *S. pneumoniae* can be differentiated because it: (1) is bile soluble, (2) has growth inhibited by optochin, (3) is pathogenic for mice and (4) exhibits a positive capsular swelling test (see Laboratory Procedures for details). The pneumococcus is a leading cause of bacterial pneumonia but may also cause endocarditis, bacteremia, otitis media, mastoiditis or meningitis.

Antigens

Streptococcus pneumoniae has a prominent polysaccharide capsule (soluble specific substance; SSS), which is responsible for the type specificity of the 82 established and several provisional serologic types (Fig. 6–8). The structures of pneumococcus types 3, 6, 8, 9 and 14 polysaccharides have been established. For example, type 3 consists of repeating cellobiuronic acid units (cellobiuronic acid is composed of repeating D-glucuronic-β1-4-D-glucose dissacharides); cellobiuronic acid is the antigenic determinant. There are cross-reactions between types 1, 3 and 8 because of a sharing of this acid. The polysaccharide capsules of *S. pneumoniae* are antigenic, and being antiphagocytic, they are the principal factor in the pathogenicity of the pneumococcus (Fig. 6–8). During a pneumococcal infection, these antigens stimulate B lymphocytes to synthesize type-specific antibodies which aid in recovery from the pneumonia. These pneumococcal polysaccharides may cross-react with antibodies to carbohydrates from other sources, as, for example, type 2 cross-reacts with

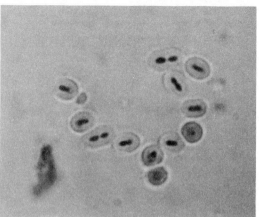

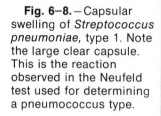

Fig. 6–8. — Capsular swelling of *Streptococcus pneumoniae,* type 1. Note the large clear capsule. This is the reaction observed in the Neufeld test used for determining a pneumococcus type.

Klebsiella pneumoniae antiserum (rhamnose is the common antigenic determinant). Type 14 reacts with antibodies to blood group A substance (galactose is the common antigenic determinant). The pneumococcal polysaccharide antigens can be detected in the blood, cerebrospinal fluid or urine of certain patients by counterimmunoelectrophoresis; their presence in these fluids forecasts a grave prognosis. The particular serologic type (1–82) is determined by the Neufeld test, in which one adds specific antiserum to the pneumococcus and observes for the presence or absence of capsular (Fig. 6–8) swelling (see Laboratory Procedures).

S. *pneumoniae* has a cell wall which contains choline in the ribitol teichoic acid. This is "C-substance" antigen. In addition, choline is found in the membrane lipoteichoic acid, which is a Forssman antigen. Serum from pneumococcal pneumonia patients contains a substance which reacts with pneumococcal C antigen in the presence of $Ca.^{2+}$ This is a nonspecific β-globulin, which is termed C-reactive protein. It also appears in serum in response to inflammatory reactions in a number of infectious and noninfectious diseases. It is detected by doing a precipitin test using the patient's serum and specific β-globulin antiserum. Its presence is used as an aid in the diagnosis of several diseases, including rheumatic fever, rheumatoid diseases and myocardial infarctions.

Hemolysins, Toxins and Enzymes

S. *pneumoniae* readily undergoes lysis in culture either spontaneously or in the presence of detergents, such as optochin, sodium lauryl sulfate or bile. Lysis is due to activation of the enzyme L-alanine-muramyl amidase.

A hemolysin, pneumolysin O, is produced and is similar to streptolysin O both antigenically and functionally. It is activated by sulfhydryl groups and inactivated by cholesterol. It causes dermonecrosis and is lethal to animals.

A neuraminidase is produced by freshly isolated cultures. This glycosidic enzyme cleaves N-acetylneuraminic acid from sugars on glycoproteins and glycolipids.

Infections

PNEUMONIA.—Pneumonia may be lobar, bronchial or interstitial and caused by bacteria, viruses, mycoplasmae or fungi. Of the bacteria, *S. pneumoniae* causes 60–80% of the cases with the remainder due to *S. pyogenes, Staphylococcus, Klebsiella, Escherichia, Pseudomonas, Haemophilus, Serratia, Francisella* or *Yersinia*. Essentially, almost any organism capable of establishing itself in the lungs can cause pneumonia. Bacterial pneumonia may be primary or secondary to virus pneumonia (particularly influenza), debilitating disease or malignancies. Also prone to develop pneumonia are patients receiving immunosuppressive therapy, mechanical respiration or long-term broad-spectrum antibiotic therapy.

Fig. 6–9.—Gram stain of sputum from a patient with pneumococcus pneumonia. Note the numerous diplococci and leukocytes.

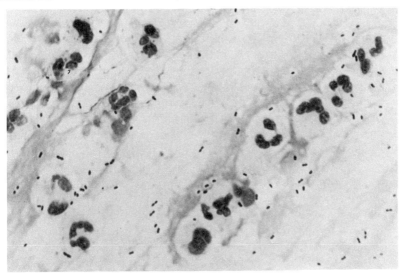

Bacteria reach the lungs through the airways or the bloodstream but most frequently by air, either as droplets (0.5–2.0 μm in diameter) or as aspirated particles (chap. 1). After bacteria reach the alveoli, macrophages may phagocytize and kill them. If the organisms are able to metabolize and survive, there is an accumulation of plasma, multiplication of the organisms and spillage of this exudate into the bronchioles and adjoining alveoli. Accompanying this is a migration of leukocytes and leakage of erythrocytes into the area with eventual coagulation of the plasma within the alveoli. Bacteria, leukocytes, and erythrocytes are trapped and air is displaced. If this consolidation (coagulation of plasma) is sufficiently extensive to interfere with pulmonary gaseous exchange, it can cause death. Clinically, there is a sudden onset of a shaking chill, high fever, pleuritic type of chest pain, and a cough, producing a thick, rusty sputum (Fig. 6–9). The prognosis is grave with involvement of more than one lobe, leukocytosis, bacteremia and a high polysaccharide titer in the blood.

In pneumococcal pneumonia, types 1–9 are most frequently involved, particularly in adults. These may also be encountered in children, but types 12, 14, 16, 18, 19 and 23 are more common. Overall mortality approximates 7% and increases with age, which is often related to the presence of other noncurable diseases. Type 3 has the highest mortality, which correlates with its large capsule and resistance to phagocytosis. Pneumococcal pneumonia tends to be multilobular, although the alveolar wall and lung parenchyma are usually not destroyed, so upon resolution and recovery the lung returns to its normal function. About 30% of the patients have a bacteremia which may result in the development of meningitis, endocarditis or arthritis. If alveoli next to the pleura are involved, the infection may extend, causing pleurisy, or purulent pericarditis.

The pneumococcus can also cause sinusitis, conjunctivitis, mastoiditis, septic arthritis, endocarditis or meningitis; it is the most common cause of acute suppurative otitis media, followed by *Haemophilus influenzae* and *S. pyogenes*. Organisms from the oropharynx gain access to the tissue of the middle ear cleft via the eustachian tube. If the infection becomes chronic, there is usually a shift in microflora to the antibiotic-resistant *Pseudomonas aeruginosa, Escherichia coli* or *Proteus* sp. In some patients, a serous otitis media develops which is nonbacterial but results from a type 1 (IgE) or type 3 (immune complex and complement) hypersensitivity (chap. 1). The aspirated fluid is either sterile or contains few bacteria.

S. pneumonia can also cause a severe corneal ulceration and peritonitis in children who have ascites due to nephrosis.

Mechanisms of Pathogenicity

The *S. pneumoniae* capsule is antiphagocytic and is the only demonstrable factor responsible for pathogenicity. Rough, noncapsulated strains are nonpathogenic. Presumably, all encapsulated types are pathogenic but the lower types (1–9) are more frequently encountered in pneumococcal infections, and type 3 with its large capsule causes the highest mortality. The other factor of pathogenicity relates directly to the ability of the organism to grow and metabolize in the lung or other organs. In so doing, it competes with tissue cells for essential nutrients; this also reduces the amount of available oxygen and increases the acidity. In the lung there is an alteration of capillary permeability with fluid accumulation and release of chemotactic factors. The enzymes or other factors which may be involved are not established. Necrosis usually does not occur, and thus, with resolution, the lung tissue readily returns to its normal structure and function. This is not always true of pneumonia due to gram-negative bacteria.

The pneumococci produce a hemolysin (pneumolysin O) similar to streptolysin O which acts on cell membranes. Its role is unknown but it may cause death of phagocytic and other cells and release lysosomal enzymes. A neuraminidase is also produced by freshly isolated strains. Its role in pathogenesis is not known. Since the glycoprotein substrate is found in tissue fluids and on membranes, it may alter physiological function of the tissue or make nutrients available to the cell.

Some, but not all, pneumococci can react nonimmunologically with the Fc portion of γ-globulin, thereby attracting phagocytes and augmenting inflammation and either phagocytosis or cell damage. Some data suggest that more virulent serotypes have less reactivity with Fc. Purified cell walls and some purified capsular polysaccharides can activate complement by the alternative pathway. Some recent work shows that lipotechoic acid may be the component responsible for complement activation. Some authors have suggested that this mechanism may aid in phagocytosis, but others have proposed that it may play a role in pathogenesis of pneumococcal glomerulonephritis and in fulminant pneumococcal disease with disseminated intravascular coagulation.

Immunity

Resistance to pneumococcal infection is a reflection of both innate and acquired immunity. Several factors, e.g., mucociliary blanket, epiglottal reflex, cough reflex and the alveolar macrophages and lymphatic system, serve to prevent infections of the lower respiratory tract. The normal flora of the upper respiratory tract may also be important by producing substances that are toxic and prevent colonization by other microorganisms. Alteration in natural resistance by prolonged bed rest, alcoholism, antibiotic therapy, drug treatment and other bacterial or viral infections predispose to infection with *S. pneumoniae*.

During infection the capsular polysaccharide of *S. pneumoniae* is released into the blood and tissues where it may persist for weeks. Antibodies can be detected during the first week of the infection. Their appearance often corresponds with the "crisis" in pneumococcus pneumonia, heralding the subsidence of symptoms and recovery. These antibodies (IgM or IgG) are type specific and react with the capsule, opsonizing it to facilitate phagocytosis and killing of the pneumococcus. Also, a nonspecific heat-labile opsonin in normal serum aids phagocytosis before the appearance of antibodies. Complement is fixed in both instances, although by different pathways (chap. 1), and aids phagocytosis.

Vaccines

A polyvalent vaccine containing the polysaccharide antigens of types 1–4, 6–8, 9, 12, 14, 19, 23, 25, 51 and 56 is now available for human use. The fourteen capsular types represent about 80% of isolates from pneumococcal disease. The purpose of immunization is to reduce the incidence of pneumonia in the aged and other selected groups, such as splenectomized individuals, those with chronic pulmonary or heart disease or other predisposing conditions, who have a high mortality and morbidity from pneumonia. Individuals vary in their immunologic response to these different antigens, but antibody titers do increase and persist for months, and the incidence of infection decreases.

Treatment

The pneumococci are susceptible to penicillin and this is the antibiotic of choice. The response of pneumococcal infection to therapy is usually rapid. Tetracyclines, cephalosporins and erythromycin may be used in patients allergic to penicillin. Recently, penicillin-resistant *S. pneumoniae* have been isolated in the United States and multiply-resistant organisms have been isolated in other countries.

OTHER STREPTOCOCCUS SPECIES

A large number of streptococci, some of which are groupable by the Lancefield method but which are usually alpha-hemolytic, are found as normal flora of the skin, oral cavity and intestinal tract. The alpha-hemolytic organisms are often termed the *viridans* streptococci.

In general, they play three important roles in human disease. They are frequently the cause of bacteremia and infective endocarditis, usually associated with some trauma to the oral cavity. *S. mutans,* in addition to causing bacteremia and endocarditis, is the cause of dental caries. Finally, there is evidence that the oral streptococci produce factors which kill other organisms, and their presence in the oral cavity may prevent establishment of other pathogenic organisms.

These organisms as well as other groupable streptococci are briefly described below.

STREPTOCOCCUS SANGUIS, GROUP H. — This species is alpha-hemolytic with different strains exhibiting considerable variation in biochemical reactions. Most produce dextran from sucrose. They have the ability to inhibit growth of other streptococci, reportedly due to H_2O_2 formation, which may also be responsible for the alpha-hemolysis. This species is a dominant organism in early dental plaque (chap. 3) and a constant inhabitant of the oral cavity, adhering particularly to the teeth and epithelial cells of the cheek. It is one of the organisms causing bacterial endocarditis.

STREPTOCOCCUS SALIVARIUS, GROUP K. — This species is nonhemolytic (some alpha) with cell wall polysaccharides as both the group and serotype antigens. This group is not as well established antigenically as the other groups. There are cross reactions with group G, and some of the serotypes do not react with the group antiserum. When this organism is grown on sucrose agar, large mucoid colonies are formed due to the production of soluble levans. *S. salivarius* is an oral inhabitant, adhering particularly to the dorsal surface of the tongue. It can cause endocarditis or bacteremia.

STREPTOCOCCUS MITIS (S. MITEOR). — This species is alpha-hemolytic, has no Lancefield group antigen, but contains a ribitol teichoic acid in the cell wall. Serotypes have been described but are not well defined. Mucoid colonies are not formed on sucrose agar. Hyaluronidase is produced. Intracellular polysaccharides are stored but not utilized as an adherence factor. *S. mitis* frequents the oral cavity but is not cariogenic. It can cause infective endocarditis.

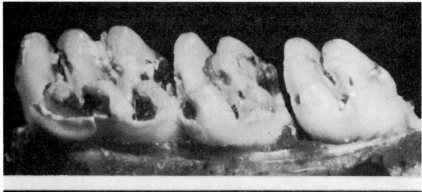

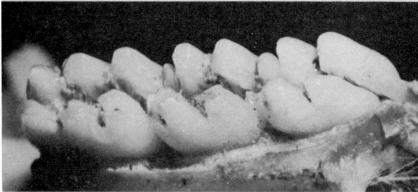

Fig. 6–10.—Pathogen-free rats infected with *Streptococcus mutans* for experimental production of caries. **Top,** buccal view showing extensive smooth surface and sulcal caries. **Bottom,** absence of smooth surface caries and reduction of sulcal caries infected with a glucan synthesis-defective mutant of *S. mutans*, indicating that adherence to the teeth is associated with virulence. (From Tanzer, J. M., Freedman, M. L., Fitzgerald, R. J., and Larson, R. H.: Infect. Immunol. 10:197–203, 1974. By permission of authors and journal.)

STREPTOCOCCUS MUTANS.—This species is nonhemolytic (some alpha or beta), does not have a Lancefield group antigen (some strains crossreact with group E), but has been divided into seven serologic types, a–g. Strains within the species vary biochemically, but all ferment mannitol and sorbitol, and produce fucosyltransferase enzymes which synthesize insoluble glucose polymers (glucan, mutan) from sucrose. These polymers are responsible for adherence to tooth or epithelial surfaces. *S. mutans* is cariogenic and a principal etiologic agent of smooth surface caries in humans (Fig. 6–10). In the production of caries there is first adherence to the tooth (chap. 3) and then demineralization of the tooth surface by the production of acids. Adherence is inhibited by specific secretory IgA antibodies. S. *mutans* may also cause bacteremia and bacterial endocarditis.

LABORATORY PROCEDURES

MATERIALS. — Since the streptococci cause a wide variety of infections, almost any type of material may be submitted for culture, but the most common are throat swabs, sputum, pus, exudate, blood and cerebrospinal fluid (see chap. 4 for methods of collection).

CULTURING. — The clinical specimen is streaked onto blood agar plates (sheep blood is preferred), incubated at 37 C in CO_2 (5–10%) and examined in 18–24 hours.

IDENTIFICATION. — The blood plates are observed for small, convex or flattened colonies with alpha-, beta- or gamma-hemolysis (see Table 6–1). Smears and gram stains are made of the colonies to be certain they are gram-positive cocci with an indication of chain formation. Catalase testing helps in differentiating streptococci from staphylococci.

ALPHA- OR GAMMA-HEMOLYTIC COLONIES. — Differential characteristics are given in Table 6–2. Because these colonies are most likely to be group D (particularly S. *faecalis*) or S. *pneumoniae*, only these organisms will be discussed. For the enterococci of group D, growth in 40% bile and 6.5% NaCl broth and aesculin hydrolysis are distinctive with identity confirmed serologically by the Lancefield or fluorescent antibody test.

To identify S. *pneumoniae*, one usually performs an optochin test. A disk containing optochin is placed on the surface of a heavily inoculated blood agar plate, and after incubation there is a zone of no growth around the disk. S. *pneumoniae* is serotyped by the Neufeld test (Quelling or Capsular Swelling test). This is done by placing a loop of the specimen (broth culture, sputum, cerebrospinal fluid or peritoneal washings from an inoculated mouse) onto a slide. A drop of antiserum containing methylene blue is added and mixed with the specimen. The preparation is observed microscopically for the presence of capsular "swelling." A combination of pooled and type-specific antisera will identify the type, e.g., S. *pneumoniae*, type 2.

BETA-HEMOLYTIC COLONIES. — Differential characteristics are listed in Table 6–1, but as S. *pyogenes* is most likely to be isolated, the use of bacitracin and serologic procedures will be discussed. Bacitracin sensitivity is determined by streaking one or more colonies onto a blood agar plate, placing a bacitracin disk (0.04 units) onto the streaked area and incubating 18–24 hours at 37 C. A 10–18-mm zone of no growth indicates a group A streptococcus. At this point most laboratories report "beta-hemolytic *Streptococcus*, presumptively group A by bacitracin sensitivity."

LANCEFIELD GROUPING AND TYPING TEST. — Beta-hemolytic colonies are transferred to Todd-Hewitt broth, incubated 24 hours and centrifuged. HCl is added to the bacterial sediment, which is boiled for 10 minutes, neutralized and centrifuged. The supernate is used in a precipitin test with specific group antisera. If the organism is *S. pyogenes*, the test is repeated using as many separate type-specific (anti-M) antisera as available; the report gives the species name and type, e.g., *Streptococcus pyogenes*, type 12. Some laboratories carry out the T-agglutination test to aid in the determination of the M types. The fluorescent antibody technique (chap. 4) can be used for the identification of groups A through G.

ANTIBIOTIC SENSITIVITIES. — Antibiotic sensitivity testing (antibiogram) is usually not done on beta-hemolytic isolates. However, resistant isolates of *S. pneumonia* have been found. Sensitivities are routinely done on streptococcal isolates from cases of endocarditis as well as alpha-hemolytic streptococci (other than *S. pneumoniae*) from other sources. The standard disk method (chap. 4) of testing is used.

ANTI-STREPTOLYSIN O TEST (ASO). — Serial dilutions of the patient's serum are made, and measured quantities of streptolysin O and red blood cells are added to each dilution, incubated at 37 C and read for the highest dilution of the patient's serum which inhibits lysis. Results are reported in terms of "Todd units" with the normal range being 85–170 Todd units. Other tests such as anti-DNase B, anti-NADase and anti-hyaluronidase measure the highest dilution of the patient's serum which neutralizes the action of these various enzymes. These have normal ranges, but of most significance is a rise in titer over a period of time.

Counterimmunoelectrophoresis. This procedure is now being used to detect antigens in cerebrospinal fluid, pleural fluids and urine of patients and provides an aid to the diagnosis of infections due to *S. pneumoniae, Neisseria meningitidis, Haemophilus influenzae,* fungi and the viruses of hepatitis B and influenza. This procedure is used for determining the presence, concentration and persistence of an antigen, such as capsular polysaccharide, in body fluids.

PROBLEM SOLVING AND REVIEW

GIVEN: — A 12-year-old boy was admitted to the hospital because of fever, shortness of breath, puffiness around the eyes and hematuria. As a young child he had had numerous sore throats and had spent much of one summer in bed because of a heart murmur; he was given penicillin to take after that but usually forgot his pills. There had been an outbreak of skin infections in his class at school, and about 2 weeks before being admitted to the hospital he developed on his arm a few vesicular lesions that became pustular. They were treated with iodine, but since then he complained of being tired with some nausea and vomiting. His temperature was 39 C and his blood pressure was normal. Red cells and granular casts were found in the urine and the BUN was increased. The presence of a heart murmur was questionable. Two small pustular lesions were present on the right arm. Blood, urine and swabs from the arm lesions were cultured. The ASO titer was low (85 Todd units), but the streptococcal anti-DNase B titer was elevated. Blood cultures were negative. The urine culture had 5,000 *E. coli* per milliliter, but direct smears were negative. Small beta-hemolytic colonies, bacitracin sensitive, were cultured from the skin lesions. The patient was placed on bed rest and penicillin therapy was started. The signs of edema subsided but microscopic hematuria was still present in 2 weeks.

PROBLEMS. — 1. What disease did the patient probably have as a young child? 2. Was this disease related to his present problem? 3. What is the cause of the hematuria and eye puffiness? 4. What is the relationship of the skin lesions to the present disease? 5. Could the kidney be infected with streptococci? 6. If a percutaneous renal biopsy had been done, stained with conjugated anti-human globulin and examined by FA, what would have been observed? 7. What is the rationale of the penicillin therapy? 8. Which serologic types of *S. pyogenes* are most likely to be involved? 9. How would you do a Lancefield grouping and typing test? 10. How do you explain the low ASO titer and the increased anti-DNase B titer? 11. What additional serologic tests could be done? 12. What is the correlation between the 5,000/ml *E. coli* count in the urine and the negative smears? (Ans. p. 123.)

SUPPLEMENTARY READING

Avery, O. T., MacLeod, C. M., and McCarty, M.: Studies on the chemical nature of the substance inducing transformation of pneumococcal types. Induction of transformation by desoxyribonucleic acid fraction isolated from pneumococcus Type III, J. Exp. Med. 79:137–158, 1944.

Baldwin, D. S.: Poststreptococcal glomerulonephritis: A progressive disease? Am. J. Med. 62:1–11, 1977.

Brogden, R. N., Speight, T. M., and Avery, G. S.: Streptokinase: A review of its clinical pharmacology, mechanisms of action and therapeutic uses, Drugs 5:357–445, 1973.

Broome, C. V., Moellering, R. C., Jr., and Watson, B. K.: Clinical significance of Lancefield groups L-T streptococci isolated from blood and cerebrospinal fluid, J. Infect. Dis. 133:382–392, 1976.

Coonrod, J. D.: Physical and immunological properties of pneumococcal capsular polysaccharide produced during human infection, J. Immunol. 112:2193–2201, 1974.

Diebel, R. H.: The group D streptococci, Bacteriol. Rev. 28:330–366, 1964.

Dorff, G. J., Rytel, M. W., Farmer, S. G., and Scanlon, G.: Etiologies and characteristic features of pneumonias in a municipal hospital, Am. J. Med. Sci. 266:349–358, 1973.

Duma, R. J., Weinberg, A. N., Medrek, T. F. F., and Kuntz, L. J.: Streptococcal infections. A bacteriological and clinical study of streptococcal bacteremia, Medicine (Baltimore) 48:87–127, 1969.

Facklam, R. R.: Characteristics of *Streptococcus mutans* isolated from human dental plaque and blood, Int. J. Syst. Bacteriol. 24:313–319, 1974.

Facklam, R. R.: Physiological differentiation of viridans streptococci, J. Clin. Microbiol. 5:184–201, 1977.

Fossieck, B., Craig, R., and Paterson, P. Y.: Counterimmunoelectrophoresis for rapid diagnosis of meningitis due to *Diplococcus pneumonia*, J. Infect. Dis. 127:106–109, 1973.

Fox, E. N.: M proteins of group A streptococci, Bacteriol. Rev. 38:57–86, 1974.

Ginsburg, I.: Mechanisms of cell and tissue injury induced by group A streptococci: relation to poststreptococcal sequelae, J. Infect. Dis. 126:294–340, 1972.

Howie, V. M., Ploussard, J. H., and Lester, R. L.: Otitis media: A clinical and bacteriological correlation, Pediatrics 45:29–35, 1970.

Merrill, J. P.: Glomerulonephritis, N. Engl. J. Med. 290:257–266; 313–319; 374–381, 1974.

Patterson, M. J., and Hafeez, A. B.: Group B streptococci in human disease, Bacteriol. Rev. 40:774–792, 1976.

Peter, G., and Smith, A. L.: Group A streptococcal infections of the skin and pharynx, N. Engl. J. Med. 297:311–317, 1977.

Tagg, J. R., Dajani, A. S., and Wannamaker, L. W.: Bacteriocins of gram positive bacteria, Bacteriol. Rev. 40:722–756, 1976.

Unger, J. D., Rose, H. D., and Unger, G. F.: Gram negative pneumonia, Radiology 107:283–291, 1973.

Wannamaker, L. W.: Differences between streptococcal infections of the throat and of the skin, N. Engl. J. Med. 282:23–31; 78–85; 1970.

Wannamaker, L. W., and Matsen, J. M. (eds.): *Streptococci and Streptococcal Diseases* (New York: Academic Press, 1972).
Weinstein, L., Rubin, R. H., and Schlesinger, J.: Infective endocarditis, Prog. Cardiovasc. Dis. 16:239–302, 1973.

ANALYSIS

1. Rheumatic fever. 2. Probably not related, although the heart valve injury makes the individual more susceptible to endocarditis. 3. All or most of the glomeruli are involved, resulting in fluid retention and escape of erythrocytes. 4. Acute glomerulonephritis is more likely to follow streptococcal skin lesions, such as pyoderma or impetigo, and it is probable that there was an outbreak of impetigo in the school. 5. Probably not, this is not a direct infection of the kidney; streptococcal antigens or complexes become fixed to the glomerular membrane, IgG accumulates and complement is fixed; leukocytes migrate into the area, releasing hydrolytic enzymes which initiate glomerular injury. 6. The lumpy-dumpy appearance due to irregular deposit of antigen-antibody reactions along the glomerular basement membrane. 7. This prevents continuation of the streptococcal infection but does not alter the course of the glomerulonephritis. 8. Serotypes 1, 4 and 12 (pharyngitis), and 49, 55, 56 and 57 (pyoderma) are nephritogenic. 9. Grow the isolate in Todd-Hewitt broth, acidify and boil the centrifuged cells, neutralize and do a precipitin test with known group A antisera. 10. Patients with streptococcal infections of the skin do not produce antibodies to streptolysin O as readily as patients with pharyngitis. 11. Anti-NADase and anti-hyaluronidase determinations. 12. Fewer than 100,000 bacteria per milliliter of urine cannot be visualized microscopically; one bacterium per high-power field is equivalent to 100,000/ml.

7 / Neisseria, Acinetobacter and Moraxella

OVERVIEW

Of the two species of *Neisseria* which cause disease in man — *N. gonorrhoeae* and *N. meningitidis* — the former is more prevalent. Approximately 1 million cases of gonorrhea are reported each year, but a reasonable estimate suggests that 3 million or more cases probably occur. This is unfortunate because, with cooperation and understanding, epidemics of gonorrhea can be prevented and the incidence of this disease markedly reduced. The primary venereal infection itself is not important, but the consequences — both social and medical — of this disease are significant. Venereal infection of the mother may allow the organism to be transmitted to the eye of the newborn and result in blindness. In women, infection can result in sterility or in closure or constriction of the fallopian tubes and ectopic pregnancy. In men, stricture of the urethra can result. Septicemia, meningitis, and arthritis can also be consequences of gonococcemia. Control of gonorrhea is likely to become even more complicated with the recent isolation of B-lactamase-resistant organisms.

N. meningitidis is still important as a causative agent of meningitis. Although it does not occur with the same frequency as in the past, occasional epidemics have been reported and the occurrence of antibiotic-resistant strains remains a problem. The development of successful vaccines against two of the common serogroups involved in disease and work which suggests that successful immunization may be accomplished with the third major group predict even better control of this organism.

NEISSERIA AND BRANHAMELLA

General Characteristics

Neisseria and *Branhamella* are gram-negative cocci (0.6–1.0 μm) which appear in pairs with adjacent sides flattened (Fig. 7–1). They

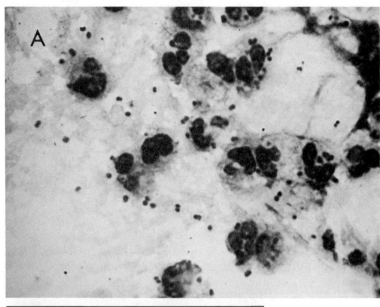

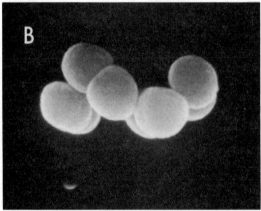

Fig. 7–1.—A, *Neisseria meningitidis* in cerebrospinal fluid. The gram-negative diplococci are located both intra- and extracellularly. **B,** scanning electron micrograph of a *Neisseria* species. (Courtesy of R. H. Ruff and P. Allender, West Virginia University Medical Center.)

are facultatively anaerobic; some have complex nutritional requirements. Growth of pathogenic species may be restricted at 37 C. *N. gonorrhoeae* requires 5–10% CO_2 for primary isolation. All species produce catalase and cytochrome oxidase. Some species produce a yellow pigment.

TABLE 7-1.—CHARACTERISTICS OF *NEISSERIA* AND *BRANHAMELLA*

	YELLOW PIGMENT	FERMENTATION: GLUCOSE	MALTOSE	SUCROSE	LACTOSE
N. gonorrhoeae	−	+	−	−	−
N. meningitidis	−	+	+	−	−
N. lactamica	−	+	+	−	+
N. sicca	+	+	+	+	−
N. flavescens	+	−	−	−	−
N. mucosa	−	+	+	+	−
N. subflava	+	+	+	±	−
Branhamella catarrhalis	−	−	−	−	−

±Pigment is yellow.

	SUPPLEMENTARY TESTS: GROWTH ON BLOOD AGAR AT 22 C	GROWTH ON NON-BLOOD AGAR AT 37 C
N. gonorrhoeae	−	−
N. meningitidis	−	−
N. lactamica	−	−
N. sicca	+	+
N. flavescens	+	±
Branhamella catarrhalis	+	+

±Some strains.

Species

Several species are found in man: *N. gonorrhoeae, N. meningitidis, N. sicca, N. subflava, N. flavescens, N. mucosa* and *N. lactamica. Branhamella catarrhalis,* formerly called *Neisseria catarrhalis,* is the only species in the genus *Branhamella.* Differential characteristics are shown in Table 7-1.

Ecology

Two species, *N. meningitidis* and *N. gonorrhoeae,* cause most of the disease associated with this genus in man. Other species, *N. sicca, N. subflava, N. flavescens, N. lactamica* and *N. mucosa,* are found as normal flora of the upper respiratory tract and have been isolated from patients with meningitis, septicemia, postpneumonectomy empyema and cellulitis. *Branhamella catarrhalis* is also a member of the normal flora of the upper respiratory tract and has been reported as causing meningitis.

Veillonella parvula and *Veillonella alkalescens* are anaerobic gram-negative cocci which are similar morphologically to the *Neisseria.* They are found as normal flora in the mouth and intestinal tract. Their role in disease is uncertain.

Cell Wall and Associated Structures

The cell wall of the *Neisseria* is typical of that described for other gram-negative organisms. It contains endotoxin and several other antigens. In *N. gonorrhoeae* and *N. meningitidis* an autolytic enzyme, N-acetylmuramyl-L-alanine muramidase, is responsible for the high rate of autolysis. Pili and capsules have also been demonstrated.

NEISSERIA MENINGITIDIS

Antigens and Toxins

Neisseria meningitidis have polysaccharide capsules that are useful in serogrouping. Seven serogroups, A, B, C, D, X, Y and Z, have been identified. Serotypes A, B, C and Y are most frequently found in disease. The capsular polysaccharide of serogroup A is a polymer of N- and O-acetylated D-mannosamine phosphate. The group B polysaccharide is composed of N-acetylneuraminic acid, whereas the group C polysaccharide is a polymer of both N- and O-acetylneuraminic acid.

Type-specific protein antigens have been isolated from the outer membrane of groups A, B and C. The group B serotype antigen is a protein found as part of a lipoprotein-lipopolysaccharide complex, and like the type-specific antigens of groups A and C, it is located in the outer cell membrane. A genus-specific protein antigen has also been described.

Pili have been demonstrated on fresh clinical isolates of *N. meningitidis* but are absent on strains cultivated for long periods in the laboratory. The function of these pili is unknown, but they probably play a role in interfering with phagocytosis and in adhering to mucosal cells.

The endotoxin of *N. meningitidis* has activities identical with those of other endotoxins and is responsible for the pathophysiologic features of meningococcal disease. The meningococcus endotoxin appears to be more effective than endotoxins from other organisms in producing purpura.

Genetics

Transformation of *N. meningitidis* has been demonstrated and the organisms undergo an S → R dissociation during growth in vitro. Nutritional auxotrophs have been demonstrated.

Infections

Neisseria meningitidis is an obligate parasite of man and is found as normal oral flora in 5–25% of the population. Meningococcal disease occurs most commonly in late winter and early spring and most frequently in young children. In the host lacking antibody, the organ-

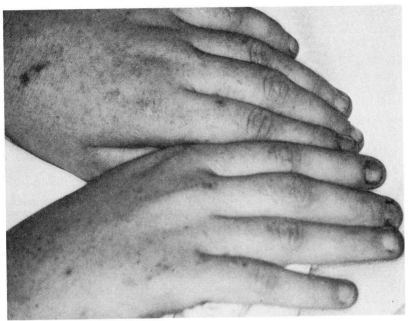

Fig. 7–2.—Skin lesions in patient with meningococcemia. (Courtesy of Dr. Edmund Flink, Department of Medicine, West Virginia University Medical Center.)

isms, acquired by inhaling droplets, lodge in the nasopharynx producing a mild inflammatory reaction and pharyngitis. Pneumonia may follow. By some means the organism enters the bloodstream, producing a meningococcemia that may be mild or fulminating. In patients with fulminating meningococcemia there is an abrupt onset with chills, headache and dizziness. In 50–65% of the patients with meningococcemia large, irregular-shaped, purpuric spots may be present on the skin (Fig. 7–2). Hemorrhage of the adrenals, vascular collapse and disseminated intravascular coagulation may then follow (Waterhouse-Friderichsen syndrome). A polyarthritis may also be produced. In a fulminating meninococcemia, death may occur in 6–24 hours.

Patients with or without evidence of meningococcemia may develop meningitis. The gram-negative coccobacilli can be demonstrated in cerebrospinal fluid (Fig. 7–1). Meningitis is an acute inflammation of the leptomeninges and may occur following head trauma, otitis media, sinusitis, mastoiditis, pneumonia and bacteremia. Some of the common etiologic agents and their frequency by age are given in Table 7–2.

TABLE 7-2.—COMMON AGENTS IN SEPTIC MENINGITIS AS
RELATED TO AGE

AGE	ETIOLOGIC AGENTS IN APPROXIMATE ORDER OF OCCURENCE
Prematures to 3 mo	E. coli, other enteric bacilli, S. agalactiae, H. influenzae, S. pneumoniae, Listeria monocytogenes
3 mo to 6 yr	H. influenzae (type b), N. meningitidis, S. pneumoniae
6 to 21 yr	N. meningitidis, S. pneumoniae
Over 21 yr	H. influenzae, S. pneumoniae, N. meningitidis

The symptoms of meningitis are due initially to infection and then to increased intracranial pressure. In early meningitis, the symptoms may be flu-like with a sore or stiff neck, headache, low-grade fever and lethargy. Classically there is fever (37.8–41.1 C), tachycardia, chills, lethargy, malaise and skin rash. Meningeal irritation (Brudzinski's and Kernig's signs), lethargy, confusion, stupor or coma may be evident.

At the extremes of age, the symptoms of meningitis may not be classic. In the elderly patient, only flu-like symptoms with slight stiffness of the neck may be recognized. In the neonate, the temperature may be slightly elevated, normal or subnormal, the fontanelles may be either full or bulging and the child may be lethargic, vomit and refuse to eat.

Untreated bacterial meningitis is fatal in 70–100% of patients. In addition, 50% of neonates with meningitis may have motor or intellectual impairment. Meningitis is a medical emergency.

Most cases of meningococcal infections are caused by serogroups A, B, C and Y. Groups B and C are the predominant causes. Group B is most common in children under 5 years of age and in adults 50 years and older. Group C predominates in children 5–14 years of age, and group Y is found primarily in persons between 15 and 29 years of age. Epidemics of disease by group A, however, have occurred in recent years.

Mechanisms of Pathogenicity

The organism is commonly found in man and as such readily colonizes the upper respiratory tract of nonimmune individuals. Attachment to mucosal cells and colonization of the upper respiratory tract may be due to the presence of pili. Antibody to the capsular polysaccharide prevents colonization and disease by permitting ingestion and destruction of the organisms by leukocytes. The ability to survive phagocytosis is primarily related to the polysaccharide capsule. An extracellular enzyme which cleaves IgA_1 between the proline-threonine bond in the IgA_1 heavy chain has been demonstrated and may be a mechanism by which the organism circumvents local immunity. In the absence of antibody, organisms colonize the host, incite an inflammatory response and then may gain access to the vascular system and produce a meningococcemia. Petechial and purpuric lesions which represent a dermal Schwartzman reaction may occur in more than half of the patients. Organisms can be cultured from the purpuric lesions and they can be demonstrated in both endothelial cells and neutrophils. Immunoglobulins, antigen, and complement also can be found in these lesions, suggesting a role for both endotoxin and immunologic factors. The vascular injury consists of endothelial necrosis, thrombosis and necrosis of other vascular wall components. In some patients shock and disseminated intravascular coagulation (Waterhouse-Friderichsen syndrome) result and are related to the action of endotoxin. Finally, the organisms may enter the cerebrospinal system and cause inflammation of the leptomeninges and resultant meningitis.

Immunity

Immunity is a reflection of IgM, IgG and IgA concentration. Immunity, passively transferred from mother to child, disappears within 4–6 months, after which the child is susceptible until immunity is again acquired through carriage or subclinical infection. This age-related susceptibility, which is due to disappearance of passively acquired immunity and lack of actively acquired immunity, is reflected in the data in Table 7–2 indicating an increased frequency of *Neisseria* meningitis in older children and young adults. A deficiency in serum bactericidal activity correlates with susceptibility to disease. IgA antibody from convalescent human serum interferes with the bactericidal activity of IgM and IgG and probably accounts for the decrease in bactericidal activity observed in some patients after infection. A similar effect has been shown in patients with chronic brucellosis. Immunization decreases the carrier rate of homologous meningococcal groups but may in fact select for carriage of other serogroups. Vaccines containing capsular polysaccharides of serogroups A and C have been used with success. Hemagglutinating and bactericidal antibodies as well as resistance to disease follow immunization. The group B capsular polysaccharide, a polymer of N-acetylneuraminic acid, is a poor immunogen, and an effective vaccine against this group of organisms has not been produced. Antibody to the type-specific antigen of group B organisms is bactericidal and suggests that these antigens might be good immunogens. Infection with group B represents a major portion of meningococcal diseases.

The carrier develops antibody after 2 weeks of carriage, and the large percentage of the population with antibody is reflected as herd immunity. Antibodies specific for the group being carried but cross-reactive with other types are produced. Thus, herd immunity is broadened as the host is exposed via colonization to other strains of N. meningitidis.

Prevention

The meningococcus is acquired by contact with a carrier or infected person. Control of the carrier is not a practical approach to prevention of disease. Chemotherapy is used in epidemics to reduce the possibility of acquisition of meningococci by susceptible people. Because the attack rate is 500- to 800-fold greater in household contacts, prophylactic chemotherapy is recommended. Immunization against group A and C organisms is now possible. These vaccines have been licensed and are recommended for use during epidemics and for protecting household contacts. Future efforts may be directed at increasing the immunity of populations at risk by immunization.

Treatment

Meningococcal disease is an acute disease and treatment must be started as early as possible. Up to 75% of group C strains and 25% of

TABLE 7-3.—CHARACTERISTICS WHICH PERMIT
DIFFERENTIATION OF MENINGITIS BY DIFFERENT
ETIOLOGIC AGENTS

TYPE OF INFECTION AND CAUSES	CSF PROTEIN	CSF GLUCOSE	CELL CONCENTRATION (per cu mm)	CELL TYPE

Acute
  S. pneumoniae
  H. influenzae
  N. meningitidis
  L. monocytogenes
  Gram-negative rods
	Marked elevation >400 mg/ 100 ml	Marked depression 0-4 mg/ 100 cc	Thousands	PMN

Subacute
  M. tuberculosis
  Cryptococcus
  Inadequately treated
    bacterial infections
	Moderate elevation 100-300 mg/ 100 ml	Moderate depression	Hundreds	Mononuclear and PMN

Aseptic Viral	Mild	Normal	Hundreds	Lymphocyte
Normal	15-45 mg/ 100 ml	50-75 mg/ 100 ml	0-5	Mononuclear

all strains are resistant to sulfadiazine. The case fatality rate with group C is higher than that of other serogroups of *Neisseria* and may be a reflection of this resistance. Rifampin and penicillin G are the drugs of choice, particularly since sulfadiazine-resistant meningococci have become common. Minocycline and a combination of minocycline and rifampin are also effective in reducing the carrier rate. Supportive measures to treat the host response to endotoxin may also be necessary.

Meningitis must be promptly diagnosed and treated. Table 7-3 shows some characteristics which permit differentiation of meningitis as caused by bacteria, fungi and viruses. These differential characteristics, along with direct observation of organisms in the cerebrospinal fluid, age and patient history, should permit a presumptive judgment as to cause and allow the physician to begin chemotherapy promptly.

NEISSERIA GONORRHOEAE

Antigens and Serology

Thermostable common antigens, lipopolysaccharide antigens and other type- and strain-specific antigens have been described. Many attempts have been made to develop a serologic basis for classification and detection of gonorrhea. Sixteen serotypes have been described based on specificity of a protein serotype antigen located in the outer membrane. In addition to antigenic cell wall-associated antigens, pili which are found primarily on virulent strains are antigenic.

Antigens of *N. gonorrhoeae* cross-react with antiserum against *N. meningitidis*. A method for epidemiologic characterization of *N. gonorrhoeae* using antisera for *N. meningitidis* has been reported. Differences in the susceptibility of various isolates to the bactericidal effect of serum permit strain differentiation.

Genetics

Transformation between strains of *N. gonorrhoeae* has been described. Competency for transformation is associated with piliated cells and certain colonial morphological features on particular media. DNA from clinical isolates has been used to transform nutritional mutants of *N. gonorrhoeae* and is suggested as a tool for detection of *N. gonorrhoeae* in man. Auxotyping, i.e., determination of the nutritional requirements of *N. gonorrhoeae*, has been used to group isolates and to study the epidemiology of these organisms.

Transfer of the penicillinase plasmid by transformation and by conjugation has been demonstrated. Transfer by conjugation is accomplished with relatively high efficiency among gonococci, and transfer to other species has also been demonstrated.

Virulence Factors

Neisseria gonorrhoeae is classified into four types based on colonial morphological features. Types 1 and 2 are virulent for man and animals, whereas types 3 and 4 are relatively avirulent. The avirulent strains produce mild, transient infections without establishment of infection in the genital tract. Pili have been demonstrated on gonococci of types 1 and 2 but are absent on types 3 and 4. Pili from different strains are antigenically distinct. Pili enhance attachment to tissues, and cells with pili are more resistant to phagocytosis than nonpiliated cells. Virulent strains of *N. gonorrhoeae* are also more resistant than avirulent strains to complement-serum-mediated killing. A capsule of unknown composition has been demonstrated both in vivo and in vitro. It appears to aid the organism in resisting phagocytosis.

There is a suggestion that the lipopolysaccharide (LPS) from the type 1 (piliated) organisms differs from that of type 4 (nonpiliated). The type 1 may be a complete LPS containing high molecular weight O polysaccharides, whereas the type 4 LPS may contain a structurally different O polysaccharide. However, some workers have not found a difference in the LPS.

Infections

Several microorganisms can cause venereal disease. Among these are *Treponema pallidum* (syphilis), *Haemophilus ducreyi* (soft chancre), *Chlamydia trachomatis* (lymphogranuloma venereum), *Donovani granulomatis* (granuloma inguinale), and *N. gonorrhoeae* (gonorrhea). In addition to bacterial agents, viruses such as herpes simplex are important venereal agents. However, gonorrhea is the most common bacterial infection.

Neonatal Disease

The neonate acquires *N. gonorrhoeae* during birth with resultant infection of the eye (neonatal gonococcal ophthalmia). The eyelids become edematous and erythematous and a purulent discharge is present. The conjunctivas are inflamed and without treatment the cornea vascularizes. This is an acute pyogenic infection which must be treated. The disease is evident within a few days after birth and can result in blindness. Gonococcal ophthalmia is prevented by instillation of penicillin or 1% silver nitrate (Credé's solution) into the eyes immediately after birth. Ophthalmia neonatorum can also be caused

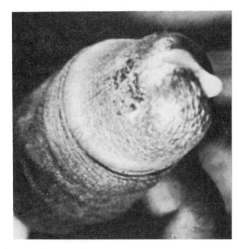

Fig. 7–3.—Mucopurulent yellow discharge in a patient with gonorrhea. (Reproduced with permission of the VD Control Division, Bureau of State Services, Center for Disease Control, Public Health Service, Department of Health, Education and Welfare.)

by other organisms, e.g., *Chlamydia, Staphylococcus, Haemophilus* and other bacteria. Gonococcal arthritis may also be found in neonates. *N. gonorrhoeae* has been isolated from orogastric aspirates of neonates with signs of sepsis.

Gonorrhea in Men

In the male, the incubation period is 2–8 days. The onset of symptoms is sudden and characterized by frequent, urgent and painful urination with a yellow mucopurulent discharge (Fig. 7–3). The anterior urethral infection may extend to the posterior urethra and involve the epididymis and prostate. The organisms (Fig. 7–4) may disseminate resulting in septicemia, arthritis, endocarditis, meningitis or osteomyelitis. Rectal and pharyngeal gonorrhea may also occur. About 10% of infected men are asymptomatic.

Gonorrhea in Women

Up to 70% of infected women may have no signs or symptoms of disease. The prepubertal child may have vulvovaginitis with symptoms of dysuria, vulvar pain, perianal soreness and discomfort on defecation. A yellowish green discharge may be found at vaginal and urethral orifices and occasionally from the anus. Vulvovaginitis also occurs in premenstrual and postmenopausal women.

Acute gonorrhea in women involves the urethra, Skene's glands, Bartholin's glands, the cervix and the fallopian tubes, resulting in purulent or chronic salpingitis. Rectal and pharyngeal infection may also occur. Pelvic inflammatory disease (PID) may follow an acute infection or be delayed for several months. In PID, both fallopian tubes may be blocked by scar tissue formed as a response to infection. This results in trapping of the purulent discharge to form a pyosalpinx and consequent peritonitis.

As in men, the gonococci may disseminate, with resultant septicemia, arthritis or meningitis. In women, the gonococcus may cause the Curtis-Fitz-Hugh syndrome, an infection resulting in jaundice, pneumonia and pleural effusion (gonococcal perihepatitis).

Gonococcal Arthritis-Dermatitis Syndrome

The two most common manifestations of gonococcal sepsis are arthritis and dermatitis, frequently referred to as the gonococcal arthritis-dermatitis syndrome (GADS). The incidence is about 3%, and the syndrome is more common in women. The symptoms are fever, chills, malaise, and arthritis or tenosynovitis. Urogenital symptoms are usually absent. The rash begins as pinpoint, erythematous macules which may progress to papular and vesiculopustular lesions with an erythematous base or to purpuric or hemorrhagic papules. The lesions tend to appear on the extremities and the palms and soles of the feet.

Mechanisms of Pathogenicity

Humans are the sole host for the gonococcus, and gonococcal infection is acquired from an infected person or a carrier. Pili (types 1 and 2 gonococci) permit attachment to the mucosa and to sperm cells and also aid the organisms in resisting phagocytosis. The gonococci have a predilection for columnar epithelium. In addition to pili, other adherence factors may exist. The microvilli of the host cell surround and may even wrap around the gonococci, indicating an intimate association between host cell surface and microbial surface. The organisms penetrate the epithelial cells and also gain access to the connective tissue through intercellular junctions. The organisms and polymorphonuclear leukocytes accumulate in subepithelial connective tissue and destroy the overlying mucosa, which is then replaced by squamous epithelium. The ciliary activity of epithelial cells within the human fallopian tubes is inhibited even though the cells are not invaded by the gonococcus.

A factor also related to virulence may be the ability of piliated gonococci to resist complement-mediated serum killing. This property is lost in conversion from virulent to avirulent morphological types by prolonged passage on agar. A second form of serum resistance acquired by growth in serum is not associated with conversion from virulent to avirulent colony types.

An extracellular IgA protease produced by the gonococci may contribute by local alteration of the immune response. Toxins other than endotoxins have not been demonstrated, so the acute inflammation and signs and symptoms associated with gonococcal septicemia are probably related to the effects of endotoxin.

Two important and interesting aspects of the pathogenesis of gonococcal infection are that (1) a number of infected persons are asymptomatic and (2) in some patients the disease disseminates. Studies on auxotyping of isolates show that a high percentage of these isolates require arginine, hypoxanthine and uracil for growth. These nutritionally dependent strains have been isolated from 89% of the patients with disseminated gonococcal infection (DGI) and from 96% of asymptomatic patients. The reasons for the relationship between nutritional dependency and disease are not known but may relate to ability to grow in certain environments or to produce a product that alters host response. In addition to nutritional dependency, strains isolated from patients with DGI are more sensitive to penicillin and resistant to bactericidal effect of serum than strains from patients with uncomplicated disease.

Immunity

Whether immunity to the gonococcus is produced is not clear. Certainly, repeated episodes of gonococcal urethritis may occur despite increases in antigonococcal serum antibody, secretory IgA and cell-mediated immunity. However, only about 35% of men experiencing a single sexual contact with an infected woman develop gonorrhea, which suggests some natural or acquired immunity. Repeated exposure increases the risk to about 75%.

In the chimpanzee, which serves as an experimental model for gonorrhea, immunity to urethritis and pharyngitis can be acquired. In addition, natural immunity of different mucosal surfaces to gonococcal infection varies, and in this animal model it is higher in the cervix and pharynx than in the urethra. Whether these findings can be translated to infection of man is questionable. In man, the incubation period for gonococcal urethritis is about 3 days, and patients usually come for treatment in 2–3 days. In the chimpanzee, the incubation period is 20–50 days. This longer incubation period in animals may be adequate for development of immunity. In humans, antibodies are produced in women with local infection of the female genital tract and in males with recurrent infection.

Increased lymphocyte blastogenesis of peripheral monocytes from persons with gonorrhea has been shown, but the role of cellular immunity is not known.

Attempts are presently being made to produce a vaccine for prevention of gonorrhea and to develop a serologic test for detection of gonorrhea. The gonococci are antigenically complex and there is apparently little correlation between serotype and immunotype, which complicates attempts to produce a vaccine and a serologic test.

Prevention and Control

The only certain method for preventing gonorrhea is abstention from sexual intercourse with infected persons. As a practical alternate, the use of mechanical prophylaxis (condoms) offers some protection.

Detection and adequate treatment of infected persons, monitored by culture of the urethra, cervix and rectum, appears to be the only effective method for control.

The results of a recent gonorrhea testing program reported an overall isolation rate of 4.4%. The rate was 1.6% in a private family group practice and 18.7% in a venereal disease testing clinic.

Control of the disease is complicated by the large percentage of men (10%) and women (up to 70%) who are asymptomatic but can transmit the disease.

Treatment

Strains of *N. gonorrhoeae* resistant in vitro and in vivo to penicillin have been isolated in the Far East and in the United States and threaten to make control difficult. About 30–40% of the *N. gonorrhoeae* isolated from selected populations in the Far East are resistant to penicillin, which is the antibiotic of choice.

The recommended treatment for uncomplicated gonococcal infection is 4.8 million units aqueous procaine penicillin G intramuscularly divided into 2 doses and injected at different sites. Probenecid (1 gm) is given by mouth just before the antibiotic. Ampicillin (3.5 gm) and probenecid (1 gm) can be used if oral therapy is preferred. If the patient is allergic to penicillin or probenecid, tetracycline hydrochloride (1.5 gm) followed by 0.5 gm, 4 times a day for 4 days, or spectinomycin (2 gm intramuscularly) is recommended for treatment of patients infected with B-lactamase-producing *N. gonorrhoeae* or who still have a positive culture after initial treatment with penicillin, ampicillin or tetracyclines.

Pregnant women should be treated with penicillin or ampicillin along with probenecid. Erythromycin (1.5 gm orally with 0.5 gm, 4 times a day for 4 days) should be used in pregnant women with penicillin hypersensitivity.

Patients with disseminated gonococcal infection should receive extended treatment with aqueous crystalline penicillin G (10 million units) intravenously each day for 3 days or until there is significant clinical improvement. Ampicillin, 500 mg 4 times a day, to complete 7 days of treatment follows. Tetracycline and erythromycin can be used in the allergic patient.

Neonatal disease such as gonococcal ophthalmia is treated with 50,000 units aqueous crystalline penicillin G (50,000 units/kg/day) in 2 or 3 doses intravenously for 7 days plus saline irrigations and instillation of penicillin, tetracycline or chloramphenicol into the eyes.

ACINETOBACTER AND MORAXELLA

Moraxella and *Acinetobacter* are taxonomically associated with the *Neisseria* and *Branhamella*.

Acinetobacter are gram-negative plump rods which are found in pairs or short chains. They are nonmotile, oxidase negative and are usually resistant to penicillin. Some strains are hemolytic.

Moraxella are rod-shaped during growth but become spherical in the stationary phase. They grow readily on simple media; they are nonmotile, oxidase positive and usually sensitive to penicillin.

Disease

Moraxella consists of several species. *M. lacunata* (Morax-Axenfeld bacillus) causes conjunctivitis in man. *M. osloensis* (previously *M. polymorpha* var. *oxidans*) has been isolated from the upper respiratory tract, urine, and secretions from the genital tract. Some species of *Moraxella*, because of morphological features and oxidase reaction, may be confused with *N. gonorrhoeae*. *Acinetobacter calcoaceticus* (previously *Herellea vaginicola* and *Mima polymorpha*) is found in soil and water and has been isolated from animals and man. It is an opportunist and has been isolated from a number of disease processes, e.g., pneumonia and other infections of the respiratory tract, urinary tract infections, wounds and meningitis.

Laboratory Procedures

Isolation: Neisseria meningitidis

The physician can, based on analysis of the cerebrospinal fluid, differentiate acute, aseptic and viral meningitis as in Table 7-3.

Specimens to be submitted may include nasopharyngeal swab, blood, cerebrospinal fluid, synovial fluid and aspirates from purpuric lesions.

Gram stains should be done on all specimens except blood, but gram stain of the buffy coat may be of value. The presence of gram-negative diplococci should be reported promptly (see Fig. 7-1). The cocci may be pleomorphic and appear swollen, particularly if the patient has received antibiotics. Fluorescent antibody stains may also help in identifying the organism, especially where they may be nonviable due to prior treatment. Counter-current immunoelectrophoresis can be used to detect capsular polysaccharide in blood, cerebrospinal fluid and synovial fluid. With cerebrospinal fluid, antigen can be detected by precipitin formation with antisera to the meningococcal groups.

All specimens except blood are inoculated onto "chocolate" agar or Thayer-Martin medium. Thayer-Martin is a selective medium containing Mueller-Hinton starch agar with hemoglobin and yeast extract as growth factors. Vancomycin, colistin and nystatin are included as

Fig. 7–4.—Smear of exudate from patient with gonococcal urethritis. Note intracellular diplococci in polymorphonuclear leukocytes. (Courtesy of R. H. Ruff, West Virginia Medical Center.)

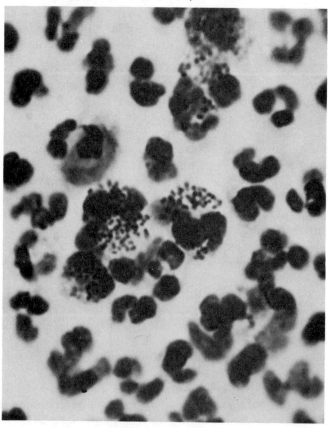

inhibitors of other bacteria. The inoculated medium must be incubated in 10% CO$_2$ and is used *only when a specimen with mixed bacterial flora is suspected.* If the specimen cannot be immediately delivered to the laboratory, the specimen is inoculated on Transgrow medium, which is bottled Thayer-Martin medium containing an overlay of CO$_2$. The bottle is placed in an upright position for inoculation to prevent loss of the CO$_2$ overlay and is tightly closed after inoculation.

Isolation: Neisseria gonorrhoeae

MEN. — Urethral discharge from the symptomatic patient and scrapings or swabs of the urethral meatus from the asymptomatic should be obtained for gram stain and cultures. A 2-mm platinum loop or small cotton-tipped applicator can be used to obtain urethral canal specimens. The urethral specimens are gram stained and observed for the presence of polymorphonuclear leukocytes containing gram-negative diplococci (Fig. 7–4). Rectal colonization is common in homosexuals, and swabs should be obtained and cultured.

WOMEN. — Cervical, vaginal, rectal and urethral cultures should be obtained. Gram stains are of limited value because of the mixed flora. Specimens should be obtained carefully so as to minimize contamination and maximize recovery of small numbers of gonococci.

In both men and women, blood, synovial fluid, cerebrospinal fluid, and pharyngeal cultures may also be necessary if pharyngitis, meningitis, arthritis or gonococcemia is suspected. Aspirates from skin lesions should be stained and cultured.

NEONATES. — Swabs of conjunctival exudate should be obtained and cultured as described. Gastric aspirates may also be cultured in infants from mothers with chorioamnionitis and neonates with signs of sepsis.

Specimens are promptly plated onto Thayer-Martin, Transgrow or Gonogrow media. A nonselective medium should also be used because some strains of *N. gonorrhoeae* do not grow on selective media. Gonogrow is a variation of Transgrow with clindamycin in addition to nystatin, colistin and vancomycin as inhibitors. An improved transport system for *N. gonorrhoeae*, the Jembec plate, is also in use. This transport medium contains a modified Thayer-Martin medium in a plastic Petri dish with a well into which is placed a CO$_2$-generating tablet. The inoculated plate is placed in an air-tight plastic bag for transport. The Jembec system is now the recommended transport system.

Identification

Colonies typical of *N. gonorrhoeae* are gram stained and tested for cytochrome oxidase. Colonies of *Neisseria* give a positive test for cytochrome oxidase and contain gram-negative diplococci. Growth from typical colonies is inoculated onto "chocolate" agar. After growth, organisms from chocolate agar are then inoculated into cystine trypticase agar containing glucose, maltose, sucrose and lactose for final identification. The reactions for *Neisseria* and *Branhamella* are listed in Table 7–1. Further supplementary testing for confirmation can be done by determining growth on nutrient and blood agar and at 22 and 37 C. Fluorescent antibody can also be an aid in identification.

PROBLEM SOLVING AND REVIEW

No. 1. GIVEN: – A 4-year-old child was brought to the emergency room by his parents, who said the child had been irritable for a few days and had cried when he was disturbed. The child had scattered petechiae on the abdomen. The child had a temperature of 39.4 C and exhibited meningismus as measured by the Kernig and Brudzinski tests. Cerebrospinal fluid was collected and the laboratory values for CSF protein were 500 mg/100 ml; for glucose, 1 mg/100 ml. Many polymorphonuclear leukocytes were seen in the cerebrospinal fluid. The physician did a gram stain on the CSF at time of collection and observed gram-negative intracellular and extracellular diplococci. Blood cultures were also sent to the laboratory.

PROBLEMS: – 1. What is your presumptive diagnosis? 2. Will you initiate treatment based on the gram stain? 3. What treatment and why? 4. What is the source of the organism? 5. What caused the rash? 6. What was initial site of infection? 7. Would you expect the blood culture to be positive? Why or why not? (Ans. p. 144.)

No. 2. GIVEN: – A 22-year-old alcoholic woman had been treated for gonococcal endocervicitis on 13 occasions. On the first day of her menstrual cycle she developed polyarthritis and "red spots," followed 3 days later by anorexia, vomiting, epigastric pain, agitation, insomnia and tremors. Over the next few days, she developed petechial lesions on the trunk and extremities, a swollen knee and hepatomegaly. She then became agitated and disoriented. The white blood cell count in cerebrospinal fluid was 3,000/cu mm (87% neutrophils). The protein was 118 mg/100 ml, and glucose was 15 mg/100 ml compared with blood glucose of 117 mg/100 ml.

PROBLEMS: — 1. What is the probable diagnosis and the cause? 2. How would you establish the diagnosis? 3. How would you culture the organism? 4. What is the antibiotic of choice? 5. Would the colony type be type 1 or type 4? 6. How does type 1 differ from type 4? (Ans. p. 144.)

SUPPLEMENTARY READING

Arko, R. J., Ducan, W. P., Brown, W. J., Peacock, W. L., and Tomizawa, T.: Immunity in infection with *Neisseria gonorrhoeae*: Duration and serological response in the chimpanzee, J. Infect. Dis. 133:441–447, 1976.
Carifo, K., and Catlin, B. W.: *Neisseria gonorrhoeae* auxotyping: Differentiation of clinical isolates based on growth responses on chemically defined media, Appl. Microbiol. 26:223–230, 1973.
Crawford, G., Knapp, J. S., Hale, J., and Holmes, K. K.: Asymptomatic gonorrhea in men: Caused by gonococci with unique nutritional requirements, Science 196:1352–1353, 1977.
Eisenstein, B. I., Lee, T. J., and Starling, P. F.: Penicillin sensitivity and serum resistance are independent attributes of strains of *Neisseria gonorrhoeae* causing disseminated gonococcal infections, Infect. Immun. 15: 834–841, 1977.
Eisenstein, B. I., Sox, T., Biswas, G., Blackman, E., and Starling, P. F.: Conjugal transfer of the gonococcal penicillinase plasmid, Science 195: 998–1000, 1977.
Frasch, C. E., and Gotschlich, E. C.: An outer membrane protein of *Neisseria meningitidis* group B responsible for serotype specificity, J. Exp. Med. 140: 87–104, 1974.
Glew, R. H., Moellering, R. C., Jr., and Kunz, L. J.: Infections with *Acinetobacter calcoaceticus (Herellea vaginicola)*: Clinical and laboratory studies, Medicine (Baltimore) 56:79–97, 1977.
Janik, A., Juni, E., and Heym, G. A.: Genetic transformation as a tool for detection of *Neisseria gonorrhoeae*, J. Clin. Microbiol. 4:71–81, 1976.
Johnson, K. H., Holmes, K. K., and Gotschlich, E. C.: The serological classification of *Neisseria gonorrhoeae*. I. Isolation of the outer membrane complex responsible for serotype specificity, J. Exp. Med. 143:741–758, 1976.
Knapp, J. S., and Holmes, K. K.: Disseminated gonococcal infections caused by *Neisseria gonorrhoeae* with unique nutritional requirements, J. Infect. Dis. 132:204–208, 1975.
Lowe, T. L., and Kraus, S. J.: Quantitation of *Neisseria gonorrhoeae* from women with gonorrhea, J. Infect. Dis. 133:621–625, 1976.
Reichert, J. A., and Valle, R. F.: Fitz-Hugh-Curtis syndrome, J.A.M.A. 236: 266–268, 1976.
Richardson, W. P., and Sadoff, J. C.: Production of a capsule by *Neisseria gonorrhoeae*, Infect. Immun. 15:663–664, 1977.
Sotto, M. N., Lander, B., Hoshino-Shimizu, S., and deBrito, T.: Pathogenesis of cutaneous lesions in acute meningococcemia in humans: Light, immunofluorescent, and electron microscopic studies of skin biopsy specimens, J. Infect. Dis. 113:506–514, 1976.

Wong, K. H., Arko, R. J., Logan, L. C., and Bullard, J. C.: Immunological and serological diversity of *Neisseria gonorrhoeae*: Gonococcal serotypes and their relationship with immunotypes, Infect. Immun. 14:1297–1301, 1976.

ANALYSIS

No. 1.

1. *Neisseria meningitidis* meningitis. 2. Yes. 3. Penicillin. Because of high mortality and to minimize brain damage. 4. Carrier. 5. Endotoxin. 6. Upper respiratory tract. 7. Yes. It is the probable route by which organisms enter the CNS.

No. 2.

1. Meningitis, arthritis and septicemia due to *N. gonorrhoeae*. 2. Culture and gram stain of CSF and synovial fluid; culture of blood. 3. Jembec plate; Thayer-Martin medium with 10% CO_2. 4. Penicillin. 5. Type 1. 6. Type 1 has pili which are adherence factors.

8 / Bacillus

OVERVIEW

The genus *Bacillus* contains the gram-positive, aerobic, spore-forming rods (50 species), which are widely distributed in nature. *B. anthracis* causes anthrax in animals and humans. Other species of the genus *Bacillus* are opportunistic, such as *B. subtilis* (eye infections, meningitis, allergic reactions, infections involving prosthetic devices), *B. megaterium* (bacteremia, meningitis), and *B. cereus* (food poisoning); see chap. 2 for a discussion of spores.

SPECIES

B. anthracis is an aerobic, gram-positive, nonmotile, encapsulated spore-forming rod (3–5 μm long) which frequently forms long chains (Fig. 8–1). It is nonhemolytic and grows well on most media forming a large irregular "Medusa's head" colony. Acid is produced from a limited number of sugars. It is highly pathogenic for laboratory animals and susceptible to most antibiotics including penicillin. *B. cereus* is similar morphologically and biochemically to *B. anthracis*.

ECOLOGY

B. anthracis is associated primarily with domestic animals, particularly cattle, horses and sheep. Spores may persist for extended periods of time on hides, hair, or wool, and in bone meal and contaminated soil. The source of infection for animals (domestic or wild) is soil, but transmission can occur by direct contact with carcasses or products from infected animals. *B. cereus* is found in soil and in raw, dried and unprocessed foods.

BACILLUS ANTHRACIS
ANTIGENS AND TOXINS

ANTIGENS.—The anthrax bacillus has at least 23 demonstrable antigens, including those associated with the cell wall, cytoplasm, spore,

145

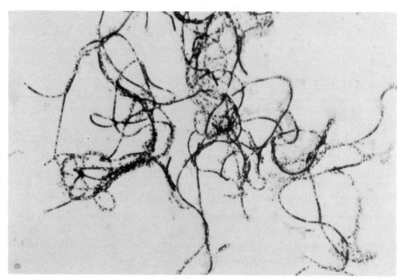

Fig. 8–1.—Gram stain of a 72-hour culture of *Bacillus anthracis*. Note the chains and that most of the cells have formed spores which appear as un-stained elliptical areas within the cell.

capsule and toxin. Only the capsule and toxin are associated with pathogenicity. The capsular polypeptide is composed of D-glutamic acid (unique among the bacteria), and although antigenic, it does not stimulate protective antibodies. It is produced in the animal body or in the presence of serum or blood but usually not on nutrient agar. Noncapsulated (R) mutants are nonvirulent.

TOXIN.—The toxin is a thermolabile protein or lipoprotein made up of at least three components which individually have little toxicity. When combined they are immunogenic, lethal, edema producing and dermonecrotic. These components are termed: (1) edema factor, (2) protective antigen and (3) lethal factor as listed in Table 8–1.

The complete toxin is synthesized by the bacterium. In vivo production of toxin is demonstrable by injecting edema fluid from infected animals into healthy animals and observing for the production of edema or death. In vitro production of the toxin in broth is promoted by the presence of serum and an increased concentration of sodium bicarbonate. The complete toxin is the principal mechanism of pathogenicity for both animals and humans. Animals differ in susceptibility, with the mouse being the most sensitive. Toxin production has not yet been shown to be phage mediated, although a phage has been isolated which will specifically lyse *B. anthracis*.

TABLE 8-1.—COMPONENTS AND ACTION OF
THE ANTHRAX TOXIN

COMPONENT	ACTION°			
	ANTIGENIC†	IMMUNOGENIC‡	EDEMA	LETHAL
Edema factor (EF)	+			
Protective antigen (PA)	+	+		
EF + PA		+	+	
Lethal factor (LF)	+			
LF + PA		+		+
EF + PA + LF	+	+	+	+

°The activities of these components are demonstrable in animals, particularly the mouse, rat and rabbit.
†Each component is antigenically specific and can be identified through the use of diffusion, complement fixation or hemagglutination procedures. The edema and protective antigens have at least two fractions.
‡This indicates protection in experimental animals against the action of the complete toxin.

ANTHRAX

Anthrax is primarily a disease of herbivorous animals—particularly cattle, sheep, horses and goats—but other mammals, birds and reptiles may acquire the disease. It is a problem in zoos and in African wildlife sanctuaries. Infection in animals results from inhalation, ingestion or, more often, direct inoculation of vegetative cells or spores into cuts or injuries. Frequently a fatal bacteremia and toxemia develop.

Human anthrax in this country is not common (222 cases, 1955–73). It is usually associated with agricultural workers (farmers, butchers, veterinarians) or those in certain industrial occupations (workers in woolen or goat hair mills, packing houses, tanneries) who have contact with diseased animals or their products and develop cutaneous, respiratory or alimentary tract infections. Cutaneous anthrax (malignant pustule), is the most common type. It starts with a cut or abrasion, usually on exposed parts of the body, which is contaminated with the organisms. The organisms multiply locally, and in 1–7 days a painless papule develops. It becomes vesicular, ruptures and a central black eschar surrounded by a rim of edema is formed (Figs. 8–2, 8–3). The lesion usually heals spontaneously, but the organisms can spread to the regional lymph nodes to produce a bacteremia and toxemia, which, without treatment, may frequently be fatal. Inhalation anthrax (wool-sorter's disease) results from inhaled, aerosolized spores being carried into the lower bronchi or alveoli where they are phagocytized by the alveolar macrophages. They are then carried via the lymphatics to the regional mediastinal lymph nodes where the spores then germi-

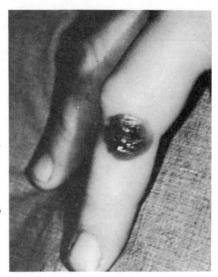

Fig. 8–2.—Early cutaneous anthrax with the typical black eschar. (Courtesy of W. A. Welton, Division of Dermatology, West Virginia University.)

nate. The vegetative cells multiply and cause an acute hemorrhagic mediastinitis. The onset is sudden with fever, dyspnea and chest pain. Death, which may be sudden, is due to respiratory failure because of the toxin, which causes a depression of the respiratory centers of the central nervous system and the development of pulmonary capillary

Fig. 8–3.—Cutaneous anthrax lesion 14 days after onset. Note the black depressed eschar with the ring of edema. Cultures were positive for *Bacillus anthracis*. (Courtesy of P. H. Brachman, Center for Disease Control, Atlanta, Ga.)

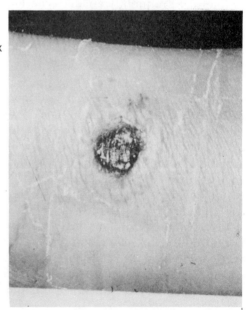

thrombi. A hemorrhagic meningitis may be a complication of either cutaneous or inhalation anthrax. Gastrointestinal anthrax is rare and has been reported in persons eating contaminated meat. After an incubation period of 2–5 days, nausea, vomiting, diarrhea with abdominal distress and even ascites are produced. The disease usually progresses to generalized toxemia, shock and death.

MECHANISMS OF PATHOGENICITY

The antiphagocytic glutamic acid capsule of *B. anthracis* allows for its establishment in the host. As the numbers of organisms increase, the complete toxin is released. The toxin alters capillary permeability and causes edema, hemorrhage and capillary thrombosis. The usual cause of death is respiratory failure due to central nervous system depression by the toxin. The toxin also injures leukocytes. In addition, *B. anthracis* must be able to metabolize and grow in competition with living tissue for the necessary nutrients which, along with the action of the toxin, contributes to tissue necrosis.

IMMUNITY AND VACCINES

Animals recovering from anthrax are immune to reinfection, and second attacks in man are rare. The immunity apparently is antitoxic, as anticapsular antibodies are protective only in certain animals.

The vaccine presently used in animals is a suspension of viable spores derived from the noncapsulated, avirulent Sterne strain of *B. anthracis*; however, it is considered unsafe for humans. The "Wright vaccine," which contains the protective antigen, has been used in field trials and is 92% effective in humans. It can be used in high-risk groups, such as woolsorters or certain laboratory personnel, but requires a yearly booster.

PREVENTION

Anthrax is an occupational disease, although cases of anthrax acquired by contact with finished materials made of animal skin have been reported. Workers at risk should be immunized. Aerosol production should be minimized, and workers involved in operations where aerosols are generated should wear respirators.

An employee education program is necessary to stress cleaning and protecting cuts and abrasions from contamination. Plant cleanliness and personal hygiene are important in preventing and minimizing the disease.

Immunization of animals in endemic areas and proper disposal of infected animals by cremation or deep burial are important to control the disease.

TREATMENT

Penicillin is the drug of choice for treatment; tetracyclines can be used as an alternate. In cutaneous anthrax the response to chemotherapy is excellent. Inhalation anthrax has a mortality of approximately 80% even with massive doses of penicillin or other antibiotics. A complicating factor is that a diagnosis is rarely made prior to the development of bacteremia and toxemia.

LABORATORY PROCEDURES

Materials usually collected include fluid and scrapings from cutaneous lesions (preferably unopened), sputum or aspirates from the lungs, blood and possibly cerebrospinal fluid. Stained smears should be made from all specimens, including blood. Anthrax is one of the few bacterial diseases in which bacteria can be demonstrated directly in the blood. Large rods, single or in short chains, and particularly if capsulated, are tentative evidence of *B. anthracis*. Blood or cerebrospinal fluid is cultured by the methods described in chap. 4. All other materials are streaked onto blood agar and incubated aerobically at 37 C. The colonies are large, irregular, "Medusa's heads," some with comma-shaped outgrowths which are nonhemolytic. Final identification is made by demonstrating a large, capsulated nonmotile rod which ferments a limited number of sugars. The demonstration of pathogenicity for mice or other laboratory animals is a singular characteristic. The fluorescent antibody technique (chap. 4), with conjugated specific antiserum, is used to identify the organism directly in smears from clinical material or from cultures (the organism should be capsulated). The laboratory must have positive identification before reporting an organism as *B. anthracis* because of difficulties in differentiation from *B. cereus* or other bacilli.

BACILLUS CEREUS

B. cereus has been recognized with increasing frequency as a cause of food-borne disease. Two clinical syndromes are recognized, both of which are associated with production of enterotoxins. One form is similar to that caused by the staphylococcal enterotoxin and results in emesis and abdominal cramps. The second form is similar to that caused by the *V. cholerae* and *E. coli* enterotoxin and is character-ized by diarrhea. The incubation period in those persons with diarrhea as the main complaint ranges from 6 to 14 hours and the ill-ness lasts 24–36 hours. The disease characterized by emesis has a shorter incubation period (2 hours) and the symptoms last up to 10 hours. Fever is uncommon. The disease is associated with eating of improperly prepared fried rice. Documentation of the etiologic agent is by isolation of 10^5 or more organisms from incriminated food.

PROBLEM SOLVING AND REVIEW

GIVEN: — A 40-year-old man was admitted to the hospital with chills, fever, severe dyspnea and cyanosis. Rales were audible in both lung fields and his blood pressure was 100/60. He was placed in oxygen and improved slightly. He remained restless and then gasped for breath and died. He worked in the local clothing mill, and during the pre-vious week had been sorting a foreign shipment of goat hair. His face mask had become obstructed so he discarded it rather than cleaning it or obtaining a replacement. Two days prior to admission he had expe-rienced severe shortness of breath with coughing. He thought he was coming down with the "flu." At autopsy, edema of the upper chest and neck, and enlarged, dark red mediastinal lymph nodes were noted. The larynx and trachea were normal. The mediastinum was occupied by a massive bloody edema; the bronchi contained bloody mucus and the lungs were markedly engorged. Gram stains from the mediastinal nodes and pulmonary exudate showed large gram-positive bacilli.

PROBLEMS: — 1. What is the source of the organisms? 2. Trace the development of the infection. 3. What is the role of the toxin in this disease? 4. Would bacteremia be the cause of death? 5. How could this disease be prevented? 6. How would you isolate and identify the organism? (Ans. p. 152.)

SUPPLEMENTARY READING

Brachman, P. S.: Anthrax, Ann. N.Y. Acad. Sci. 174:577–582, 1970.

Christie, A. B.: The clinical aspects of anthrax, Postgrad. Med. J. 49:565–570, 1973.

Lincoln, R. E., and Fish, D. C.: Anthrax Toxin, in Montie, T. C., Kadis, S., and Ajl, S. J. (eds.): *Microbial Toxins*, vol. III: *Bacterial Protein Toxins* (New York: Academic Press, 1970), pp. 361–414.

Nungester, W. J.: Conference on progress in the understanding of anthrax, Fed. Proc. 26:1491–1571, 1967.

Terranova, W., and Blake, P. A.: Bacillus cereus food poisoning, N. Engl. J. Med. 298:143, 1978.

ANALYSIS

1. The goat hair imported from a country where anthrax is endemic. 2. Spores are inhaled during the cleaning and handling of the goat hair; they are phagocytized by alveolar macrophages and carried to mediastinal nodes, where they germinate, produce toxin and invade the bloodstream. 3. The toxin is probably the principal factor in causing edema, altering capillary walls and allowing blood to escape and producing anoxia, all of which cause pulmonary and cardiac embarrassment, resulting in inhalation anthrax. The toxin also causes depression of the CNS respiratory center. 4. Bacteremia may be a contributing factor and result in abscess formation in various organs, but animals can be cleared of bacteremia with antibiotics and still die of toxemia. 5. By improving working conditions and by using safety devices to eliminate inhalation of spores; vaccination is possible. 6. *B. anthracis* forms a large, irregular, nonhemolytic colony on blood agar; large, gram-positive, capsulated, spore-forming rod. It is nonmotile and pathogenic for laboratory animals. Identifiable by the fluorescent antibody technique.

9 / Clostridium and Other Anaerobes

OVERVIEW

By the late 1800s, the anaerobes were recognized as the cause of putrefaction and infections in man associated with tissue necrosis, gas bubbles in tissues and a foul odor. The various wars stimulated interest in gram-positive spore-forming rods *(Clostridium)*, and the diseases—gas gangrene, tetanus and botulism—caused by these organisms were extensively studied. There continued to be references to the fact that anaerobes were involved in peritonitis, deep abscesses or ulcerative oral lesions, but little definitive diagnostic microbiology was done. In the 1960s there was renewed interest in the anaerobes, resulting in the development of an adequate anaerobic technology now available to any clinical laboratory.

As the result of these advances it is now recognized that non-spore-forming anaerobes frequently cause or complicate infections. *Bacteroides* (particularly *B. fragilis*), *Fusobacterium*, *Peptococcus* and *Peptostreptococcus* are most frequently involved, although *Bifidobacterium*, *Eubacterium*, *Lactobacillus* and *Veillonella* may contribute to these infections. Such infections are polymicrobial, i.e., caused by a mixture of different anaerobes with or without facultative anaerobes, such as *Escherichia*, *Klebsiella*, *Proteus*, *Pseudomonas*, *Haemophilus*, *Staphylococcus* or *Streptococcus*. In some pulmonary and brain abscesses *Actinomyces* are encountered, but usually when these organisms are the etiologic agent they cause the identifiable disease of actinomycosis, which involves the cervicofacial, thoracic or abdominal regions of the body (chap. 12).

The symptoms of tetanus and botulism are due to specific exotoxins. The major cause of tissue necrosis in gas gangrene is lecithinase C, but other enzymes may also contribute to the symptoms. The non-spore-forming anaerobes cause infections that may involve almost any tissue or organ and are characterized by tissue necrosis, but specific exotoxins are not produced.

153

ANAEROBIOSIS

Numerous concepts have been advanced to explain "life without air," but the process is still not entirely understood. It was established that molecular oxygen, O_2, is toxic for anaerobes, although they do require and use oxygen atoms obtained through various processes of reduction in their metabolism. Toxicity has been attributed to the absence of catalase, which would expose the bacteria to toxic concentrations of hydrogen peroxide. This is not a major factor as catalase is produced by some anaerobes; also, a number of aerobes do not produce catalase. More recently it has been demonstrated that superoxide (O_2^-), a highly reactive and toxic radical, is produced by a number of biological systems (catalytic activity of cytochromes, ionized radiation of water). Most bacteria, as well as plant and animal cells, contain the enzyme superoxide dismutase, which destroys superoxide; a deficiency in this enzyme may be an important factor in the lethality of oxygen for the anaerobes.

Another important factor which determines growth of anaerobes is the oxidation-reduction potential (O-R) — the capacity of various compounds in the environment to accept or donate electrons. The O-R potential is affected by pH and by oxygen, hydrogen and other oxidizing and reducing chemicals. It is frequently considered as a measure of the amount of available oxygen and is expressed (as E_h) in millivolts over a range of $+400$ to -400. Anaerobic bacteria possess electron carriers and enzymes which function only at a low E_h and, therefore, grow best at potentials of -400 to -150 mv, although some survive at $+150$ mv. Circulating blood has an O-R potential ranging from $+125$ to $+250$ mv, which approximates the range within the various tissues; anaerobes do not grow under these conditions. The intestinal tract, necrotic tissue and abscess cavities have an E_h of -150 to -250 mv, which represents less than 10 ppm of dissolved oxygen and readily supports the growth of anaerobes.

Bacteria may be classified relative to their oxygen requirements as follows: (1) strict or obligate anaerobes which can metabolize, grow and divide through successive transfers in a suitable medium in the absence of molecular oxygen but not in the presence of molecular oxygen; (2) facultative anaerobes which metabolize, grow and divide in the absence or presence of molecular oxygen and (3) strict aerobes which do not grow in the absence of oxygen. It is doubtful that strict aerobes survive in an area of inflammation or necrosis. The majority of the facultative organisms grow best in the presence of oxygen, and most human pathogens are in this group.

TABLE 9–1.—CHARACTERISTICS OF ANAEROBES DIRECTLY OR INDIRECTLY INVOLVED IN HUMAN INFECTIONS

GENERA	STAINING MORPHOLOGY					HABITAT				PATHOGENESIS				COMMENTS
	GRAM	RODS	COCCI	FILAMENTS	SPORES	ORAL CAVITY	INTESTINAL TRACT	GENITOURINARY TRACT	SKIN	% ISOLATED°	PATHOGENIC	NECROSIS†	TOXIGENIC	
Actinomyces	+	+		+		+	+	+		0.1	+	+		Branching filaments, Y, V forms
Bacteroides	−	+				+	+	+		37.0	∓	+		Rounded ends, pleomorphic
Bifidobacterium	+	+				+	+	+		2.0				Y, V, and bifid forms
Clostridium	+	+			+	+	+	+		8.0	+	+	+	Blunt or rounded ends; spores, usually subterminal
Eubacterium	+	+				+	+	+		3.0	∓			Pleomorphic, pairs, chains
Fusobacterium	−	+		+		+	+	+		2.0	+	+		Pointed ends, nonbranching filaments
Lactobacillus	+	+				+	+	+		0.1	∓			Pleomorphic, sometimes chains
Peptococcus	+		+			+	+	+		17.0	+	+		Single, pairs, clumps
Peptostreptococcus	+		+			+	+	+		9.0	+	+		Pairs and chains
Propionibacterium	+	+				+	+	+	+	21.0	∓			Y, V forms
Veillonella	−		+			+	+	+		1.0	∓			Pairs, irregular clumps

°Percentage of isolates from 27,588 clinical specimens (Mayo Clin. Proc. 49:300, 1974).

†Necrosis is used to indicate either cell necrosis or accumulation of pus.

GENERA

The anaerobic organisms associated with disease in man fall into two large groups. One group is the gram-positive spore-forming rods which are in the genus *Clostridium* (Table 9–1). The second group, the non-spore-forming organisms, is a complex group with several genera of widely different characteristics (Table 9–2). One group comprising the gram-negative rods contains the genera *Bacteroides* and *Fusobacterium*. The genera containing gram-positive rods are

TABLE 9–2.–SELECTED CHARACTERISTICS OF REPRESENTATIVE SPECIES OF NON-SPORE-FORMING ANAEROBES*

ORGANISM	MORPHOLOGY AND CULTURE REACTIONS												END PRODUCTS†					
	GRAM	MOTILITY	CATALASE	GLUCOSE	LACTOSE	MANNITOL	SUCROSE	XYLOSE	ESCULIN	NITRATE	INDOLE	10% BILE‡	ACETIC	BUTYRIC	FORMIC	LACTIC	PROPIONIC	SUCCINIC
Bacteroides§																		
fragilis	−	−	−	+	+	±‖	±	+	+	±	±	+	+	−	±	±	+	+
melaninogenicus	−	−	−	+	+	−	+	−	+	−	−	−	+	−	±	−	−	+
Bifidobacterium																		
bifidum	+	−	−	+	+	−	−	±	−	−	−	−	+	−	±	+	−	−
Eubacterium																		
lentum	+	−	−	−	−	−	−	−	−	+	−	+	±	−	±	±	−	±
Fusobacterium																		
mortiferum	−	−	−	+	+	−	−	−	−	−	−	−	+	+	±	±	+	−
necrophorum	−	−	−	±	−	−	−	−	−	−	+	−	+	+	±	±	+	±
nucleatum	−	−	−	±	−	−	−	−	−	−	+	−	+	+	±	±	+	+
Lactobacillus¶																		
catenaforme	+	−	−	+	±	−	+	−	+	−	−	−	±	+	±	+	−	±
Peptococcus																		
asaccharolyticus	+	−	−	−	−	−	−	−	−	+	+	−	+	+	±	±	−	±
Peptostreptococcus																		
anaerobius	+	−	−	+	−	−	−	−	−	−	−	−	+	±	−	−	−	−
Propionibacterium																		
acnes	+	−	+	+	−	±	−	−	−	+	+	−	+	−	±	±	+	±
Veillonella																		
parvula	−	−	−	−	−	−	−	−	−	+	−	−	+	−	−	−	+	−

*In general, the species listed are those most frequently isolated in the clinical laboratory and associated with human infections. However, in each genus 1–15 other species are described in Bergey's *Manual* or in references listed at the end of this chapter.
†The end products from the fermentation of glucose or peptone utilization (if glucose is not fermented) as determined by gas chromatography techniques. The ± indicates that they are minor products which are sometimes produced.
‡+ indicates growth in 10% bile.
§There are 5 subspecies of *B. fragilis* and 3 of *B. melaninogenicus*, each of which differs somewhat in its biochemical reactions.
‖± indicates that approximately 10% of the strains of a species complete that particular reaction.
¶The majority of lactobacilli are facultative and nonpathogenic.

Bifidobacterium, Eubacterium, Lactobacillus and *Propionibacterium* and *Actinomyces*. The *Actinomyces* are discussed in chap. 12. The third group contains the anaerobic cocci. One genus, *Veillonella*, contains the gram-negative cocci. The *Peptococci* are gram-positive cocci and by gram stain resemble staphylococci. The *Peptostrepto-cocci* are also gram-positive cocci and resemble the *Streptococcus* on gram stain.

NON-SPORE-FORMING ANAEROBES

Ecology
The non-spore-forming anaerobes are found in normal flora of the mouth, skin, and intestinal and genitourinary tracts of man and these sites represent the source of infection (Table 9–1).

Although man usually lives in happy symbiosis with these millions of oral and intestinal bacteria, they can be harmful or even life threatening. For example: (1) an injury (perforation, wound, surgery) to the intestinal tract may result in peritonitis, intra-abdominal abscess or bacteremia; (2) dental manipulations in the oral cavity frequently result in bacteremia; (3) structural abnormalities (strictures, fistulas, adhesions) may increase the bacterial population in the ileum, resulting in deconjugation of bile salts, which in turn causes malabsorption of fat and steatorrhea and (4) certain bacteria in the large intestine may convert bile acids, bile steroids or proteins to carcinogens or co-carcinogens, such as deoxycholic acid, polycyclic aromatic hydrocarbons and nitrosamines. Epidemiologic studies indicate that the incidence of colon cancer is higher in Western Europe and North America than in Japan and India, which correlates with the presence of certain intestinal bacteria and a greater intake of fats and animal proteins.

Genera and Species of Non-Spore-Forming Anaerobes
The characteristics of this group are listed in Tables 9–1 and 9–2. Capsules have now been described for *Bacteroides* but not for other genera. All genera are nonmotile. The morphology shows that the organisms are pleomorphic, but these differences are useful in separating the species (Table 9–2). Colonial morphological features are not characteristic. *B. melaninogenicus* is an exception in that most isolates form tan colonies that become black upon further incubation. They vary in their ability to ferment carbohydrates and in the end products produced by fermentation of carbohydrates and peptone utilization, and this is the basis for differentiation. The following brief discussion of these genera can be augmented by the references listed at the end of this chapter.

GRAM-NEGATIVE RODS. — Several species of *Bacteroides* are associated with human infection. The following three species are most frequently isolated. *B. fragilis* (subspecies *distasonis, fragilis, ovatus, thetaiotaomicron* and *vulgatus*) grows in 10% bile and produces β-lactamase, resulting in resistance to penicillin and cephalosporins (other species are usually susceptible). It has limited pathogenicity for animals. *B. melaninogenicus* (subspecies *asaccharolyticus, intermedius* and *melaninogenicus*) produces black colonies on blood agar that fluoresce under UV light. It is proteolytic and requires menadione (vitamin K) or hemin for growth. *B. corrodens* is a slow-growing organism that causes small pits on the surface of agar media. Other species include *B. oralis, B. hypermegas* and *B. putredinis*.

There are 14 recognized species of *Fusobacterium*, but the three most frequently isolated from human infections are as follows. *F. mortiferum* is highly pleomorphic producing many bizarre forms. Colonies are translucent and nonhemolytic with a raised center on blood agar. *F. necrophorum (Sphaerophorus necrophorus)* on gram stain are usually broad with rounded ends. They may be short or long and filamentous and may have bulbous swellings. Small beta-hemolytic colonies are produced on blood agar; it is the only species producing lipase. *F. nucleatum (F. fusiforme)* usually appears on smears as long, thin filaments with pointed ends. White, convex colonies, which may be alpha-hemolytic, are produced on blood agar.

Fusobacteria are demonstrable in direct smears and can be isolated from ulcerative gingivitis, undermining ulcers of the oral cavity and skin, and pulmonary and brain abscesses. Most of these infections are polymicrobial and the etiologic relationship of the fusiforms to such lesions is not well established.

GRAM-POSITIVE RODS. — The *Bifidobacterium* are designated as "bifid or divided ones." The ends of the bacilli and the bifid forms may be swollen, particularly if grown on special media. Colonies are usually circular, convex, white and nonhemolytic. There are 11 established species, but only *B. bifidum* is listed in Table 9–1. Other species include *B. adolescentis, B. infantis, B. breve, B. longum, B. globosum, B. ruminale, B. suis, B. asteroides, B. indicum* and *B. coryneforme.* There is a question as to whether or not these species are pathogenic, but they have been isolated from a variety of human infections.

The *Eubacterium* appear as coccobacilli and contain several species. *E. lentum*, the species most frequently isolated from clinical material, is characterized by forming pinpoint, nonhemolytic colonies on blood agar; it does not ferment carbohydrates. Other species include *E. aerofaciens, E. cylindroides, E. limosum* and *E. rectale.*

There are at least eight species of *Propionibacterium,* but the only one frequently associated with man is *P. acnes (Corynebacterium acnes),* which has a diphtheroid morphology, produces indole, liquefies gelatin and has two serologic types. This organism is a normal inhabitant of the skin and has been isolated from a wide variety of infections as well as blood cultures. It is usually considered a contaminant.

Most species of *Lactobacillus* are facultative. They are widely distributed in nature and economically important in causing milk to sour. *L. catenaforme* is anaerobic and frequently forms chains. It ferments a variety of carbohydrates, grows at 45 C and has been isolated from pulmonary and other types of abscesses.

COCCI. — The *Peptococcus* appear singly or in pairs, in tetrads or in irregular masses but not in packets. They have been isolated from patients with bacteremia, osteomyelitis, septic arthritis and appendicitis, but pathogenicity is not well established. Species include *P. asaccharolyticus* (Table 9 – 2), *P. niger, P. aerogenes* and *P. activus.*

The *Peptostreptococcus* occur in chains. Gas and a foul odor are produced in both cultures and tissue. They have been isolated from patients with septic abortion, abscesses, myositis, endocarditis and bacteremia; infection is often associated with putrid odor and gas. Species include *P. anaerobius* (Table 9 – 2), *P. productus, P. lanceolatus, P. micros* and *P. parvulus.*

The *Veillonella* are gram-negative, small diplococci. Some strains require putrescine or cadaverine for growth. They appear as small, white, soft nonhemolytic colonies on blood agar. *V. parvulus* is catalase negative and usually does not require cadaverine or putrescine. There are three subspecies which differ antigenically. *V. alcalescens* is catalase positive, usually requires cadaverine or putrescine for growth and has three subspecies with different polysaccharide antigens. These organisms have been isolated from the oral cavity, genitourinary tract and intestinal tract of man and animals.

Infections Caused by Non-spore-forming Anaerobes

In considering infections due to the aerobes, one thinks immediately of gas gangrene, tetanus and botulism. Yet it is now evident that anaerobes, other than clostridia, are more frequently involved. Infections caused by non-spore-formers are the most misdiagnosed of all bacterial diseases, and not until the advent of improved cultural techniques was there a realization that these organisms often caused infections of soft tissue, internal organs or any other areas. Any one of the non-spore-forming anaerobes but most frequently *Bacteroides, Fusobacterium* and *Peptostreptococcus* are associated with disease.

SKIN AND SOFT TISSUE INFECTIONS.—These occur following an injury, wound, surgery or bite that has been contaminated with anaerobes, most frequently from the oral cavity or intestinal tract. Such infections tend to burrow through subcutaneous tissue, discharge gas and have a putrid odor. The bacterial flora is usually a facultative-anaerobe mixture.

INFECTIONS OF THE ORAL CAVITY.—Ulcerative lesions, harboring a mixture of facultative and anaerobic organisms that provoke gas formation and a foul odor, may develop following dental manipulation or trauma. Other types of infections, including periapical abscesses, root canal infections and peritonsillar abscesses, are usually caused by anaerobes and frequently result in bacteremia. Although necrotizing ulcerative gingivitis (Vincent's angina) is referred to as a "fuso-spiro-chetal" disease, other oral anaerobes are present so the exact cause remains in doubt. *Bacteroides melaninogenicus* are highly proteolytic and present in large numbers in the oral cavity. These species are probably active in many oral infections.

LUNGS AND PLEURAL CAVITY INFECTIONS.—Anaerobes frequently cause infections of the pleuropulmonary region, including pulmonary abscesses, pneumonitis, necrotizing pneumonia and empyema. These infections are usually subacute or chronic with symptoms of fever, weight loss, cough and a foul-smelling sputum; mortalities approximate 15%. Factors predisposing to such an infection include aspiration, bronchiectasis, periodontal disease, penetrating chest wound, diabetes, and extrapulmonary anaerobic infection or a tumor. The infection may be superimposed on a tumor and be responsible for the initiation of diagnostic work leading to the detection of the malignancy. A single anaerobe may be involved, with *B. fragilis* being the most frequent, although two or more anaerobes or a mixture of anaerobes and facultatives may be present. The associated facultative anaerobes could include *Klebsiella, Pseudomonas, Proteus, Staphylococcus, Streptococcus* or *Haemophilus*. These organisms lower the E_h through oxygen utilization, which aids the growth of anaerobes. Specimen collection is a major problem with these infections as sputum is contaminated with oral anaerobes; thus transtracheal or percutaneous transthoracic aspiration (chap. 4) or thoractomy should be used. The normal tracheobronchial tree is bacteria-free below the larynx, and isolation of any organism from such specimens is significant. Prolonged antibiotic therapy, based on sensitivities of the organisms, in conjunction with adequate surgical drainage, is necessary for patient recovery, which at best is very slow.

INTRA-ABDOMINAL INFECTIONS.—Reports indicate that over half of the liver abscesses are due to anaerobes. *Peptostreptococcus* is most often isolated, but mixed infections with enterics and staphylococci are frequently encountered. Such abscesses may result from appendicitis, intestinal perforation, malignancies, cholecystitis, cholangitis or pyelophlebitis. Liver scans are aids in diagnosis and blood cultures are frequently positive. The role of bacteria in the development of cholecystitis and gallstones is still debated, but gallstones frequently harbor bacteria, including *Bacteroides, Actinomyces* and enterics. Even though appendicitis is a common acute abdominal condition, the microbial cause is not well established. There is frequently a blockage of the appendix lumen with a fecalith, followed by a marked increase in the bacterial flora, particularly the anaerobes. This causes inflammation and necrosis of the appendiceal wall, which may rupture and result in peritonitis and abscess formation. Peritonitis or abscesses may also result from contamination of the abdominal cavity with intestinal contents after traumatic or surgical perforation, diverticulitis or malignancies. Anaerobes are one of the causative agents of anorectal infections, which are often associated with rectal fistulas.

GENITOURINARY TRACT INFECTION.—The most serious genitourinary tract infection is clostridial, causing endometritis and myometritis, leading to perforation, peritonitis and bacteremia. This may follow an attempted abortion with contamination of the fetus, membranes or endometrium with vaginal or fecal flora. Anaerobes may cause infections involving the vulva, Bartholin's gland, Skene's gland, fallopian tubes or ovaries. These infections may develop during pregnancy or after prolonged labor, abortion, malignancy, irradiation or surgery. *B. fragilis* and *B. melaninogenicus* are frequently isolated, but most infections are mixed with facultatively anaerobic organisms without a single identifiable etiologic agent. The genital tract may be the source of these organisms. In one survey 70% of the cervical cultures were positive for anaerobes with the most frequent isolates being *Bacteroides, Peptostreptococcus* and *Clostridium.*

OTHER TYPES OF INFECTIONS.—Bone infections are not common, but purulent arthritis and osteomyelitis can occur. About 4% of the cases of endocarditis are caused by anaerobes, although this percent-

age is higher following dental treatment or oral surgery. Chronic sinusitis, otitis media or mastoiditis may be due to anaerobes which
through contiguous spread can also invade the central nervous system
or brain. In one series of nontraumatic brain abscesses, anaerobes
were isolated from 89% and included (in decreasing incidence) *Peptostreptococcus, Bacteroides, Veillonella, Fusobacterium* and *Actinomyces.*

The bloodstream is a common route of spread of bacteria within the
body, and there is accumulating evidence that bacteria take this route
more frequently than previously considered. In a recent study in
which the blood of patients was sampled immediately after tooth extraction, positive cultures of anaerobes were reported in 23 of 25 patients. *Bacteroides, Fusobacterium* and *Peptostreptococcus* were isolated most frequently. Transient bacteremia with anaerobes following
barium enemas has also been demonstrated. Reports on the use of
anaerobic blood culture techniques indicate that approximately 12%
of bacteremias involve anaerobes. Complications associated with such
bacteremia include (1) septic thrombophlebitis, particularly of the
pulmonary and pelvic veins, and (2) septic shock and disseminated
intravascular coagulation due to the endotoxins of the gram-negative
anaerobes, particularly *Bacteroides.*

Mechanisms of Pathogenicity

The mechanisms of pathogenicity for this group are poorly understood. These organisms are opportunists and infections do not occur
unless appropriate conditions exist in the host. These conditions are
that (1) the organisms must find an environment which is anaerobic
and thus permits growth, and (2) the organisms must escape from their
usual ecological niche (intestinal tract, oral cavity, genital tract) and
locate in the susceptible area. *B. fragilis* contains superoxide dismutase and is more aerotolerant than other anaerobes, which may account for its more frequent role as a human pathogen. *B. fragilis* and
B. melaninogenicus contain an antigenic polysaccharide capsule. The
importance of this capsule is not known, but it may account for these
organisms being the major non-spore-forming organism associated
with disease.

These gram-negative organisms contain endotoxins which correlate
with the production of shock and DIC. Peptidoglycan in the gram-
positive organisms probably plays a similar if not identical role in infections caused by these organisms.

F. necrophorum produces a hemolysin and leukocidin. By infer-
ence, these probably have an effect by damaging leukocytes and pre-

venting phagocytosis. The lysosomal enzymes released may contribute to tissue damage.

A collagenase is produced by *B. melaninogenicus*, but its role in pathogenesis is unknown.

Treatment

The primary treatment for infections due to non-spore-forming anaerobes is drainage of abscesses and debridement of necrotic tissue combined with antibiotic therapy. If the infection is severe or life threatening, antibiotics are administered before receiving laboratory reports, but one should use the direct gram stain as a guide to therapy. Penicillin G is the choice for gram-positive anaerobes, and either clindamycin or chloramphenicol for gram-negatives. Metronidazole is also effective in treating anaerobic infections. Combinations of antibiotics are used for mixed infections. The regimen is then altered, depending on laboratory reports and the clinical response of the patient. Antitoxin, toxoid and hyperbaric oxygen are of no value in treating these infections.

SPORE-FORMING ANAEROBES

Genera and Species of Clostridium

The clostridia are gram-positive, anaerobic, endospore-forming rods. The spores are larger than the cell and may be central, subterminal or terminal in location; most are subterminal. All human pathogens except *C. perfringens* are motile. Some species form capsules and all are catalase negative, although there are exceptions among the nonpathogens. The majority of species ferment a variety of carbohydrates and are frequently proteolytic. Clostridia grow well on blood agar; most species are hemolytic.

All the pathogenic species produce enzymes or toxins, some of which are responsible for the pathogenicity of the organism. It is common to refer to these as "exotoxins," even though many of the enzymes are not demonstrably related to pathogenicity. The extracellular toxins diffuse through the cell wall of young cells, but the protoplasmic toxins are released only by older (3–5 day), altered or lysed cells. Although most of the toxins are fully active when released, some have to be activated by a proteolytic enzyme such as trypsin and are referred to as prototoxins. These differentiations become important in the laboratory because in attempts to prove that an isolate produces toxins, one must test young and old cultures with and without adding dilute trypsin.

Ecology

The principal habitat of all species of *Clostridium* is the soil. The populations are greater in cultivated soils (1,000–50,000 *C. perfringens* per gram of soil). They are present in all types, including desert sands and marine sediments. The clostridia can persist for years as spores in these environments, and when growth conditions are favorable the spores germinate. The vegetative cells carry out processes of decay, making basic elements as carbon and nitrogen available to plants and indirectly to animals. Soil serves as a major source of the clostridia in the contamination of wounds, cuts, abrasions and food. The clostridia and a wide variety of other anaerobes are present in the oral cavity, female genital tract and intestinal tract of humans (chap. 3). They are also widely distributed in animals.

Species of Clostridium Causing Gas Gangrene

There are five species of *Clostridium* which either singly or as mixtures may cause gas gangrene in humans. Listed in the order of frequency of involvement, these are *C. perfringens, C. novyi, C. septicum, C. sordellii* and *C. histolyticum*. One species, *C. perfringens*, is discussed in some detail with information on the others included primarily in chart form (Tables 9–3, 9–4, 9–5, 9–6).

C. perfringens, also referred to as *C. welchii*, is a large (0.8–1.5 μm wide and 2–4 μm long) encapsulated rod (Fig. 9–1). The capsule is antiphagocytic but apparently plays little or no part in pathogenicity. This is the only nonmotile *Clostridium* pathogenic for man. The endospores are subterminal but are not easily demonstrable in laboratory cultures. This species is more aerotolerant than the other pathogens and grows at +230 mv at pH 6 but not on successive transfers. On

TABLE 9–3.—CHARACTERISTICS OF THE *CLOSTRIDIUM* OF GAS GANGRENE

SPECIES	HEMOLYSIN	LECITHINASE	LIPASE	GLUCOSE	LACTOSE	MALTOSE	SUCROSE	INDOLE	MOTILITY	CAPSULE	% ISOLATION FROM GAS GANGRENE°
C. perfringens	+	+	−	A	A	A	A	−	−	+	39–83
C. novyi	+	+	+	A	−	A	−	−	+	−	32–48
C. septicum	+	−	−	A	A	A	−	−	+	−	0–24
C. sordellii	+	+	−	A	−	A	−	+	+	−	4–55
C. histolyticum	+	−	−	−	−	−	−	−	+	−	0–6

°Compiled from reports of 298 cases during World War II. In the majority of the cases more than one species was isolated.

TABLE 9-4.—DEMONSTRABLE ACTIVITY OF THE "TOXINS" OF
CLOSTRIDIUM PERFRINGENS ENZYMATIC OR
BIOLOGICAL ACTIVITY

NAME OF TOXIN	LECITHINASE C	NECROTIZING	NEUROTOXIC	HEMOLYTIC	INTESTINAL PERMEABILITY	CAPILLARY PERMEABILITY	COLLAGENASE	HYALURONIDASE	DEOXYRIBONUCLEASE	PRODUCED BY TYPES	COMMENTS
Alpha	+	+		+		+				A,B,C,D,E	Principal toxin of type A
Beta		+	±							B,C	Causes intestinal necrosis
Gamma°										B,C	Little is known of action
Delta				+	+					B,C	Inflammation of intestines
Epsilon		+			+					B,D	Intestinal permeability
Eta°										A	Little is known of action
Theta		+		+						A,B,C,D,E	Blood cell hemolysis, necrosis
Iota		+				+				E	Capillary permeability, necrosis
Kappa							+			A,B,C,D,E	Collagenase
Lambda°										B,D,E	Proteolytic
Mu								+		A,B,C,D,E	Hyaluronidase
Nu									+	A,B,C,D,E	Deoxyribonuclease

°There is insufficient information about the activities of these toxins.

TABLE 9-5.—TOXINS OF THE CLOSTRIDIUM
CAUSING GAS GANGRENE°

NAME OF TOXIN	C. perfringens TYPE A	C. novyi	C. septicum	C. sordellii	C. histolyticum
Alpha	+	+	+	+	+
Beta		+	+	+	+
Gamma		+	+		+
Delta		+	+	+	+
Epsilon		+			+

°These toxins have been demonstrated for each species, although their role in pathogenicity is not always clear. The alpha toxin of each species has been shown to be lethal and causes necrosis in animals.

TABLE 9-6.—BIOLOGIC ACTIVITIES OF
THE *CLOSTRIDIUM* TOXINS°

SPECIES	ALPHA				BETA					GAMMA					DELTA†		EPSILON	
	LECITHINASE	NECROTIZING	HEMOLYSIN	LEUKOCIDIN	LECITHINASE	NECROTIZING	HEMOLYSIN	DEOXYRIBONUCLEASE	COLLAGENASE	LECITHINASE	NECROTIZING	HEMOLYSIN	HYALURONIDASE	PROTEASE	HEMOLYSIN	ELASTIN	LIPASE	HEMOLYSIN
C. perfringens, A	+	+	+															
C. novyi					+	+	+			+	+	+			+		+	
C. septicum	+	+	+						+			+			+			
C. sordellii‡					+		+								+			
C. histolyticum	+								+					+		+		+

°Taken primarily from Smith, L. D., and Holdeman, L. V.: *The Pathogenic Anaerobic Bacteria* (Springfield, Ill.: Charles C Thomas, Publisher, 1968).

†These hemolysins are oxygen labile and there is a close serologic relationship between these as well as to the theta hemolysin of *C. perfringens*, the hemolysin of *C. tetani* and streptolysin O of *S. pyogenes*.

‡*C. sordellii, C. novyi* and *C. septicum* produce a lethal alpha toxin, but other activities have not been demonstrated.

blood agar, the low convex colonies in 24 hours are 1-3 mm in diameter with a small zone of hemolysis. Mucoid and dwarf colonies have been described, and when grown in the presence of penicillin, L-forms are produced which remain quite stable on subculture.

The other four species of *Clostridium* that cause gas gangrene are morphologically similar, except that they are motile and do not produce capsules. Certain differential cultural reactions are listed in Table 9-3. *C. novyi*, which is difficult to isolate, forms a large hemolytic colony, and is divided into types A, B, C and D on the basis of toxins synthesized. It produces severe infections with excessive amounts of edematous fluid. *C. septicum* is actively motile and swarms over the surface of solid media as well as over the surface of organs. *C. sordellii* (*C. bifermentans*) forms a large number of spores in culture and produces a marked edema in human infections. *C. histolyticum*, which ferments no sugars, forms small colonies with a narrow zone of hemolysis. It is the most proteolytic of the clostridia, and perhaps of any bacterium, and produces an extensive degree of muscle necrosis in human infections although it is seldom involved.

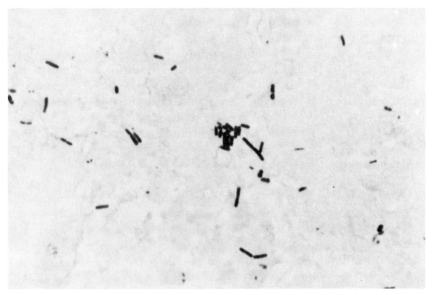

Fig. 9–1.—A gram stain of a direct smear from a patient with gas gangrene of the leg. Note the large gram-positive rods and the absence of leukocytes. *Clostridium perfringens* was isolated.

Enzymes, Hemolysins and Toxins

C. perfringens is divided into types A, B, C, D and E on the basis of toxin production, with type A the principal human pathogen, although types C and D have been implicated as a cause of enterotoxemia of man in Europe and New Guinea. Collectively, these five types produce 12 identifiable "toxins," although none produces all of them. They are designated by Greek letters as indicated in Table 9–4. Type A synthesizes alpha, eta, theta, kappa, mu and nu toxins, with alpha principally involved in human or experimental infections as demonstrated by the fact that experimental infections can be successfully treated with anti-alpha antiserum. Little is known about eta, but the others may play a supportive role in pathogenicity.

Lecithinase C (alpha toxin; phosphatidylcholine cholinephosphorylhydrolase) is an acidic protein which hydrolyzes both lecithin and sphingomyelin. There are two components, A and B, which have similar activities with molecular weights of 54,000–60,000. Zinc seems to be necessary for activation of the enzyme. As phospholipids are common constituents of cell membranes, lecithinase C can alter the membrane structure, resulting in permeability changes, along with cell lysis and extensive necrosis. This is the probable mechanism for red cell lysis (hot-cold) as observed around colonies of the organism and for in vivo hemolysis.

Another hemolysin (theta toxin) produces a clear zone of hemolysis on a blood plate. Its action is inhibited by cholesterol, and it is related to the oxygen-labile hemolysins of S. *pyogenes* and other organisms, but its role in pathogenicity has not been established. Collagenase (kappa toxin) causes a breakdown in collagen fibers, resulting in the loss of texture in muscle and connective tissue, and plays a role in pathogenicity.

Hyaluronidase (mu toxin) depolymerizes the hyaluronic acid and may facilitate spread of the organisms or their metabolic products through the tissue. Deoxyribonuclease (nu toxin) hydrolyzes DNA and may cause death of tissue cells and macrophages. *C. perfringens* also produces a neuraminidase which hydrolyzes gangliosides and a mucinase which depolymerizes glandular mucin. Recently it has been recognized that an enterotoxin is produced which can cause food poisoning (see *C. perfringens*, Type A, Food Poisoning in the next section).

C. novyi, C. septicum, C. sordellii and *C. histolyticum* also produce extracellular enzymes or toxins which, individually or collectively, are responsible for their pathogenicity. These toxins are designated by Greek names (Table 9–5), but confusion is compounded by the fact that the same name is applied to cell products that have different biologic activities. For instance, the term beta toxin may indicate lecithinase, DNase or collagenase (Table 9–6). With all the species, the alpha toxin has been shown to be lethal to animals. Presumably this is the principal toxic product responsible for human infections, but this has not been clearly demonstrated with species other than *C. perfringens* type A.

Infections

INFECTIONS OF THE GAS GANGRENE TYPE. — These are divided into three categories: simple contamination, cellulitis and gas gangrene.

Simple contamination. — This is a mixed infection involving toxigenic clostridia along with nontoxigenic or saprophytic clostridia and other organisms such as anaerobic streptococci. Characteristically, there is a brownish seropurulent discharge with an odor of putrefaction. This type of infection usually remains uncomplicated and heals, but sometimes a progressive pyogenic infection develops or there is an extension by the toxigenic clostridia.

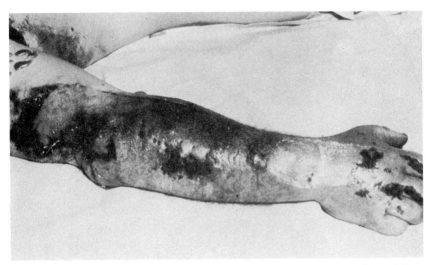

Fig. 9–2. — Anaerobic cellulitis following an injury to the elbow. *Clostridium perfringens* was isolated. (From Willis, A. T.: Some Infections due to Anaerobic Sporeforming Bacilli, in Balows, A. (ed.): *Anaerobic Bacteria: Role in Disease* [Springfield, Il.: Charles C Thomas, Publisher, 1974]. By permission of author and publisher.)

Anaerobic cellulitis. — This may result from an extension of a simple contamination or it may be an initial infection caused by the clostridia. The incubation period is 3 – 4 days. The organisms multiply in the connective tissue spaces, producing gas which opens the spaces permitting extension of the bacteria with the development of a brownish discharge and a foul odor. The gas extends between the muscle groups, but not into the muscle, and may bubble out of the wound. This infection may remain localized or become quite extensive. There is usually little constitutional involvement or pain (Fig. 9 – 2).

Gas gangrene (malignant edema, clostridial or anaerobic myositis, clostridial or anaerobic myonecrosis). — The incubation period may be as short as 4 – 6 hours or as long as 6 weeks. The onset is acute with an early sense of increasing weight of the involved area, followed by pain in the region of the wound. The patient appears critically ill, pale, sweaty and may be delirious, maniacal or very apathetic. Shock may develop at any time. Initially, there is little change at the injury site other than tenderness and edema with serosanguineous discharge but usually without gas or foul odor. Gas does develop with bubbles between the muscle fibers, and palpitation reveals crepitation. Untreated, there is rapid development of toxemia, hemolytic anemia, and

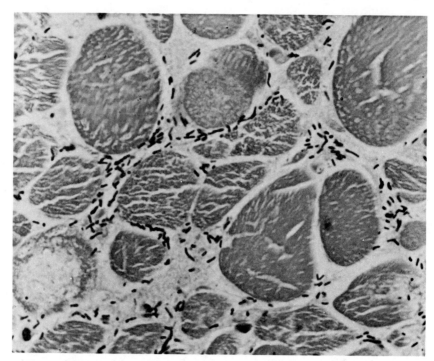

Fig. 9–3.—Experimental gas gangrene in a sheep due to *Clostridium novyi*. Note the organisms have penetrated the muscle fibers and there are indications of myonecrosis. Gram stain of section of muscles. (From Boyd, N. A., Walker, P. D. and Thomson, R. D.: J. Med. Microbiol. 5:459–465, 1972. By permission of authors and journal.)

renal shutdown due to tubular necrosis, and death follows (Fig. 9–3).

Such clostridial infections are not limited to the skin or muscle but may involve the lungs, pleural cavity, eye, brain, liver or uterus. Anaerobic puerperal sepsis may occur secondarily to instrumentation of the genital tract, as in an attempted abortion. This is an anaerobic myositis of the uterus with a sudden onset and rapid progression, which, even with ideal treatment, has a high mortality.

C. perfringens, Type A, Food Poisoning. Enteritis caused by *C. perfringens* is now recognized as one of the major causes of food poisoning in this country. This gastroenteritis has an average incubation period of 12 hours followed by symptoms of abdominal cramps and diarrhea. Nausea, vomiting, headache, chills and fever are not common. The disease is usually self-limited. It is usually over in 24 hours and mortalities are rare. In this country most outbreaks have been associated with restaurant, dormitory or bulk food preparation and not with home cooking. Invariably the food has been cooked, poorly refrigerated and then inadequately reheated or served cold.

Mechanisms of Pathogenicity

Gas Gangrene

The clostridia do not grow in living tissue with an O-R potential of +150 to +250 mv. However, in cellulitis and gas gangrene the O-R is initially lowered to +70 to −150 mv by: (1) a decreased blood supply; (2) release of sulfhydryl groups or oxidases by traumatic injury (wound, foreign body, tourniquet) or (3) diseases with injury to the vascular system, as in diabetes or arteriosclerosis. This decrease in O-R potential, along with the amino acids, carbohydrates, salts and vitamins released from the injured tissue, supports the metabolism and growth of these bacteria. After or in conjunction with the injury, the site must be contaminated with clostridial vegetative cells or spores from the soil, dust (including hospital dust), air, skin, feces or clothing. In this suitable environment they begin to multiply and synthesize their various enzymes and toxins. These products spread into adjacent tissue and lymph spaces, killing cells and extending the nutritious anaerobic environment. This process can spread rapidly, involving an entire thigh in a few hours. The patient may develop bacteremia and toxemia which may lead to hemolytic anemia, circulatory failure, renal shutdown and death.

The toxin of major importance in clostridial infection is the alpha toxin. This toxin causes lysis of membranes and thereby causes cellular destruction with release of lysosomal enzymes. The action of lecithinase C and released lysosomal enzymes results in necrosis as well as red cell lysis, destruction of platelets and damage to the capillary endothelium. Lecithinase C is probably responsible for the marked hemolysis which is observed in some patients. The production of hyaluronidase also facilitates spread of the organism within the organ and may, via depolymerization of hyaluronic acid, provide the organisms with a source of fermentable carbohydrate.

The physiologic activities of the organism result in fermentation of carbohydrates with production of gas, which disrupts tissue and compresses blood vessels so as to extend the anaerobic environment. Collagenase production then contributes to further spread of the organism and destruction of tissue.

Although the action of the toxins is stressed in these infections, it can be shown that if washed cells are injected intraperitoneally into a guinea pig, the animal dies in 5–12 hours with symptoms of profound shock due to hypovolemia. Toxins are not formed, nor is death prevented by antitoxin. Bacteria growing in the peritoneal cavity release an oxidase that reduces the oxygen as fast as it diffuses in from the blood, and thus depletes the supply necessary for tissue respiration of the animal.

Food Poisoning

The sequence of events is that foods become contaminated with clostridia from the soil, preparation environment, or personnel. The initial cooking kills the vegetative cells but heat-shocks the spores to initiate germination. As the vegetative cells form spores, toxin (may be a spore-coat protein) is synthesized and then released as the cells undergo autolysis to free the mature spores. This enterotoxin is an antigenic, heat-labile protein which then acts on the intestinal mucosa. The mechanism of action is not known, but from studies using the ligated ileal loop in rabbits, it can be shown that after a small quantity is introduced, fluid starts to accumulate in 30 minutes, reaching a maximum in 7 hours. It does not activate adenyl cyclase. In addition, there is evidence of vasodilation, increased capillary permeability and increased intestinal motility but without necrosis so the intestinal mucosa recovers rapidly. These all relate to symptoms in humans. The toxin is detectable by electroimmunodiffusion techniques in culture supernates of food in concentrations as low as 1.0 μg/ml. The enterotoxin is identified by: (1) producing erythema but not necrosis in the skin of a rabbit; (2) inducing fluid accumulation when injected into the ileal loop of a rabbit; (3) being lethal for mice and (4) being cytotoxic for tissue culture cells.

Prevention and Treatment

Prevention of myonecrosis requires early and adequate debridement of wounds to remove foreign bodies which result in inflammation, tissue damage and an anaerobic environment suitable for anaerobic growth. Penicillin may be of help in preventing infection.

Treatment requires an aggressive approach: all necrotic tissue must be debrided, even if this means amputation of the limb. Penicillin must also be given. Antitoxin is available but is of questionable value and is not frequently used. Hyperbaric oxygen (100% oxygen at 3 atm pressure) therapy is sometimes used in conjunction with debridement and antibiotic therapy. Five to seven exposures of hyperbaric oxygen are used to raise the O-R potential, thus inhibiting growth and toxin production.

Food poisoning is a self-limiting disease that requires only supportive treatment to replace lost fluids and salts.

Clostridium Tetani

C. tetani is a slender rod, 3–6 μm in length, with a terminal spore that causes the end of the cell to bulge and is thus described as a "drumstick" shape (Fig. 9–4); a capsule is not produced. The organism produces a convex, gray irregular colony with a narrow zone of hemolysis. Some strains swarm over the surface of the agar and this property may aid isolation from a clinical specimen (Fig. 9–5). Carbohydrates are not fermented. Gelatin and coagulated serum are slowly liquefied. Lecithinase and lipase are not produced. *C. tetani* has somatic, flagellar and spore antigens. The flagellar antigens are used to designate serotypes 1–9 with the first five being more frequently isolated from wounds or soil. The antigenicity of the neurotoxin does not vary with the serologic type. The fluorescent antibody technique, which depends on somatic antigens, can be used to specifically identify *C. tetani* in culture or clinical material.

Tetanus toxin (tetanospasmin). *C. tetani* synthesizes this proto-

Fig. 9–4.—Terminal spores of *Clostridium tetani*. Note the bulging of the end of the cell causing the "drumstick" shape. Phase contrast of a 72-hour culture. (From Hoeniger, J. F. M., and Taushel, H. D.: J. Med. Microbiol. 7:425–432, 1974. By permission of author and journal.)

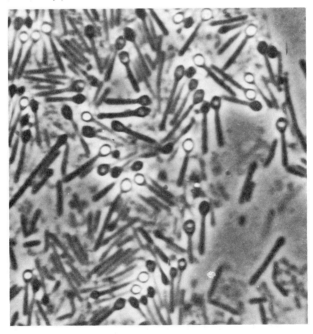

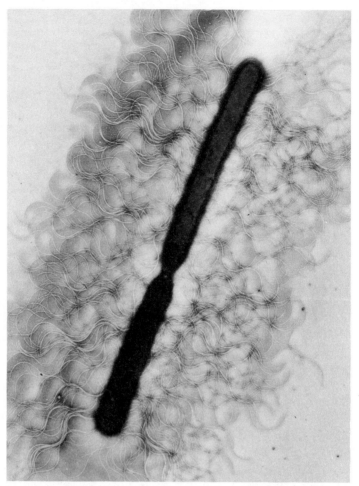

Fig. 9–5. — Peritrichous flagella of *Clostridium tetani*. Prepared from the edge of a 12-hour swarming surface colony. Electron micrograph, negatively stained. (From Hoeniger, J. F. M., and Taushel, H. D.: J. Med. Microbiol. 7:425–432, 1974. By permission of authors and journal.)

plasmic neurotoxin which is released as the cell undergoes lysis. The toxin is a protein with the major amino acids being aspartic acid, glutamic acid, isoleucine, leucine, lysine and tyrosine. Nothing about the composition of the amino acid explains its affinity for nerve tissue or toxicity, although histidine, tyrosine and tryptophan seem to be associated with toxicity. There is still disagreement as to the molecular weight of the toxin, but indications are that the native toxin is a dimer with a MW of 146,000. The dimer contains two monomers, composed of two subunits, one with a MW of 21,000, and the other with a MW of 52,000, linked together with an $-S-S-$ bridge.

To obtain toxin for laboratory or commercial use, one grows *C. tetani* anaerobically in an infusion broth (Mueller-Miller medium) for 72 hours and then extracts the toxin from the collected cells with hypertonic saline. The toxin is purified by a series of precipitation and concentration procedures. Toxins with a potency of 200 million mice minimum lethal doses per milligram nitrogen have been produced.

Tetanus

The incubation period (time from infection to onset of trismus) varies from 3 to 21 days, and delays of several months have been recorded. The longer incubation times might be due to: (1) spores being harbored at the injury site for prolonged periods before germination; (2) slow growth of the organism or (3) delay in lysis of the cells and release of toxin.

Tetanus is a highly variable disease but it can be divided into three forms: local, cephalic and generalized (includes tetanus neonatorum).

LOCAL TETANUS.—In local tetanus there is persistent rigidity of the mucles near the infection. The toxin is fixed in the area of the spinal cord innervating the involved muscle. The rigidity may persist for weeks but usually abates without residual paralysis. In some instances it may progress to generalized tetanus.

CEPHALIC TETANUS.—This is usually associated with an injury to the face or head in which there is dysfunction of cranial nerves, most frequently the seventh. There is a short incubation period before the onset of trismus; the prognosis is grave and mortalities are high.

GENERALIZED TETANUS.—Generalized tetanus implies a toxemia with the toxin ascending to the spinal cord via a number of neural pathways. The initial symptom is usually trismus, often combined with dysphagia along with pain and stiffness of the neck, back and abdomen. Generalized spasms start with a sudden jerk, and every muscle is thrown into an intense tonic contraction that may last from a few seconds to several minutes. If these start within a few hours after trismus the case is severe and the prognosis is poor (time between trismus and first major spasm is called the onset period). The spasms may cause opisthotonos, a fixed facial expression called the sardonic smile (risus sardonicus), and interference with respiration (Figs. 9–6, 9–7). In severe cases there is often increased blood pressure and tachycardia, indicating a sympathetic nerve dysfunction. Death

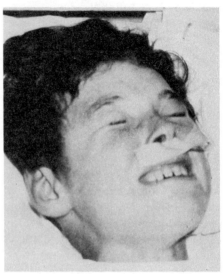

Fig. 9–6. – Risus sardonicus in a young boy with clinical tetanus. The eyebrows and corners of the mouth are drawn up to this fixed smile. (From Willis, A. T.: Some Infections due to Anaerobic Sporeforming Bacilli, in Balows, A. (ed.): *Anaerobic Bacteria: Role in Disease* [Springfield, Ill.: Charles C Thomas, Publisher, 1974]. By permission of author and publisher.)

Fig. 9–7. – Opisthotonos in child with clinical tetanus. Arching of the back is due to rigidity of the muscles of the back. (From Willis, A. T.: Some Infections due to Anaerobic Sporeforming Bacilli, in Balows, A. (ed.): *Anaerobic Bacteria: Role in Disease* [Springfield, Ill.: Charles C Thomas, Publisher, 1974]. By permission of author and publisher.)

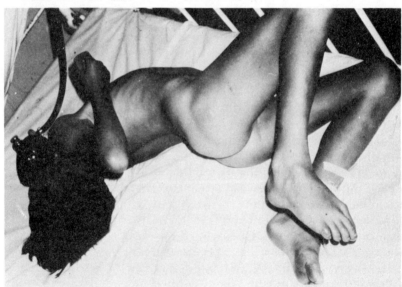

may be due to respiratory failure, cardiac failure or pulmonary complications such as aspiration pneumonia or pulmonary embolism.

TETANUS NEONATORUM. — Tetanus of the newborn results from contamination of the umbilicus at birth. In countries or areas where medical facilities are not available, the umbilical cord may be cut with a rock or piece of glass and daubed with mud or cow dung to stop bleeding. Contamination with tetanus bacilli may result in severe generalized tetanus with violent convulsions, respiratory paralysis and a high mortality. The principal means of prevention is by active immunization of the mother.

Before 1960, about 500 cases of tetanus were reported each year; since then reported cases have declined to about 120 per year. However, the reported mortality still approximates 50%. Most of these cases occur in persons who have not been vaccinated.

Mechanisms of Pathogenesis

C. tetani is introduced (usually as spores, sometimes as vegetative cells) into human tissue from soil, feces or clothing, during or following a cut, abrasion, burn, compound fracture, gunshot wound, criminal abortion, severed umbilical cord or puncture from the drug-addict's needle. In many instances the injuries are minor and may completely heal prior to the onset of symptoms. The local O-R potential is lowered by released tissue enzymes, ischemia or other contaminating bacteria permitting the spores to germinate. The resulting vegetative cells or those already present begin to synthesize the protoplasmic neurotoxin, which is released upon autolysis of the cells. The toxin from the local site, bloodstream, or both penetrates the peripheral nerve endings and ascends from the site to the CNS via retrograde intraaxonal transport. In the cat the rate of travel is 0.5–1.0 mm/hour. In the CNS it is fixed to gangliosides and acts on the presynaptic apparatus, disturbing the release of inhibitory transmitters in both the spinal and peripheral synapses. This results in hyperactivity of motor neurons, causing local or generalized spastic paralysis. The route by which the toxin reaches the central nervous system has been controversial. Recently, direct evidence for retrograde intraaxonal transport of the toxin from the inoculation site to the CNS has been obtained (Fig. 9–8).

The receptors for the tetanus toxin within the spinal cord and brain tissue are gangliosides which contain two sialosyl residues attached to a lactosyl moiety with a terminal galactose residue. The bond between the two sialic acids is sialidase (neuraminidase) sensitive. Within the spinal cord the tetanus toxin is fixed to the gray matter

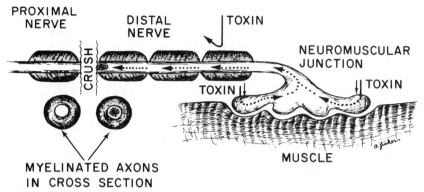

PROXIMAL NERVE   DISTAL NERVE   TOXIN   NEUROMUSCULAR JUNCTION   TOXIN   CRUSH   TOXIN   MUSCLE

MYELINATED AXONS IN CROSS SECTION

Fig. 9–8.—Schematic drawing of experimental model with interpretation of results. ^{125}I-Tetanospasmin, injected into the muscle of a mouse *(solid arrow),* is presumably taken up at nerve terminals rather than along axon and carried by retrograde axonal transport *(dotted arrows)* to the crush where it accumulates in distal segment. Grains are depicted as dots in distal segment of crushed axon; radioactivity was not demonstrated in nerve segments proximal to the crush. (From Price, D. L.: Science, 188:945–947, 1975. By permission of author and journal.)

which has the greatest concentration of gangliosides (Wassermann-Takaki phenomenon). After the toxin is fixed to the gangliosides, it acts on the presynaptic apparatus, disturbing the release of inhibitory transmitters in both spinal and peripheral synapses. The exact mechanism of inhibition is not yet known, but it probably acts on the presynaptic membrane. The toxin produces no observable pathologic changes, and electron microscopy studies show only the presence of synaptic vesicles in the presynaptic apparatus. The inhibitory transmitters interfered with include both γ-aminobutyric acid (present particularly in gray matter) and acetylcholine from cholinergic nerve terminals. Interference with these inhibitors results in hyperactivity of motor neurons, causing skeletal muscle spasms, which lead to spastic paralysis. Paralysis of the respiratory muscle is a frequent cause of death.

If an animal is injected intravenously with tetanus toxin, and then if tetanus antitoxin is injected intramuscularly within 10 hours, the toxin rapidly disappears and is not detectable in either the blood or cerebrospinal fluid. This indicates that the antitoxin binds directly to the toxin in the bloodstream and prompts its removal, probably by phagocytosis. If the antitoxin injection is delayed for 48 hours, the toxin is not neutralized and it is demonstrable in the spinal cord. Once the toxin is bound to the gangliosides it is not neutralized by the antitoxin. One reason is that the antitoxin does not pass the blood-brain barrier. Secondly, there is evidence that the toxin binding sites are masked as a result of binding.

TETANUS TOXOID.—The details of preparation vary, but in general, tetanus toxin is mixed with formalin to inactivate the toxin. The formalinized product is used either (1) without further treatment or (2) precipitated or absorbed with alum, aluminum phosphate or aluminum hydroxide. This latter product is labeled "adsorbed tetanus toxoid" and is considered to be a more effective immunizing agent.

TETANUS ANTITOXIN.—Immune globulin is obtained from sera of horses immunized with tetanus toxoid. Human γ-globulin is also available. Plasma is collected from random individuals, or selected persons are given booster injections of toxoid, bled and their plasma collected. The immune globulins are precipitated, purified, standardized and distributed as human hyperimmune globulin or "tetanus immune globulin." The principal advantages in the use of human globulin are that: (1) it eliminates the problems of serum sickness and hypersensitivity reactions and (2) a single intramuscular dose containing 3,000–6,000 units can be given and usually does not have to be repeated as the half-life of this antitoxin is about 25 days.

PREVENTION.—Immunization should begin at 2 months of age with three intramuscular injections 4 weeks apart and a final injection at 1 year. Adults are given two intramuscular injections 1 month apart and a final in 1 year. Both should then receive boosters every 10 years. Indications are that 0.01 unit of antitoxin per milliliter of serum provides immunity to clinical tetanus. Such a concentration is frequently detectable within 1 month after the initiation of immunization and persists for 10 years or more. Of equal importance is that if a 0.5-ml booster is given every 10 years after the initial series, there is a rapid rise in the antitoxin level beginning in 2–5 days and continuing for approximately 3 weeks. Thus, tetanus toxoid is a most effective immunizing agent, although excessive immunization can lead to a hypersensitivity to the toxoid. Recovery from the natural disease does not provide immunity, probably because the antigenic sites on the fixed toxin are not available to the antibody-synthesizing lymphocytes.

TREATMENT.—Depending on the site, extent of the injury and severity of the tetanus, treatment may include any combination of the following: debridement, antibiotic therapy, administration of toxoid or antitoxin, tracheostomy, intermittent positive pressure respiration or use of muscle relaxants (diazepam or curare) coupled with good nursing care.

Debridement removes injured or dead tissue and restores circulation; this prevents anaerobiosis and curtails growth of C. *tetani*. Antibiotics (penicillin is first choice) are given to both inhibit growth and kill vegetative cells so as to prevent synthesis of the toxin. Toxoid is injected intramuscularly if there is no history of immunization during the previous year (or during the preceding 10 years according to some experts). Antitoxin is given to increase the concentration of circulating antitoxin. If equine antitoxin is used, the first step is to perform a skin test on the individual with horse serum to be certain he is not sensitive to horse proteins, thereby eliminating the possibility of anaphylaxis. However, this does not alter the hazards of serum sickness or crippling neurologic complications. These life-threatening side effects are eliminated by the use of human hyperimmune antitoxin. If used, antitoxin should be administered as soon as possible as effectiveness depends primarily on neutralizing circulating toxin. Animal experiments demonstrate complete protection within 10 hours decreasing to no protection in 48 hours. Dosage schedules vary but some authors recommend a single dose of 3,000–6,000 units intramuscularly of human globulin. With equine antitoxin, 25,000 units is given intramuscularly, and if tolerated then additional doses are given as necessary.

Clostridium Botulinum

C. *botulinum* is a large (up to 1.2 μm wide and 6 μm long) grampositive motile rod (Fig. 9–9) which produces subterminal spores but no capsule. It forms circular, convex hemolytic colonies 4–8 mm in diameter on blood agar. Glucose and maltose are fermented but not mannitol or lactose. Gelatin is liquefied but its action on other protein substrates is variable. Catalase and lecithinase are not produced but lipase is produced. On the basis of neurotoxin antigenicity, C. *botulinum* is divided into seven types, types A to G. Types A, B and E are the principal human pathogens, F is seldom involved in human disease, and G has not yet been reported. They contain somatic, spore and flagellar antigens, but these have not been adequately studied. Nontoxic strains of C. *botulinum* are difficult to distinguish from C. *sporogenes*.

Neurotoxins

These protoplasmic toxins are the most poisonous substances known to man. The toxicities range from 8×10^7 to 3×10^8 LD_{50}/mg N in mice. Man is highly susceptible to the toxin, and there are doc-

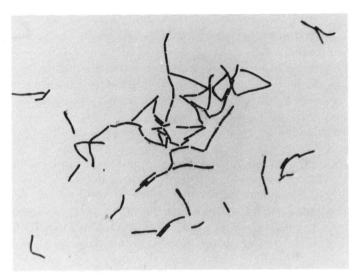

Fig. 9–9.—Gram stain of *Clostridium botulinum*. A 48-hour broth culture, note the large rod and the growth in chains.

umented fatal cases in which the person ate only a bean or a pepper or just tasted the food. Upon release from the cell, the toxicity of the toxin is increased by proteolytic enzymes, probably through some structural alteration of the toxin molecule. Although there are conflicting reports on the inactivation of the toxin by trypsin and pepsin, the toxin is not inactivated in the stomach.

Originally, the molecular weight was reported at 900,000; however, the toxin is composed of two proteins—one possesses hemagglutinating activity but is nontoxic, and the other is a toxic protein. The latter has a molecular weight of 150,000 and contains a light- and heavy-chain polypeptide held together by disulfide bonds. All the different antigenic types of botulinum toxins have a similar structure. A diagrammatic structural arrangement has been proposed indicating that the toxic protein is a cylinder 9 nm in diameter around which is coiled the nontoxic protein. There have been detailed studies of the amino acid composition and physical characteristics of the toxin, but these have not provided an explanation of the extreme toxicity.

Although bacteriophages have been isolated from each of the various types, only types C and D require a prophage for toxin production. If cultures of types C and D are cured of their prophages, they become nontoxic. These cells can then be converted to either type, depending on whether type C or D phage is used to lysogenize the cells.

Botulism

When *C. botulinum* (types A, B, E or F) grows under anaerobic conditions in home-processed or commercially processed food, it synthesizes and, upon lysis, releases the neurotoxin. Primarily, home-canned foods, including vegetables, fruit, meat or fish products, have been involved. Commercially processed foods such as tuna, mushrooms, peppers and vichyssoise have been sources of botulism in recent years. Such food usually shows no sign of decay and thus is not suspected of containing the toxin. However, these foods should not be "taste-tested," as microgram quantities of the toxin can be lethal. The best preventative, other than discarding the food, is to denature the toxin by heating food at 80 C for 10 minutes.

The incubation period varies from 6 hours to 8 days, most commonly being from 12 to 48 hours. The presenting complaints usually include ptosis, blurred or double vision, dysphagia and a dry, sore throat, with vital signs usually being within a normal range. Nausea and vomiting are uncommon. Weakness or paralysis, frequently of a descending type, may progress to quadriplegia and respiratory failure. There are usually no sensory changes and mental processes are clear. Mortalities have approximated 60%, but in recent years have decreased to about 30%.

WOUND BOTULISM.—Fifteen cases of wound botulism have been reported in the United States from 1951 through 1974. In all instances there was a wound, cut or injury, usually with evidence of contamination from the soil but not necessarily an obvious infection. The incubation period ranges from 4 to 14 days with initial symptoms of blurred or double vision, ptosis, and difficulty with speech and swallowing, followed by the development of descending motor paralysis (often symmetrical). There is no sensory deficit and the cerebrospinal fluid is normal. Electromyograms indicate a decreased amplitude of the muscle action potential after a single supramaximal nerve stimulation which, with the above symptoms, is of diagnostic value. This procedure is also of diagnostic value in food botulism. In the first nine cases there was laboratory confirmation of type A by culture or by demonstration of the toxin in the blood. There were four deaths. Type B has been isolated from two recent cases.

INFANT BOTULISM.—Recently, a number of cases of botulism have been reported in infants 3–20 weeks of age. How the disease is acquired is unclear, but it appears that it does not result from ingesting botulinum toxin in food. Instead, the disease is due to production of *C. botulinum* in the intestinal tract. Whether the *C. botulinum* is acquired through food or represents unrestricted production of toxin by *C. botulinum* found as normal flora is still unknown.

PREVALENCE AND DISTRIBUTION. — From 1899 through 1973 there were 689 outbreaks of botulism reported in the United States with 1,787 cases and 980 fatalities. In those cases where the type involved has been determined (31%), 22% were A, 6% B, 3% E and 0.3% F. The first cases of type E in the United States were reported from Michigan in 1963 and involved canned tuna. Since then there have been a number of outbreaks with the highest incidence in Alaska among the Eskimos eating raw marine products and salmon eggs. Overall, there have been 26 proven outbreaks related to fish products since 1899, with 5 involving type A, 2 B, and 19 E.

C. botulinum is widely distributed in soils throughout the world. In the United States type A is more common in the West and B in the East. Type E has been found particularly around the Great Lakes and in Alaska. Type E predominates in Russia where such intoxications were first reported, and in all areas it seems to be associated more frequently with marine sediment and fish. Type C apparently is widely distributed in the alkaline flats of the Midwest, and toxin in the water has caused the death of thousands of ducks. Neither C nor D is toxic to man. Presently, little is known about type G.

MECHANISMS OF PATHOGENESIS. — Except for wound botulism, botulism is an intoxication, not an infection. After food containing the botulinum toxin is ingested, the toxin enters the bloodstream from the intestinal tract and becomes fixed to some component of the nerve terminals at neuromuscular junctions. The mechanism of fixation is not yet known. The toxin prevents the release of the transmitter, acetylcholine, from peripheral cholinergic nerve terminals, thereby causing flaccid paralysis due to skeletal muscle and parasympathetic failure. This blocking is done without affecting nerve conduction or the sensitivity of the muscle membrane to acetylcholine. There are no observable histopathologic features, although electron microscopy studies show disorganization and fragmentation of myofilaments at the neuromuscular junction. In animals it has been shown that recovery from transmitter blockage is by axonal sprouts growing out from the intact nerve terminal and forming new end-plates to restore muscle function.

Wound botulism results from contamination of a wound with *C. botulinum*. The local processes of inflammation and necrosis reduce the O-R potential, providing an environment for growth, synthesis and release of the neurotoxin. The toxin circulates via the bloodstream, becoming fixed to the peripheral nerve endings and causing the same type of symptoms as seen in botulism derived from foods.

PREVENTION AND TREATMENT. — First, the stomach contents should be removed to eliminate residual toxin, then a blood sample taken for toxin titration and a skin test done for hypersensitivity to horse proteins. If symptoms warrant, antitoxins should be administered without delay. A trivalent antitoxin containing 7,500 units of type A antitoxin, 5,500 units of B and 8,500 units of E is available from the Center for Disease Control in Atlanta, Ga., and a polyvalent A, B, E and F antitoxin is available from the Serum Institute in Copenhagen, Denmark. A tracheostomy and the use of a respirator may be necessary. These, combined with good nursing care, usually insure recovery without residual neurologic damage. Antibiotics are indicated only if a pulmonary or urinary tract infection develops.

Treatment of wound botulism usually consists of thorough debridement of the wound plus antibiotics, with penicillin the antibiotic of choice. Tracheostomy is frequently necessary and polyvalent antitoxin has been administered in the majority of cases. Recovery is slow but usually complete.

LABORATORY PROCEDURES FOR ANAEROBE CULTIVATION

ANAEROBIC JARS. — To facilitate cultivation of the anaerobes, investigators have developed a variety of specially designed jars with sealed tops (McIntosh-Fildes, Brown, Brewer, Torbal) in which palladium is activated by heat or electricity to catalyze the removal of oxygen. More recently a cold-catalyst activated by hydrogen (GasPak) has been introduced which will provide O-R potentials approximating − 250 mv and which can be used in jars to culture anaerobes in liquid media or on the surface of solid media (Fig. 9 – 10).

THIOGLYCOLLATE. — Brewer in 1940 introduced the use of the reducing agent sodium thioglycollate. This was added to an infusion broth containing 0.05% agar and facilitated the growth of anaerobes in tubes or flasks without anaerobic jars or special equipment. This medium is useful for growing or maintaining pure cultures but not for primary isolation from clinical specimens.

PREREDUCED MEDIA, ROLL-TUBES AND THE GLOVE-BOX. — It is now recognized that the vegetative cells of many anaerobes are very sensitive to oxygen, and exposure of clinical material or cultures to air − even for a short time − may result in death of the organism and a

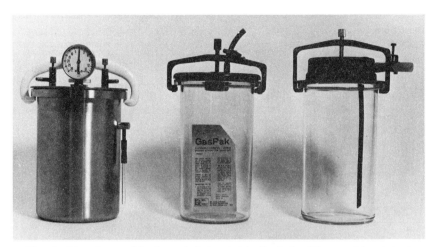

Fig. 9–10.—Anaerobic jars, left to right: Torbal with a cold-catalyst, a gauge and a side arm for an indicator solution; Gas Pak, which utilized a cold-catalyst activated by hydrogen; and the Brewer jar in which palladium is activated by electricity to remove the oxygen. (From Sutter, V. L., Attebery, H. R., Rosenblatt, J. E., Bricknell, K. E., and Fingold, S. M.: *Anaerobic Bacteriology Manual* [Los Angeles: University of California, 1972]. By permission of authors and publisher.)

negative culture. This has resulted in the design of procedures to provide and maintain an aerobic environment from the time of collection of material through identification and determination of antibiotic sensitivities of the isolates.

In 1950 Hungate introduced a roll-tube technique to grow anaerobes from the rumen fluid of cattle. Moore later modified and expanded the procedure at the Virginia Polytechnical Institute. For this technique: (1) the ingredients of a medium are mixed in a flask; (2) oxygen is removed by boiling; (3) cysteine is added; (4) the medium is dispensed into tubes under a stream of nitrogen and (5) the tubes are stoppered, autoclaved and stored. Before use the agar is melted and the tube is spun in a mechanical device, causing the solidifying agar to form a thin film over the inner surface of the tube. For inoculation of this prereduced medium, the stopper is removed, and under a stream of oxygen-free gas, a loop of the inoculum is placed near the bottom of the tube and drawn up toward the mouth while the tube is slowly rotated. The stopper is replaced and the tube is incubated. This procedure can be used for isolation as well as for determination of the biochemical reactions of pure cultures.

The anaerobic glove-box consists of a vacuum-tight plastic cabinet with glove ports. The air is evacuated and the chamber filled with oxygen-free gas. The glove-box is entered through an air lock and provides an adequate working space for streaking plates, picking colonies and inoculating prereduced media under completely anaerobic conditions. There no doubt will be numerous modifications of these methods designed to make it possible to inoculate anaerobic media at the bedside and to facilitate identification and determination of antibiotic sensitivities of the anaerobes.

Collection, Transportation and Identification

SPECIMENS. — Any type of specimen can be cultured for anaerobes, although throat swabs, sputum, gastric contents, feces, urine or vaginal swabs are not routinely cultured without a clinical reason. A brief statement about the disease and the appropriate specimens follows.

GAS GANGRENE, CELLULITIS OR INFECTIONS DUE TO NON-SPORE-FORMERS. — There is usually adequate exudative material which is best collected by aspiration; percutaneous transtracheal aspiration is used to collect sputum, and suprapubic aspiration is used for urine.

TETANUS. — In most instances tetanus is a clinical diagnosis and treatment is initiated before laboratory reports are received. Frequently the injury is healed. In this case a specimen can be obtained only by injecting sterile saline into the site and then aspirating material.

BOTULISM. — In food botulism one should try to demonstrate the toxin in the blood, gastric contents or feces of the patient or in the food. Particulate matter is removed by centrifugation and the supernate is used without filtration for animal inoculations. In wound botulism the patient's blood is used, but the wound site can also be cultured for isolation and identification of C. botulinum.

COLLECTION. — The first consideration in collecting any specimen is to avoid contamination with normal flora bacteria by an adequate skin preparation, a reliable collection procedure, or both. The needle and syringe (with all air expelled) is excellent for: (1) abscess or wound aspiration, (2) percutaneous transtracheal aspiration, (3) suprapubic aspiration, (4) spinal tap or (5) blood cultures. Swabs should not be used for collection if it can be avoided. Sections of tissue can be used. After collection, *the specimen should not be exposed to air.*

TRANSPORTATION. — Ideally, the specimen should be inoculated onto or into an anaerobic medium immediately after collection, which is always possible for blood cultures. Otherwise, the syringe containing the material should be capped and taken directly to the laboratory or the specimen injected into a transport container. A transport container may be a rubber-stoppered vial containing: (1) oxygen-free N_2 or CO_2, (2) a solution containing thioglycollate or cysteine or (3) a semisolid medium containing a reducing agent.

PRELIMINARY EXAMINATION.—The first step is a microscopic examination by gram stain and darkfield microscopy. The gram stain should be done on all suitable specimens and is of utmost importance, as the size, shape and staining characteristics of the organisms may lead to the tentative assumption that anaerobes are involved. These characteristics include large, square-ended rods; long, slender pointed rods; irregularly stained, pleomorphic organisms or cocci of different sizes. The smear can also provide a quantitative estimate of the numbers of organisms present and may be a guide to the use of certain selective media (Fig. 9–1). The darkfield should be more widely used because the size and shape of organisms (particularly *Fusobacterium*) as well as motility are more easily determined.

CULTIVATION AND IDENTIFICATION.—The specimen is then inoculated onto a variety of media, which are: (1) nonselective (blood agar, Brain Heart Infusion agar), (2) selective (kanamycin-vancomycin-blood agar) and (3) enriched (thioglycollate broth plus sterile rabbit serum or chopped meat–glucose broth). The method of inoculation and incubation can include: (1) the prereduced medium-roll-tube method, (2) the glove-box technique or (3) an anaerobic jar. The cultures are incubated 48–72 hours at 35–37 C and the plates are examined for colonial morphological features and the presence or absence of hemolysis.

Identification is dependent on the combination of gram stain, colony morphology, biochemical reactions and determination of end products from glucose fermentation. The last is done by inoculating peptone-yeast extract-glucose broth and determining end products by gas chromatography. Lecithinase production is useful for identifying *C. perfringens*, and the fluorescent antibody technique can be used to specifically identify *C. perfringens*, *C. tetani* and other anaerobes. As with all bacteria, identification of the genus and the species depends on the results of a combination of many characteristics and the same is true for the anaerobes. The final identification procedures may be time-consuming and sometimes questionable in relation to patients' needs, but this is the only way specific causative agents can be determined and correlations established between cause and clinical symptoms.

TOXIN DETERMINATION. — Identification of an isolate or toxin in the patient's blood can aid in the diagnosis of the disease. The procedures depend on specific toxin-antitoxin reactions as demonstrable by immunodiffusion, hemagglutination, complement fixation or animal protection tests. The procedural details are beyond the scope of this chapter, but the mouse-toxin neutralization tests for tetanus and botulism will be briefly described.

For *tetanus,* mouse inoculations can be done by using emulsions of clinical material, patient's blood, broth culture or suspensions of organisms (use young and old cultures). First, one passively immunizes two mice by injecting 0.5 ml of antitoxin intraperitoneally 1 hour or more before testing. Then these and two nonimmune mice are injected intramuscularly into the thigh with 0.2 ml of the specimen. Usually within 8–12 hours stiffness of the inoculated leg is noticeable, which progresses to rigidity of the limb and hindquarters and death in 24–48 hours. The immunized mice do not develop paralysis and survive. This specifically identifies the tetanus toxin and the organism as *C. tetani.*

For *botulism,* the patient's blood, gastric contents or feces, or samples of food or cultures can be used. Separate mice are passively immunized as above with types A, B, E and F antitoxin and then injected intraperitoneally with 0.5 ml of the test material, which should include trypsinized and non-trypsin-treated materials. Nonimmunized mice are also injected with test material. The mouse receiving the homologous antitoxin will survive (i.e., if the type A antitoxin mouse survives, then the toxin is type A); the others, including the controls, will die in 12–48 hours. This is the most sensitive and recommended procedure for botulism.

Antibiotic Sensitivities

The methods for performing these procedures are described in chap. 4; however, there is still no standardized procedure for the anaerobes, and many laboratories use their own modification of the broth or disk technique.

PROBLEM SOLVING AND REVIEW

GIVEN: — A 47-year-old man was admitted to the hospital with increasing trismus for 48 hours along with rigidity and spasms of the right leg. He was acutely distressed, sweating profusely with shallow respiration due to rigidity of the muscles of chest and abdomen. Eight days previously he had stepped on a stake in his garden which penetrated his foot at one side. The injury did not seem too severe, so he continued working but washed and cleansed the area that night. The site stayed tender and seemed to be healing, but some numbness and pain began about 4 days later. He had been vaccinated for tetanus some 20 years earlier when he was discharged from the Army. Because of the severity of the disease, a tracheostomy was performed and intermittent positive pressure instituted. His skin test with normal horse serum was negative, so 10,000 units of equine antitoxin was given intravenously along with penicillin. His spasms became more generalized with excruciating pain, and he died the following day.

PROBLEMS: — 1. What is the organism involved? 2. Give the pathogenesis of this disease. 3. Why was a horse serum skin test done? 4. Why did the patient fail to respond to the antitoxin? 5. How could tetanus have been prevented? 6. How would you identify this organism? (Ans. p. 190.)

SUPPLEMENTARY READING

Bartlett, J. G., and Finegold, S. M.: Anaerobic pleuropulmonary infections, Medicine (Baltimore) 51:413–450, 1972.
Black, R. E., and Arnon, S. S.: Botulism in the United States, 1976, J. Infect. Dis. 136:829, 1977.
Boroff, D. A., and Das Gupta, B. R.: Botulinum Toxin, in Ajl, S. J. (ed.): *Microbial Toxins*, vol. II (New York: Academic Press, 1971).
Chow, A. W., and Guze, L. B.: *Bacteroidaceae* bacteremia: Clinical experience with 112 patients, Medicine (Baltimore) 53:93–126, 1974.
Curtis, D. R., Felix, D., Game, C. J. A., and McCulloch, R. M.: Tetanus toxin and the synaptic release of GABA, Brain Res. 51:358–362, 1973.
Gorbach, S. L., and Bartlett, J. G.: Anaerobic infections, N. Engl. J. Med. 290: 1177–1184; 1237–1245; 1289–1294; 1974.
Gorbach, S. L., and Thadepalli, H.: Isolation of *Clostridium* in human infections, J. Infect. Dis. 131S:81–85, 1975.
Holland, J. W., Hill, E. O., and Altemeier, W. A.: Numbers and types of anaerobic bacteria isolated from clinical specimens since 1960, J. Clin. Microbiol. 5:20–25, 1977.
Hill, M. J., and Drasar, B. S.: Bacteria and the Etiology of Cancer of the Large Intestine, in Balows, A. (ed.): *Anaerobic Bacteria; Role in Disease* (Springfield, Ill.: Charles C Thomas, Publisher, 1974).
Holdeman, L. V., and Moore, W. E. C.: *Anaerobe Laboratory Manual* (Blacksburg, Va: V.P.I. Anaerobe Laboratory, 1973).
Martin, W. J.: Isolation and identification of anaerobic bacteria in the clinical laboratory, Mayo Clinic Proc. 49:300–308, 1974.
Merson, M. H., and Dowell, V. R.: Epidemiological, clinical and laboratory aspects of wound botulism, N. Engl. J. Med. 289:1005–1010, 1973.
Merson, M. H., Hughes, J. M., Dowell, V. R., Taylor, A., Barker, W. H., and Gangarosa, E. J.: Current trends in botulism in the United States, J. A. M. A. 229:1305–1308, 1974.

190   CLOSTRIDIUM AND OTHER ANAEROBES

Nobles, R. R.: *Bacteroides* infections, Ann. Surg. 177:601–606, 1973.
Poupard, J. A., Husain, I., and Norris, R. F.: Biology of the bifidobacteria, Bacteriol. Rev. 37:136–165, 1973.
Price, D. L., Griffin, J., Young, A., Peck, K., and Stocks, A.: Tetanus toxin: Direct evidence for retrograde intraaxonal transport, Science 188:945–947, 1975.
Smith, L. D. S.: *Botulism: the Organism, its Toxins, the Disease* (Springfield, Ill.: Charles C Thomas, Publisher, 1977).
Smith, L. D. S. and Holdeman, L. V.: *The Pathogenic Anaerobic Bacteria* (Springfield, Ill.: Charles C Thomas, Publisher, 1968).
Smyth, C. J., and Arbuthnott, J. P.: Properties of *Clostridium perfringens* Type A α-toxin (phospholipase C) purified by electrofocusing, J. Med. Microbiol. 7:41–66, 1974.
Weinstein, L.: Tetanus, N. Engl. J. Med. 289:1293–1296, 1973.
Weinstein, L., and Barza, M. A.: Current concepts: Gas gangrene, N. Engl. J. Med. 289:1129–1131, 1973.

ANALYSIS

1. *Clostridium tetani.* 2. Injury; contamination of site; growth of the organism and synthesis of toxin; intraaxonal ascent of the toxin to the CNS; fixation of the toxin to gangliosides in the gray matter; interference with inhibitory transmitters, GABA and acetylcholine; hyperactivity of voluntary muscles resulting in spastic paralysis. 3. To test for hypersensitivity and to minimize allergic reactions. 4. Once the toxin is bound to the gangliosides, the receptor sites for the antitoxin are masked. 5. The patient should have received a booster shot of tetanus toxoid every 10 years. 6. Gram-positive anaerobic rod, terminal spore, motile, ferments no carbohydrates and produces an exotoxin which is specifically neutralized by tetanus antitoxin.

10 / Corynebacterium and Listeria

CORYNEBACTERIUM

Overview

In the 1700s there were clinical descriptions of "throat distemper" or diphtheria (leather), but the pathogenicity of *Corynebacterium diphtheriae* was not established until Loeffler demonstrated infectivity in guinea pigs in 1884 and proposed that a toxin was responsible for the lesions. Within the next 40 years the exotoxin was identified and an immunizing toxoid produced. During this period a number of other species were described on the basis of morphological similarity to the diphtheria bacillus; some of the species were pathogenic for man or animals, but none caused a clinical entity as distinct as diphtheria.

General Characteristics

All *Corynebacterium* are gram-positive rods without spores, flagella or capsules. The cells often contain granules of polymetaphosphate (Babès-Ernst granules) which stain deeply with basic dyes such as methylene blue and give the appearance of barring. A snapping division causes the cells to assume X, Y, V or palisade arrangements described as "diphtheroid or coryneform" (Fig. 10–1). The cell wall contains meso-diaminopimelic acid (m-Dap) and the sugars arabinose and galactose. Mannose and glucose may be present. Most species have corynemycolic acid in the cell wall. Acids are produced from a number of carbohydrates and catalase is formed. They are facultative anaerobes growing best aerobically and often forming a pellicle on liquid mediums (Table 10–1).

Species

C. diphtheriae (Klebs-Loeffler bacillus) can be divided into three biotypes designated as *gravis, intermedius* and *mitis* on the basis of colony morphology on tellurite medium; originally it was believed that there was a relationship between severity of the disease and colonial morphology, but this is not true.

C. pseudodiphtheriticum (C. hofmannii) and *C. xerosis* are both

191

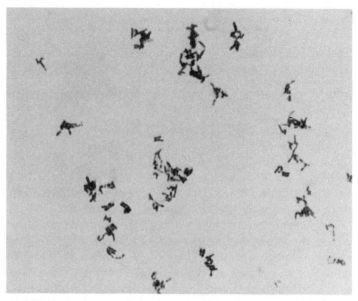

Fig. 10–1.–Gram stain of *Corynebacterium diphtheriae*. Note the variation in length of the cells, irregular staining and the arrangement of cells side by side or in palisades. These characteristics are described as diphtheroid or coryneform.

TABLE 10–1.–CHARACTERISTICS OF *CORYNEBACTERIUM* ASSOCIATED WITH HUMANS

SPECIES	GLUCOSE	MALTOSE	SUCROSE	NO₃ REDUCTASE	GELATINASE	EXOTOXIN	PATHOGENICITY FOR HUMANS	INFECTIONS
C. diphtheriae	+	+	−	±	−	+	+	Diphtheria
C. pseudodiphtheriticum (*C. hofmannii*)	−	−	−	±	−	−	−	Sometimes in compromised host
C. xerosis	+	+	+	+	−	−	−	Sometimes in
C. ulcerans	+	+	−	−	+	+	+	compromised host
C. pseudotuberculosis (*C. ovis*)	+	+	∓	±	∓	+	+	Pharyngitis Lymphadenitis
C. haemolyticum	+	+	±	−	−	−	+	Pharyngitis,
C. minutissimum	+	+	∓	∓	−	−	+	cutaneous ulcers Erythrasma

found on the skin, in the upper respiratory tract and on the conjunctivas. Morphologically, these organisms resemble *C. diphtheriae* and
are referred to as "diphtheroids," but they differ serologically and
biochemically from *C. diphtheriae*. Exotoxins are not produced. *C.
pseudodiphtheriticum* can cause infections in the compromised host,
but they are generally considered as nonpathogenic (see Fig. 10–3).

C. ulcerans is closely related to *C. diphtheriae* and produces a toxic
protein that differs from the diphtheria exotoxin. It can be lysogenized
with tox⁺ phage to synthesize the diphtheria exotoxin. It has been isolated from the throat and can cause a pharyngitis in humans.

C. pseudotuberculosis (*C. ovis*, Preisz-Nocard bacillus) causes ulcerative lymphadenitis in sheep and other animals and also can infect
humans. It produces a distinct exotoxin but can also be lysogenized
with tox⁺ phage to produce diphtheria exotoxin.

C. haemolyticum can cause acute pharyngitis and cutaneous lesions. It produces beta-hemolytic colonies on blood agar resembling
those of *S. pyogenes* (see Table 10–1).

C. minutissimum is a diphtheroid which forms colonies that fluoresce coral red under UV light, as do the scaly plaques removed from
the skin of individuals with erythrasma. This superficial infection of
the skin is often limited to the areas around the genitals or toe-webs
but may disseminate to internal organs. For years this was considered
to be a fungus disease, until it was determined that it did not respond
to griseofulvin but did respond to erythromycin. *C. minutissimum*
was isolated and the disease was produced in volunteers.

C. acnes has now been reclassified as *Propionibacterium acnes* primarily on the basis of serology, cell wall analysis and glucose fermentation end products (chap. 9). Other species include *C. belfantii, C.
bovis, C. equi, C. hoagii, C. kutscheri* and *C. renale*.

Ecology
C. diphtheriae is found only in the upper respiratory tract of humans. The reported carrier rate varies from 2% to 40%, being higher
in young age groups; however, there has been no extensive study in
recent years. Transmission is primarily through droplets. *C. pseudodiphtheriticum* and *C. xerosis* are common inhabitants of the skin, upper respiratory tract and eyes. *P. acnes* normally inhabits the skin in
the anaerobic areas of the hair follicles and sebaceous gland ducts.
Little is established about the habitat of the other species.

Cell Wall and Antigens
The peptidoglycan of the corynebacteria contains glutamic acid,
alanine and meso-diaminopimelic acid. The terminal D-alanine links

directly to the m-Dap, so there are no additional cross-linking amino acids. Coupled to the peptidoglycan is an arabinogalactan containing arabinose and galactose; this is the group antigen (O antigen), which cross-reacts with mycobacteria and nocardia. Included in this wall complex are a variety of lipids such as mycolic acid, glycolipid and phospholipid. The corynemycolic acid is an α-branched, β-hydroxy acid, having $C_{32}-C_{36}$ carbon atoms. Similar acids are present in *Nocardia* and *Mycobacterium*. The toxic glycolipid, a 6-6' diester of trehalose, is similar to the cord factor of *M. tuberculosis*, and the phospholipid is the complex dimannophosphoinositide. There is also a cell wall-associated, heat-labile protein "K antigen," which is responsible for the serologic types of *C. diphtheriae*. The K antigens also are important in antibacterial immunity.

Bacteriophage and Genetics

Freeman in 1951 made the important discovery that nontoxigenic *C. diphtheriae* (β tox$^-$) became toxigenic when infected with temperate phage β; infection with other bacteriophages does not cause toxin production. Corynebacteriophage β tox$^+$ has DNA as its nucleic acid, and the structural gene for diphtheria toxin production resides in the phage genome. Toxin is produced during phage replication (lytic cycle). In cultures, both toxin synthesis and release may be inhibited by increased amounts of inorganic iron (10 μg/ml). There is evidence that when iron is present, a protein binds the iron and then binds to the β phage to prevent the expression of the diphtheria toxin gene.

This process of cells harboring latent phage genomes is called lysogeny. The bacterium is said to be lysogenic when it harbors a phage; the phage capable of initiating lysogeny is termed a temperate phage. *C. diphtheriae* phage β lysogeny can be quite stable, and one strain (Park-Williams 8; PW8) has remained lysogenic and toxigenic for 77 years. Lysogenic bacteria are immune to lytic infection with the bacteriophages of the type they harbor as a prophage, but these cells remain sensitive to other phage strains.

Lysogenization of some bacteria with certain temperate phages results in a phenotypic change in the bacterial cell; this process is called phage conversion. A classic example of this process is the phage conversion of nontoxigenic strains of *C. diphtheriae* to toxigenic strains. Other examples include erythrogenic toxin production by *Streptococcus pyogenes*, enterotoxin production by *Staphylococcus aureus* and changing of the O antigens of *Salmonella anatum* from 0-3,10 to 0-3,15, converting it to *S. newington*. A phage-converted bacterium can be experimentally "cured" of the prophage by exposure to UV light; the phage-free cell loses those traits associated with the pro-phage (e.g., toxigenicity) and as a result becomes susceptible to infec-tion with the original phage (e.g., β tox$^+$). UV light induces the lytic cycle in the cell retaining the prophage, resulting in phage DNA syn-thesis, assembly and cell lysis. Approximately 20–100 mature phages are produced per cell with each carrying the same gene (e.g., tox$^+$). Phage β will also lysogenize *C. ulcerans* and *C. ovis*, which will then produce the diphtheria toxin. Phage conversion has biologic signif-icance in that the bacterium acquiring the new genetic information produces new extracellular enzymes, which alter in some cases its pathogenicity and in other cases its identity. A process analogous to lysogenic conversion also occurs in animal cells. Infection of nor-mal cells with a tumor virus results in the transformation of slow-growing cells to rapidly reproducing malignant cells.

C. *diphtheriae* can be divided into 19 phage types, but these do not correlate either with the serotypes or with toxigenicity. Phage typing has been useful in epidemiologic studies, even though only 75% of the isolates may be typable.

Enzymes and Hemolysin

Deoxyribonuclease is produced by most species. *C. diphtheriae* does not produce a diffusible hemolysin, but on blood agar the red cells immediately around or under the colony may be lysed, giving a narrow zone of hemolysis. None of these cellular products plays a demonstrable role in pathogenicity.

Diphtheria Toxin

This was the first bacterial toxin proved to cause disease and has been the subject of almost continuous investigation since the late 1880s. The toxin is synthesized as an intact polypeptide of 62,000 dal-tons, which is toxic for man, guinea pigs and rabbits in doses of 130 ng/kg body weight; mice and rats are quite resistant. If the toxin is treated with trypsin and reduced, the polypeptide chain is broken (nicked) into two fragments, A and B (Fig. 10–2).

Both fragments are necessary for toxicity. The B fragment binds to a receptor site on the cell surface (antibodies to B prevent the binding), and the enzymatically active A fragment penetrates the cell. The mechanism of penetration is not known, nor is it established whether or not the toxin is nicked with a protease outside or inside the cell. Complete separation of the fragments is not necessary for A to be en-zymatically active. Within the eukaryotic cell, the A fragment (probably separated from B) inhibits protein synthesis by inactivation of the peptidyl-tRNA translocation factor, elongation factor 2 (EF2).

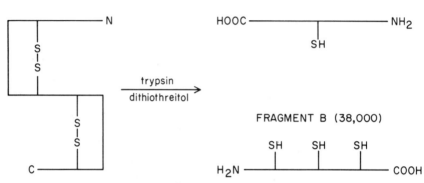

Fig. 10-2.—A schematic representation of the intact diphtheria toxin with two disulfide bridges. If treated with trypsin and reduced, the toxin is "nicked" to provide the enzymatically inactive, heat-labile B and the enzymatically active A fractions.

This is accomplished by the A fragment catalyzing the transfer of the adenosine diphosphoribose (ADPR) portion of NAD^+ to an amino acid residue on EF2 as follows:

$$NAD^+ + EF2 \rightleftharpoons ADPR\text{-}EF2 + \text{nicotinamide} + H^+$$

Inhibition of the translocation of polypeptidyl-tRNA from the acceptor to the donor site on the ribosome results in inhibition of protein synthesis.

The toxin can be inactivated by treatment with formalin. The resulting toxoid retains immunogenicity and can be used to immunize susceptible persons.

A toxin with a similar mode of action has been described for *Pseudomonas aeruginosa*.

Diphtheria

Diphtheria occurs most frequently in children, developing as an upper respiratory tract infection after an incubation period of 2–7 days. There is usually a low-grade fever and a mild sore throat. The initial lesion is usually on the tonsils and oropharynx. A grayish pseudomembrane is located over the superficial layers of the mucosa, which becomes leathery and may extend up into the nasopharynx or down into the pharynx and trachea. Similar membranes may be observed in streptococcal pharyngitis, candidiasis, Vincent's infection or infectious mononucleosis, and it is important that diphtheria be differentiated from these other diseases. The diphtheritic membrane results from a seroexudative response to the exotoxin and organism, and consists of a fibrous exudate containing leukocytes, red cells, epithelial cells and bacteria. It may extend into the bronchi or break loose and plug the bronchi, resulting in death from asphyxiation. *C. diphtheriae* does not invade the deeper tissues, although a cervical lymphadenopathy with soft tissue swelling may occur. There is no bacteremia; however, a toxemia develops with generalized distribution of the toxin, which preferentially localizes in the kidneys, heart and peripheral or cranial nerves. This localization may result in the development of interstitial nephritis, myocarditis due to necrosis of the myocardium or polyneuritis. In the last case, there is a segmental demyelination due to inhibition of synthesis of myelin protein. This causes a decrease in nerve conduction velocity, resulting in various degrees of paralysis and anesthesia. In certain cases the patient may recover from the infection but then have late cardiac or neurologic complications. Death may result from asphyxiation, cardiac failure or respiratory paralysis.

Extrarespiratory infections may involve the ear, conjunctiva or genitalia. Wound diphtheria occurs when a wound, cut or abrasion becomes contaminated with a toxigenic (tox+) *C. diphtheriae*. Production of toxin in the wound results in the formation of a local membrane, and the other symptoms of the toxemia may follow as described above. In the tropics, indolent chronic skin ulcers harboring toxigenic organisms also occur, but for some unknown reason systemic symptoms are uncommon.

Mechanism of Pathogenicity

Man is the only natural host for *C. diphtheriae*. The organism is transmitted by droplets and lodges on the mucous membranes of the upper respiratory tract (tonsils and oropharynx). The organism survives probably because of K surface antigen, which is antiphagocytic.

The principal mechanism of pathogenicity for *C. diphtheriae* is the exotoxin. The organisms themselves have limited invasive power, but they grow on the surface of the mucous membrane or in a wound, synthesizing and releasing the exotoxin. The B fragment of the toxin binds to the surface of the local tissue cells, the toxin is nicked, and fragment A penetrates the cell where it catalyzes the inactivation of the elongation factor, inhibiting cellular protein synthesis. This results in cell death and eventually areas of necrosis. A cellular infiltrate consisting of polymorphonuclear leukocytes, lymphocytes, erythrocytes and an exudate is produced. This acute inflammatory response results in development of the pseudomembrane, which can cause death by mechanical obstruction. Toxin produced by organisms growing in the pseudomembrane enters the bloodstream via the lymphatics and binds to tissue cells. Either there is a predilection for the kidney, heart muscle and nerves, or these organs are more sensitive than others to the effects of the toxin. The inhibition of protein synthesis by binding of the A fraction to EF2 then causes local areas of necrosis, and the cumulative effect interferes with organ and body metabolism.

Immunity

Active

Recovery from diphtheria or immunization with the toxoid results in active immunization of the individual. Children should be immunized with DPT (diphtheria, pertussis, tetanus) vaccine at 6 weeks to 3 months of age. Three 0.5-ml injections intramuscularly are given at 4- to 6-week intervals. Boosters are given at approximately 1 and 6 years of age and then at 10-year intervals. This maintains a protective concentration of 0.01 units of antitoxin per milliliter of serum. Nonimmunized adults are usually given two injections of a monovalent toxoid (see Tetanus Toxoid, Antitoxin and Treatment for a further discussion of these topics).

Passive

Diphtheria was the first disease (1890) to be successfully treated with an antitoxin. This is still the principal means of treatment. Antitoxin is produced commercially by immunizing horses with diphtheria toxoid, collecting the blood and fractionating the serum to obtain the γ-globulin or diphtheria antitoxin. However, before being used commercially, the antitoxin must be standardized in terms of units per milliliter as follows: A preliminary in vitro titration is made by preparing serial dilutions of the antitoxin and adding these to a fixed amount of diphtheria toxin. The dilution which is first to show flocculation contains the L_f (L = limes or limit; f = flocculation) dose of antitoxin. L_f relates to the combining and protective power of the antitoxin. The final titration is done in guinea pigs. Dilutions containing the L_f dose (in 1 ml) as well as one lower and one higher dilution are then mixed with an L^+ dose of diphtheria toxin contained in 2 ml. The L^+ dose is that amount of toxin which when combined with 1 unit of standard antitoxin and injected subcutaneously into a 250-gm guinea pig will cause its death in 4 days. Each of these 3-ml mixtures is injected subcutaneously into separate 250-gm (240–280 gm) guinea pigs.

The dilution which causes the death of the animal in 4 days has the same protective power as 1 unit of standard diphtheria antitoxin. Thus, if the dilution is 1:2,000, the antitoxin has 2,000 units/ml.

Schick Test
    This test is used to determine whether an individual is susceptible or immune to diphtheria. One-tenth milliliter of toxin (0.0006 μg toxin protein) is injected intradermally and the site observed for 4 to 5 days for the development of an area of inflammation and induration. This is a positive Schick test and indicates susceptibility. The absence of a reaction indicates immunity as the toxin was neutralized by circulating antitoxin. Sensitization to the toxin protein from repeated injections of toxoid can occur. This can be determined by an intradermal injection of 0.1 ml of a 1:10 dilution of toxoid (Maloney test); the development of a local reaction indicates sensitivity. The Schick test is seldom used at the present time.

Treatment

Diphtheria is treated by injecting 20,000 –80,000 units of antitoxin, either intramuscularly or intravenously. *This must be done as early in the disease as possible.* First, a skin test is performed with dilute horse serum to be certain there is no sensitivity to horse proteins. If the patient is sensitive, then desensitization can be carried out using very dilute solutions of the antitoxin injected subcutaneously, followed by increasing amounts intramuscularly, and finally giving the required dosage of antitoxin intravenously. A syringe containing epinephrine should always be available for immediate use in case of an anaphylactic reaction. The antitoxin contains antibodies against both the A and B fragments, but apparently neutralization of the B fragment to prevent binding to the tissue cell membrane is the important protective reaction. Once the A fragment is in the cell, it is not affected by the antitoxin. Human hyperimmune antitoxin has been used but at present is not generally available.

Antitoxin therapy is usually supplemented by antimicrobial therapy using penicillin or erythromycin. This has no effect on the released toxin, but bacterial growth as well as continued toxin synthesis are inhibited. Treatment also prevents the possible spread of the organisms to other sites and eliminates the carrier state.

Laboratory Procedure

Materials
    Swabs (preferably duplicate) are used to collect material from the membrane, surface of the tonsils and uvula, and wounds.

Culturing

A Loeffler's slant, tellurite plate (contains cystine and potassium tellurite) and a blood agar plate are inoculated and incubated 12–24 hours at 37 C. Loeffler's medium is noninhibitory and supports the growth of *C. diphtheriae* as well as numerous other organisms; the growth is often translucent and difficult to see. The tellurite medium is quite selective for *C. diphtheriae*, which forms grayish black colonies that vary in size, texture and color. The black color results from production of H_2S from cystine, which reacts to produce tellurium sulfide. If there is growth on the blood agar and not on the tellurite, it is probably not *C. diphtheriae*, but the tellurite plate should be incubated an additional 24 hours.

Isolation and Identification

Smears should be made from Loeffler's and from each colony type on tellurite and stained with methylene blue. If organisms morphologically resembling *C. diphtheriae* are present, a preliminary report to that effect can be made. However, a preliminary diagnosis should not be based on the smear because other nonpathogenic corynebacteria give the same appearance. The smear can be used to rule out Vincent's infection.

Suspected colonies from tellurite are picked, emulsified and transferred to a Loeffler's slant. The growth from Loeffler's is streaked onto tellurite for subsequent pure culture isolation if necessary. Pure cultures are used for determining both culture reactions (see Table 10–1) and toxigenicity by an in vitro or in vivo method.

Toxigenicity

The usual in vitro test is the Elek immunodiffusion method. A strip of filter paper saturated with diphtheria antitoxin (100 units/ml) is pressed onto the surface of an agar plate containing animal serum. Then heavy, single-line streaks of the culture (growth from Loeffler's or a colony from tellurite) are made at right angles to and across the paper strip. Four or more cultures with a known tox+ and tox− *C. diphtheriae* control can be tested on each plate. The inoculated plate is incubated 24–48 hours at 37 C and observed for a white line of antigen-antibody precipitate starting at the junction of the inoculum and the paper strip and angling upward from the strip. A similar line is formed from the tox+ control, and if these two lines meet, they form an arc of identity (Fig. 10–3).

For the in vivo test, two guinea pigs are used. One is injected intraperitoneally with 250 units of diphtheria antitoxin and allowed to rest for 2 hours; then both animals are injected subcutaneously with a sus-

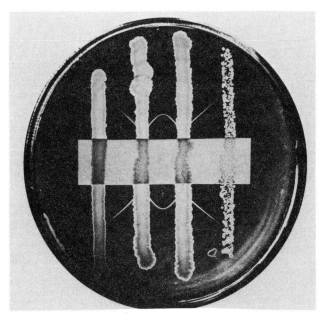

Fig. 10–3. — The Elek test. The two inner streaks are toxigenic *C. diphtheriae,* and between the two streaks the lines of precipitate meet in an arc of identity. The outer streaks are nontoxigenic corynebacteria serving as controls. (From King, E. D., Frosbisher, M., and Parsons, E. I.: Am. J. Public Health, 39:1314, 1949. By permission of author and journal.)

pension of the organism to be tested. The unprotected guinea pig will die in 24 to 96 hours if the isolate is a tox⁺ *C. diphtheriae.*

An alternative in vivo test uses either rabbits or guinea pigs. A subcutaneous injection (0.2 ml) of organisms from a 48-hour culture is made. Four hours after injection of the culture, 500 units of antitoxin are given intravenously. Thirty minutes later the same organisms are injected into different sites. The appearance of necrosis at the first site of injection but not at the second site indicates a tox⁺-producing *C. diphtheriae.* This method has the advantage that several isolates can be tested in a single animal.

LISTERIA

Overview

In 1924 an organism was isolated from an epizootic of septicemia in rabbits. Because the infection caused a monocytic response, the bacterium was named *Listeria monocytogenes.* Similar large monocytes are at times demonstrable in human infections, which resulted in the proposal that this organism caused infectious mononucleosis; however, the latter disease is now known to be caused by the Epstein-Barr virus. In man, *L. monocytogenes* most frequently causes a bacteremia leading to meningitis or meningoencephalitis. An intrauterine infection resulting in abortion or stillbirth is also produced. A variety of infections are produced in animals.

Characteristics, Species and Ecology

L. monocytogenes is a small, gram-positive, non-acid-fast rod resembling a diphtheroid, but it can occur as a short chain or even filament. It produces a characteristic tumbling motility at 22 C but not at 37 C; neither spores nor capsules are produced. It is a facultative anaerobe and produces catalase; a small hemolytic colony is produced on blood agar (resembling that produced by *S. pyogenes*). Acid is produced from a variety of carbohydrates with lactic acid as the major product from glucose fermentation. It is sensitive to most antibiotics including penicillin and tetracyclines. There are three other species but they are not pathogenic for man.

The organism is widely distributed in nature. It has been isolated from animals, birds, fish and insects, but primarily from its plant-soil environment; transmission from animals to humans has been established. Healthy human intestinal carriers also occur.

Cell Wall and Antigens

The cell wall contains diaminopimelic acid with major amounts of aspartic acid and leucine. Teichoic acids have not been reported. On the basis of flagellar (H) and somatic (O) antigens, *L. monocytogenes* is divided into four groups and 11 serotypes. Types 1 and 4 are most common in human infections. The antigens do not relate to pathogenicity or to habitat. The antigens are shared with a number of other organisms, causing serologic cross reactions, which makes it difficult to interpret serologic responses in man.

Listeriosis

This disease in humans is found worldwide with the source of infection usually being organisms from the patient's intestinal tract. The intestinal carrier rate in a random population is 1% but has been reported as 26% for household contacts of a patient with listeriosis. The infection occurs in persons of all ages, but more frequently in the young and the aged. The disease is also found in hosts whose immune status is compromised because of preexisting disease or drug treatment. It usually begins as a bacteremia, which then develops into a meningitis or a meningoencephalitis. Listeriosis can also be secondary to leukemia, Hodgkin's disease, diabetes, renal transplant or a malignancy. *L. monocytogenes* can also cause endocarditis, pneumonia, generalized abscesses, cutaneous infections, conjunctivitis or urethritis. In addition, an intrauterine infection can occur, resulting in an abortion or stillbirth, or an infant who is born healthy and then develops meningitis or septicemia 1–4 weeks postpartum. Granulomatous sepsis of the newborn, characterized by miliary granulomata in the lung, liver, spleen, intestine and central nervous system, results from intrauterine infection of the fetus by *L. monocytogenes*. In such instances the mother may have been asymptomatic or have complained only of fever or diarrhea during pregnancy. Vaginal or cervical cultures may be positive, and there is evidence that some women are long-term carriers. Some work shows that cases of repeated abortion may be due to genital colonization with *L. monocytogenes*. If listeriosis is untreated mortalities can approach 70%, but most cases respond to antibiotics (ampicillin, penicillin, tetracyclines). This organism is an intracellular parasite and the antibiotic dosage must be high and the treatment prolonged.

Mechanisms of Pathogenicity

The virulence of *L. monocytogenes* seems to depend on the organism's ability to grow and metabolize within the mononuclear phagocytes (Fig. 10–4). Avirulent strains do not survive in phagocytes. Intracellular survival permits viable organisms to remain in the tissue and act as a source of dissemination. A nontoxic lipid is responsible for the monocytic response. The hemolysin, which is both hemolytic and lipolytic, is cytotoxic and could be a factor in causing death of phagocytes. The hemolysin is lethal for animals and has a cardiotoxic effect. As yet, neither exotoxins nor endotoxins have been reported. Thus, a pathogenicity factor is the ability of the organism to survive in tissue and to compete successfully for cell nutrients, resulting in inflammatory reactions and necrosis. In mice it has been demonstrated that early in an experimental infection there are changes in hepatic carbohydrate and energy metabolism, which are probably due to impairment of oxidative phosphorylation in liver mitochrondria; such metabolic changes in the host resulting from an infection may also be factors of pathogenicity.

Immunity

L. monocytogenes provokes an immune response resulting in an acquired cell-mediated immunity. Initially there is a sensitization of lymphocytes, and when these cells come in contact with the sensitizing antigen they release macrophage activation factors. These activated macrophages have an enhanced antibacterial activity against not

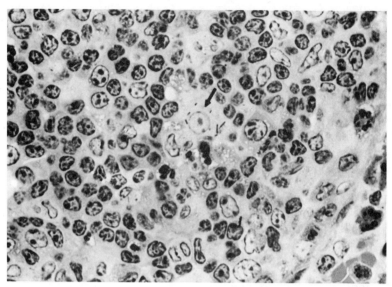

Fig. 10–4.—Intracellular *Listeria monocytogenes* within a mononuclear phagocyte *(arrow).* From experimental lymphadenitis in a guinea pig. Tissue section using Richardson stain. (From Racz, P., Kaiserling, E., Tenner, K., and Wuthe, H. H.: Virchows Arch. [Pathol. Anat.] 363:135, 1974. By permission of author and journal.)

only *Listeria* but also antigenically unrelated organisms such as *C. albicans, B. abortus, M. tuberculosis* and certain protozoa, and even against tumor cells. This acquired resistance can be passively transferred with sensitized T lymphocytes. In experimental animals, a delayed hypersensitivity develops, which correlates with the onset of the cell-mediated immunity (chap. 11). Humoral antibodies are produced, but they apparently play no role in immunity to this infection.

Laboratory Procedures

The usual materials collected are blood and cerebrospinal fluid (chap. 4), but others include swabs, pus, tissue, feces or meconium. The culture procedures for blood (chap. 4) and cerebrospinal fluid (chap. 6) are the same as are used for other organisms. Blood agar is streaked with the other materials and incubated at 37 C; heavily contaminated specimens can be placed in broth, refrigerated at 4 C and subcultured at intervals even up to 3 months. At this temperature, *L. monocytogenes* will survive and even multiply, thus facilitating isolation. Gram stains should be done on all suitable material and observed for gram-positive short rods; the fluorescent antibody technique (chap. 4) can be done directly on any suitable clinical material or culture isolates. After incubation, the blood plates are observed for small beta-hemolytic colonies which when smeared and stained show a diphtheroid morphology. This morphology, along with motility, provides a presumptive identification of *L. monocytogenes*. Identity is confirmed on the basis of biochemical reactions, agglutination tests with specific H and O antiserums, FA and animal pathogenicity studies. Pathogenicity tests can be done in mice. Death follows intraperitoneal injection. Instilling a suspension of the organisms into the conjunctivas of rabbits results in a purulent conjunctivitis (Anton test).

PROBLEM SOLVING AND REVIEW

GIVEN: — An 11-year-old boy was admitted to the hospital with sore throat and difficulty in both breathing and swallowing. His temperature was 38.8 C, and examination of his throat showed bilateral tonsillar hypertrophy and a yellowish gray exudate covering an adherent membrane. Smears were made from the exudate. A portion of the membrane was removed and left a raw bleeding surface. The smears were stained with methylene blue with the exudate showing a few cocci, but the membrane smear showed numerous club-shaped rods arranged in palisades with numerous granules. Throat swabs were taken for culture. A skin test with horse serum was done which was negative; 20,000 units of antitoxin were given intravenously along with intramuscular penicillin. The hospital course was uneventful; electrocardiograms were normal and the patient was discharged in 10 days after three negative throat cultures. The child had been immunized as an infant, but the family had moved frequently and no boosters had been given.

PROBLEMS: — 1. What is the likely diagnosis? 2. What organisms might cause such an infection? 3. Why was a skin test done? Would a Schick test have been of value? 4. What is the rationale of using both penicillin and antitoxin? 5. How does the toxin act? Why was an electrocardiogram done? 6. Why were throat cultures done before discharge? 7. Should epidemiologic studies have been done? 8. How would you isolate and identify this organism? (Ans. p. 206.)

SUPPLEMENTARY READING

Barksdale, L.: *Corynebacterium diphtheriae* and its relatives, Bacteriol. Rev. 34:378–422, 1970.
Barksdale, L., and Arden, S. B.: Persisting bacteriophage infections, lysogeny and phage conversion, Annu. Rev. Microbiol. 28:265–299, 1974.

Bottone, E. J., and Sierra, M. F.: Listeria monocytogenes: Another look at the "Cinderella" among pathogenic bacteria, Mount Sinai Med. J. 44:42–59, 1977.

Brooks, G. F., Bennett, J. V., and Feldman, R. A.: Diphtheria in the United States, 1959–1970, J. Infect. Dis. 129:172–178, 1974.

Cummins, R. S., Lelliott, R. A., and Rogosa, M.: Genus Corynebacterium, in Buchanan, R. E., and Gibbons, N. E. (eds.): Bergey's Manual of Determinative Bacteriology, vol. 8 (Baltimore: Williams & Wilkins Co., 1974).

Evans, A. S.: The history of infectious mononucleosis, Am. J. Med. Sci. 267: 189–195, 1974.

Freeman, V. J.: Studies on virulence of bacteriophage-infected strains of Corynebacterium diphtheriae, J. Bacteriol. 61:675–688, 1951.

Gill, D. M., Pappenheimer, A. M., and Uchida, T.: Diphtheria toxin, protein synthesis and the cell, Fed. Proc. 32:1508–1515, 1973.

Gray, M. L., and Killinger, A. H.: Listeria monocytogenes and listeric infections, Bacteriol. Rev. 30:309–382, 1966.

Kandell, J., Collier, R. J., and Chung, D. W.: Interaction of fragment A from diphtheria toxin with nicotinamide adenine dinucleotide, J. Biol. Chem. 249:2088–2097, 1974.

Moore, R. M., and Zehmer, R. B.: Listerosis in the United States, 1971, J. Infect. Dis. 127:610–611, 1973.

Weis, J., and Seeliger, H. P. R.: Incidence of Listeria monocytogenes in nature, Appl. Microbiol. 30:29–32, 1975.

ANALYSIS

1. Diphtheria. 2. *Corynebacterium diphtheriae*, but a similar clinical picture can be observed in *Streptococcus pyogenes, Candida albicans* or fusospirochetal infections. 3. To determine hypersensitivity to horse globulin; if sensitive, then the patient must be desensitized prior to administration of antitoxin (human hyperimmune antitoxin, if available, can be given without a skin test). Schick test would probably have been of little value as the child did not have an adequate immunity to prevent the infection. 4. Penicillin prevents continued growth and toxin synthesis by the diphtheria bacillus; antitoxin neutralizes the circulating toxin. The toxin seems to have a predilection for cardiac tissue. 5. The toxin inhibits protein synthesis by catalyzing transfer of ADPR moiety of NAD to EF-2. 6. To make certain the individual was not a carrier. 7. Yes. Members of the family should have been cultured and immunized; also, a report to the Health Department would have instituted an examination of the other school children. 8. Throat swabs are inoculated onto Loeffler's agar and tellurite plates. Identification is on the basis of an irregularly staining rod with a palisade arrangement which is toxigenic as demonstrated by using the Elek immunodiffusion plate or by animal inoculation.

11 / Mycobacterium

OVERVIEW

The mycobacteria are the etiologic agents of two ancient diseases, tuberculosis and leprosy. *M. tuberculosis* causes a deformity of the spine, referred to as Pott's disease, which has been observed in Egyptian and Peruvian skeletons, indicating that the disease is at least 10,000 years old. These two diseases have caused the deformity, incapacitation or death of millions of persons and continue to be major world-wide health problems. Saprophytic mycobacteria have been recognized for decades and were referred to as "atypical acid-fast bacilli." However, in 1951 Pollak and Buhler reported on two fatal cases caused by such organisms, and several species are now identifiable as human pathogens. They resemble the tubercle bacillus in both cell and colony morphology, although the colonies may be smooth and more pigmented. Infections caused by these organisms are referred to as mycobacterioses and are often problems in regard to both diagnosis and therapy. Like *M. tuberculosis*, the "atypical acid-fast" mycobacteria cause granulomatous infections involving the skin, lymph nodes or internal organs.

GENERAL CHARACTERISTICS

The various species of *Mycobacterium* (fungus rod) are slender, acid-fast rods, 2–4 μm long, which are sometimes slightly bent. They are considered to be gram positive, but this stain is rarely used. The organisms do not contain flagella, spores or capsules. They have a cell wall with a higher lipid content (60%) than other bacteria (1–20%). These lipids are responsible for the acid-alcohol fastness; they serve as an endogenous energy source and play a role in pathogenicity. Most species will grow in a chemically defined medium with glycerol and ammonium salts, but for isolation from clinical material a more complex medium is used. Growth on any medium is comparatively slow with *M. tuberculosis* requiring 4–6 weeks. Even the "fast grow-

207

ers" commonly require 4–7 days. Pigmentation, when present, is usually yellow to orange due to carotenoids. The organisms are catalase positive; β-lactamase may be produced. Acid is produced from various carbohydrates. Fermentation and other biochemical tests used with most bacteria have limited use for identifying mycobacteria.

SPECIES

There are at least 30 identifiable species of *Mycobacterium*, and 10 or more can cause infections in humans. *M. tuberculosis, M. bovis* and *M. leprae* cause severe diseases throughout the world and will be considered separately, followed by a discussion of the ubiquitous "atypicals." Differential characteristics are found in Table 11–1.

TABLE 11–1.—DIFFERENTIAL CHARACTERISTICS OF CERTAIN PATHOGENIC MYCOBACTERIA

SPECIES	RATE OF GROWTH	NIACIN	NITRATE REDUCTION	CATALASE 68 C	ARYLSULFATASE	NaCl TOLERANCE	SEROTYPES°	SOURCE
M. tuberculosis	4–6 wk	+	+	–	–	–	–	Humans
M. bovis	4–6 wk	–	–	–	–	–	–	Cattle
I. Photochromogens†								
M. kansasii	1–2 wk	–	+	+	–	–	1	Water?
M. marinum	1–2 wk	–	–	±	–	–	1	Water
II. Scotochromogens								
M. scrofulaceum	1–2 wk	–	–	+	–	–	3	Soil?
III. Nonphotochromogens								
M. intracellulare	1–2 wk	–	–	+	–	–	17	Soil
M. avium	1–2 wk	–	–	+	–	–	3	Soil
								Birds
M. xenopi	1–2 wk	–	–	+	±	–		?
IV. Rapid growers								
M. fortuitum	2–7 da	–	+	+	+	+	2	Soil
M. chelonei	2–7 da	–	–	+	+	±	?	Soil

°The agglutination test is used as most atypicals yield smooth suspensions of cells. Serology is not applicable to *M. tuberculosis* or *M. bovis*.

†Group names: *Photochromogens*—grow the organisms in the dark (no pigment produced) then expose to light for 1 hr, reincubate and the growth will change to yellow-orange in 8–24 hr. *Scotochromogens*—produce pigments whether grown in dark or light. *Nonphotochromogens*—produce no pigment whether grown in dark or light. *Rapid growers*—grow in 2–7 days and may or may not produce pigments, not photo-activated.

M. tuberculosis, isolated by Koch in 1882, is a slender, acid-fast rod varying from 2 to 4 μm in length. It grows best at 37 C and requires 4–6 weeks for visible growth (generation time is 12–15 hours). Growth is stimulated by 5%–10% CO_2. On solid media the colonies are raised and rough with a wrinkled surface varying in color from off-white to buff to yellow-orange. Rough colonies are virulent, which correlates with the presence of an identifiable lipid. Microcolonies can be observed in 5–14 days and have a textured pattern due to growth as cords (Fig. 11–1). When the organism is grown in broth, a thick wrinkled pellicle is formed which initially was thought to be fungus-like and is the source of the prefix *Myco*. Characteristics that aid in identification are listed in Table 11–1. This species is pathogenic for mice, guinea pigs, hamsters and monkeys; it is relatively nonpathogenic for rabbits, cattle or fowl. *M. tuberculosis* has a degree of increased resistance to chemical agents, particularly to chlorine and quaternary ammonium compounds, and it persists for extended periods in dried sputum. However, phenolics and iodides are effective disinfectants for the tubercle bacillus.

M. bovis, in comparison to the human tubercle bacillus, is usually shorter, thicker and straighter. It does not form a pellicle on liquid media and initially it grows poorly in glycerol broth. Experimentally it is highly pathogenic for rabbits, guinea pigs and calves, but less

Fig. 11–1.—Microcolonies of virulent *Mycobacterium tuberculosis* after 2 weeks of incubation. Note the irregular or serpentine growth pattern. This cording appearance correlates with the presence of the cord factor. (Courtesy of H. E. Morton, William Pepper Laboratory, University of Pennsylvania.)

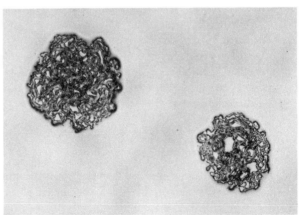

so for most other animals. It is nonpathogenic for fowl and a primary pathogen for cattle. Humans directly or indirectly contract the disease from these animals, although such infections are now quite rare in the United States due primarily to the near eradication of bovine tuberculosis. In France, a strain of *M. bovis* referred to as bacillus Calmette-Guerin, or BCG, was maintained on a low-nutrient medium for 13 years and 231 successive transfers and gradually lost its virulence for the guinea pig. This attenuated mutant is now used under certain circumstances to immunize humans against tuberculosis.

M. leprae is an acid-fast rod resembling the tubercle bacillus. Throughout the years, there have been reports of successful cultivation of *M. leprae* in vitro, but these reports have not been confirmed. Skinsnes and co-workers recently reported growth of *M. leprae* on a hyaluronic acid-based medium. The report needs confirmation. *M. leprae* can be maintained in the footpads of mice, where it will multiply and invade muscle and neural cells. Experimental infections have also been produced in the armadillo.

A large and complex group of mycobacteria commonly referred to as anonymous, unclassified or atypical are also important in disease of man. Runyon and his colleagues introduced a system of dividing these organisms into groups I, II, III and IV based on pigmentation when grown in the presence and absence of light and on growth rate (see Table 11–1). With additional studies, many of these organisms have been differentiated and assigned species names. In general, these organisms differ from *M. tuberculosis* in growing faster, being more pathogenic for mice than for guinea pigs and having an increased resistance to antitubercular drugs. Clinically they can produce either extrapulmonary or pulmonary infections in humans. The latter may be indistinguishable clinically, radiologically and histologically from tuberculosis. The term *mycobacteriosis* is often used to describe such infections. It should be emphasized that the establishment of the etiologic role in such infections requires repeated isolation or histologic evidence of the organisms combined with clinical or radiologic evidence of the disease.

ECOLOGY

Humans are the only established source of *M. tuberculosis*. The organisms are transmitted among humans via droplets or aerosols or by direct contact. *M. bovis* causes tuberculosis in cattle, and humans can contract the disease by ingestion of milk or by direct contact with the infected animal. *M. leprae* is exclusively a human parasite acquired by contact with a leper, particularly someone with lepromatous leprosy; the exact mechanism of transmission is not established. Other mycobacteria responsible for human disease are widely distributed in the soil and have been isolated from soil, water, plants, birds, rodents, as well as from domestic and cold-blooded animals. A number of these species have been isolated from house dust. Man-to-man transmission has been reported but is rare.

CELL WALL

The mycobacterial cell wall differs from that of most bacteria in at least two respects: (1) the peptidoglycan contains N-glycolylmuramic acid instead of N-acetylmuramic acid, and (2) lipids constitute about 60% of the dry weight of the cell wall, in contrast to 1–20% in other bacteria. These lipids are esterified to an arabinogalactan (6-0-β-D-arabinofuranose), which in turn is coupled to the N-glycolylmuramic acid by a phosphodiester linkage. This in its entirety makes a complex unit consisting of lipids, peptides and carbohydrates. This cell wall has unique biologic properties: (1) it acts as an immunizing agent in experimental animals, (2) it exhibits adjuvant properties and (3) it promotes nonspecific resistance in animals to such organisms as *Salmonella*, *Klebsiella* and certain viruses.

Lipids

Interest in the role of mycobacterial lipids in pathogenicity began soon after the discovery of the tubercle bacillus. These lipids, primarily associated with the cell wall, are glycolipids, fatty acids and phospholipids. These compounds probably have several functions within the cell. These may include (1) an endogenous source of energy; (2) a transport system for metabolites across the cytoplasmic membrane; (3) a regulator of water content within the cell; (4) a means for providing resistance to penetration of dyes, enzymes and antibiotics because of increased hydrophobicity and (5) a role in promoting the tissue response of the host to the tubercle bacillus.

The mycolic acids are β-hydroxy acids with aliphatic chains branching at the α-position. At least four mycolic acids with 60–90 carbon atoms, e.g., $C_{87}H_{174}O_3$, have been isolated from *M. tuberculosis*. Mycolic acids with fewer carbons are found in *Nocardia* (C_{40}–C_{60}) and in *Corynebacterium* (C_{28}–C_{40}). In the mycobacteria they are necessary, but not entirely responsible, for the acid-fast staining characteristic. This is evidenced by the fact that if the integrity of the cell is broken by grinding, they become non-acid-fast even though mycolic acid is still present in the cell fragments. Thus, the mycolic acids may function as a permeability barrier to the acid-alcohol. The mycolic acids have not yet been demonstrated to play a role in pathogenicity. Isoniazid, a chemotherapeutic agent used in treatment of tuberculosis, inhibits mycolic acid synthesis resulting in eventual death of the cells.

Included among the glycolipids are the cord factor, sulfatides, wax D and the mycosides.

Koch, in examining growth of the tubercle bacillus in broth, noted that they sometimes grew in strands or "cords." Later this serpentine growth was shown to be related to virulence, and eventually the cord factor was identified as trehalose-6'-dimycolate (see Fig. 11 – 1). Cells which phenotypically lose the cord factor become avirulent, although the mechanism is not understood. The cord factor exhibits certain biologic properties: (1) inhibition of leukocyte migration, (2) stimulation of an acute granulomatous response in the lungs of mice when dissolved in oil and injected intravenously and (3) disintegration of mouse liver mitochondrial membranes, which interrupts the membrane-associated respiration and phosphorylation processes. The cord factor has a molecular weight of 2,900 and is a haptene. This antibody-to-cord factor can act in vivo and in vitro to neutralize the toxic effect of the cord factor. The determinant of serologic specificity is α-D-trehalose.

The sulfatides (sulfolipids) are a group of trehalose sulfate derivatives or trehalose glycolipids which are strongly acidic, and because of this anionic character they may interact with cationic sites on the lysosomal hydrolases of the macrophages and either immobilize or inactivate these enzymes. In addition, they affect mitochrondrial membranes of animal liver and spleen cells causing distortion, swelling and interference with the electron transport system, resulting in disruption of oxidative phosphorylation. Such actions on hydrolases and on mitochondria may well aid in the intracellular survival of the tubercle bacillus. These trehalose glycolipids may act on the phagosomal membranes, allowing release of hydrolases into the cytoplasm of the cell with detrimental effects on the macrophage. The sulfatides do not contain mycolic acids, but they enhance the toxicity of the cord factor. These compounds are the basis for the neutral red test used in the identification of *M. tuberculosis*.

Wax D is an ether-soluble complex containing mycolic acids, glycolipids (trehalose-6-monomycolate) and peptidopolysaccharides. It has multiple biologic properties: it can enhance the immunogenicity of Freund's adjuvant, produce an allergic arthritis and delayed hypersensitivity in rats, stimulate interferon production and have antileukemic or antitumor potential. Cycloserine inhibits the synthesis of wax D.

The mycosides have been classified A, B, C and G depending on the carbohydrate covalently linked to the lipid moiety of the molecule. Mycoside A is found in *M. kansasii*, B in *M. bovis*, G in *M. marinum* and C in a number of other pathogenic mycobacteria. These are apparently located close to the cell surface and influence colonial morphology. Mycoside C from *M. smegmatis* has been shown to be a bacteriophage receptor, and this might be a general property of these compounds. No toxic or antigenic properties have been demonstrated for these compounds, so any role in pathogenicity is questionable.

The phospholipids, which include diphosphatidylglycerol, phosphatidylinositol and mannosides, are found primarily in the cytoplasmic membrane but also in the cell wall. These are among the more active antigenic substances produced by *M. tuberculosis* and have been used as antigens in various serologic tests designed to aid in the diagnosis of tuberculosis. So far, such tests have had only limited application. Crude phospholipid preparations in rather large amounts will evoke a cellular response in animals resembling a tubercle which will undergo caseation necrosis. Such reactions are presumably due to phthienoic acids and other branched-chain fatty acids.

ANTIGENS

The mycobacteria are antigenically complex and share antigens, not only among the various species, but also with the nocardiae and corynebacteria. At least 18 antigens have been identified by gel diffusion and immunoelectrophoresis. Two-dimensional immunoelectrophoresis has identified as many as 60 immunoprecipitates. This procedure permits quantitation of the antigens and provides a two-dimensional pattern which indicates that the reactions are species-specific (Fig. 11–2). Even with all this detailed and exacting work, there is still no serologic procedure to identify *M. tuberculosis*. It seems probable that such a procedure will not be developed, and the quantity of antigens as visualized in an overall antigenic profile will provide the clue to identity.

MYCOBACTERIOPHAGES

Three phage types exist and are designated as A, B and C. The majority of isolates are phage type A, but this is not differential as type A includes strains of both *M. tuberculosis* and *M. bovis*. Phage typing

214   MYCOBACTERIUM

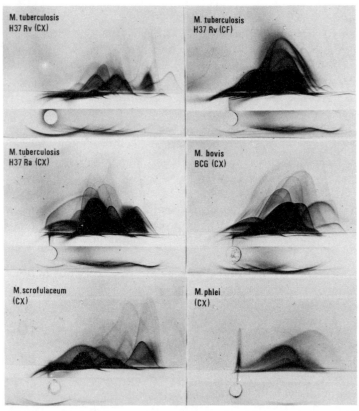

Fig. 11–2.—Two-dimensional electrophoresis of *Mycobacterium* antigens. A one-dimensional pattern is below each well. Cell extract (CX) and culture filtrate (CF) antigens from virulent *M. tuberculosis* are compared with the cell extracts of the other indicated species. Note the complexity of antigens with at least 36 precipitin peaks. (From Wright, G. L., and Roberts, D. B.: Am. Rev. Respir. Dis. 109:306, 1974. By permission of authors and journal.)

has been used in attempts to trace sources of infection. As indicated above, mycosides are the probable phage receptor sites. It is of interest that mycobacteriophages contain lipids that have not been demonstrated in other bacteriophages. Species-specific phages have also been described for the atypicals.

Genetics

With *M. tuberculosis*, bacteriophages have been used primarily for typing, but studies with *M. phlei* and *M. smegmatis* have demonstrated both lysogenic conversion and transduction. Colony changes from rough to smooth in *M. smegmatis* accompany phage infection. It has been postulated that the so-called atypicals are genetic mutants of the tubercle bacillus, but as yet there is no experimental proof for such a concept.

TUBERCULOSIS

The usual portal of entry of *M. tuberculosis* is the lung, with transmission via droplets in the air, although the organisms can penetrate the mucous membranes or skin through breaks or abrasions. Once in the lung, the organisms multiply locally, creating a small area of inflammatory exudate, and are then carried to the regional lymph nodes; this combination is referred to as the primary complex. The extent to which the disease then develops is variable, depending on such factors as: (1) size of the inoculum, (2) physical state of the individual (malnourished are more susceptible), (3) presence or absence of hypersensitivity and (4) presence or absence of cell-mediated immunity. In the previously healthy, tuberculin-negative individual, tuberculosis is usually a self-limiting asymptomatic disease with the principal evidence of infection being tuberculin conversion. A positive tuberculin test indicates the presence of viable tubercle bacilli which are necessary for continued sensitization of the lymphocytes. Pulmonary tuberculosis is divided into primary and reactivation tuberculosis.

Primary Tuberculosis

This is the first infection to occur in either a child or an adult. The tubercle bacilli are usually disseminated by a sputum-positive individual and the droplet nuclei $(1-5 \mu m)$ are inhaled. Transmission by ingestion may also occur. These bacilli bypass the normal defense mechanisms of the upper respiratory tract and lodge in the alveoli or along alveolar ducts, and most are phagocytized by alveolar macrophages. These macrophages vary in their enzyme content and microbicidal ability, and if both are high they kill the bacillus in a short time. If the cell is low in both, the bacterium multiplies, kills the phagocyte and the infection becomes established. A localized inflammatory reaction with an increased concentration of macrophages and a tubercle develops. In most instances the host is able to confine the organisms and the lesion heals. However, the organisms may spread and involve adjacent tissue to the extent that the lesion can be visualized roentgenographically. The organisms can also enter the lymphatics, probably by macrophage transportation, and be carried to the hilar and mediastinal lymph nodes where inflammatory foci develop.

Tubercle bacilli enter the bloodstream via the thoracic duct or directly into pulmonary capillaries. The organisms disseminate hematogenously to any organ, including the lungs. There seems to be a predilection for lymph nodes, kidneys, brain, bones and joints. If excessive numbers or repeated showers of bacilli enter the bloodstream, this may result in wide-spread metastic lesions or miliary (millet seed) tuberculosis. Such lesions in the brain, or meninges, may lead to tuberculous meningitis. Both of these conditions are more apt to occur in children. The host's response to the inflammatory lesion is variable, depending on such factors as numbers of organisms, growth and multiplication of the tubercle bacilli, effectiveness of phagocytosis and state of health and resistance of the individual. As indicated above, in most instances the primary lesions heal and may even be completely resolved.

In 2 to 12 weeks after infection the host becomes hypersensitive or tuberculin test positive. However, the tuberculin test can revert to negative when the primary infection is treated shortly after tuberculin conversion. In the tuberculin-positive host, mycobacterial antigens become attached to precommitted, thymus-dependent lymphocytes (T cells) and cause these cells to undergo blast transformation, resulting in committed lymphocytes, which are the effectors of tuberculin hypersensitivity. Clones of these cells persist for years or even a lifetime and continue to be capable of initiating the localized reaction of the tuberculin test. These cells play an important role in cellular immunity, but the mechanisms for initiating such responses are not yet fully understood.

Concurrent with the development of hypersensitivity are the cellular changes characterizing the granulomatous lesion or tubercle. The polymorphonuclear leukocytes are replaced by macrophages with increased phagocytic and killing power and apparently can transform into epithelioid cells and giant cells, both of which are phagocytic. Lymphocytes accumulate and fibroblasts are formed (Fig. 11–3). The components of this granulomatous lesion then function to kill the tubercle bacillus through increased killing power of the phagocytic cells and inhibit spread through fibroblast proliferation and eventual fibrosis. Caseating necrosis, apparently associated with hypersensitivity, can develop in which there is death of host cells (primarily macrophages) and the formation of a semisolid cheesy mass. This caseous material may persist for years becoming encapsulated and calcified, or the mass may undergo liquefaction causing erosion into adjacent tissue. If a bronchus is eroded, the contents of the lesions drain and carry

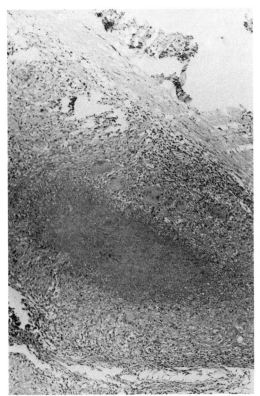

Fig. 11–3. – A tubercle from a human lymph node. Note the central area of caseous necrosis surrounded by a zone of epithelioid cells and fibroblasts with some lymphocytes. There are a number of giant cells in the peripheral area. (Courtesy of W. A. Albrink, Department of Pathology, West Virginia University.)

tubercle bacilli into the surrounding lung tissue, or if swallowed the contents can initiate infections of the oral cavity, larynx, middle ear or gastric mucosa. Drainage of the lesion results in cavity formation with the presence and growth of the tubercle bacilli in the cavity wall. This is a continuing source for spreading the infection within the patient and for aerosols which transmit the organisms to other individuals. The processes that bring about caseation and liquefaction are not understood, but they involve enzymes released by macrophage disintegration, which is initiated by lymphotoxins or mycobacterial lipids.

Reactivation Tuberculosis (Post-primary, Disseminated, Reinfection)

In this form of the disease, a tuberculin test-positive individual without signs or symptoms of the disease develops active tuberculosis. In the past, this was considered to indicate reinfection via droplets. This can occur, but rarely does. Epidemiologic studies have shown that reinfection occurs at least five times more frequently in tuberculin-positive than in tuberculin-negative individuals. These findings led to the present concept that post-primary tuberculosis is a reactivation of an endogenous source of the tubercle bacillus. This means that the viable but metabolically inactive organisms present in the tubercles (usually caseous) begin to multiply and spread. This provokes an intense cellular response in the hypersensitive individual that may result in the onset of symptoms.

Symptoms

Commonly, persons with tuberculosis do not have symptoms until there is considerable tissue involvement. Frequently there is evidence of hypersensitivity as measured by skin testing before the appearance of symptoms, including malaise, anorexia, fatigue, weight loss, a fever as high as 40 C and night sweats. There may be little or no cough when the lesions are small, but as the lesions increase the cough becomes obvious. The sputum is usually mucopurulent and there is hemoptysis. As the infection spreads, the patient may develop shortness of breath and pleural pain.

The disease may spread to other organs, e.g., larynx, lymph nodes, eye, tonsils, adenoids, mastoid, bones, joints, intestinal tract, urinary tract, genital tract, adrenals, heart, brain, spleen and liver. The lymph nodes may suppurate and drain through sinus tracts. Infection of the spine may result in vertebral destruction and a paravertebral abscess (Pott's abscess). Persons with tuberculosis of the kidney are asymptomatic until there is extensive disease. Dysuria, pyuria and hematuria are associated with kidney tuberculosis as well as with other bacterial infections of the kidney.

Miliary tuberculosis may be present as a severe acute disease with toxemia or as a chronic disease with persistent fever.

It should be pointed out that the symptoms are not specific and are similar to those seen in many acute and chronic bacterial and fungal diseases.

Incidence of Tuberculosis

Within the United States an estimated 15 million persons are infected with the tubercle bacillus. From 1962 to 1972 the active cases declined from 179,000 to 80,382; the death rates for these two years were 5.1 per 100,000 and 2.2 per 100,000 population, respectively. The disease occurs twice as frequently in men as in women. The incidence is highest in: (1) groups with low socioeconomic conditions as occurs in the ghettos of large cities and on certain Indian reservations; (2) the malnourished; (3) persons with chronic lung diseases such as silicosis; and (4) persons with other chronic wasting disease, such as lymphoma or diabetes or those receiving treatment with steroids.

OTHER MYCOBACTERIA PATHOGENIC FOR MAN

A number of other mycobacteria cause diseases indistinguishable from those caused by *M. tuberculosis*. They differ in that they are not communicable from person to person and they are more resistant than *M. tuberculosis* to chemotherapeutic agents. Thus it is important that they be considered in the differential diagnosis. For discussion, they have been divided into groups as proposed by Runyan. (For a definition of the group names see Table 11 – 1.)

Group I. Photochromogens

M. kansasii causes pulmonary infections and may disseminate to cervical lymph nodes, bones or joints; response to antitubercular therapy is variable. The organism is pathogenic for mice and hamsters but has limited pathogenicity for guinea pigs. The source of the organism has not been established, although it has been isolated from water but not from soil.

M. marinum (M. balnei) causes granulomatous lesions on the skin of ankles, knees and elbows that may resemble sporotrichosis, a fungal infection. The abraded skin is infected from contaminated water such as in fish tanks or swimming pools, hence the name "swimming pool granuloma." The lesions usually heal spontaneously but some are quite persistent, although they usually respond to treatment with rifampicin. Pathogenicity for laboratory animals is limited, but infections can be produced in the footpads of mice as well as in fish, amphibians and reptiles. Growth in the laboratory is best at 25 C but some strains may adapt to 37 C.

Group II. Scotochromogens

M. scrofulaceum has been associated particularly with cervical lymphadenitis in children (scrofula) but rarely with pulmonary infections; infections usually respond to treatment with antitubercular drugs (Fig. 11 – 4). Initial isolates sometimes take 3 – 4 weeks to grow, forming yellow-orange colonies. They have seldom been isolated from the soil. Other species in this group are *M. flavescens* and *M. gordonae*.

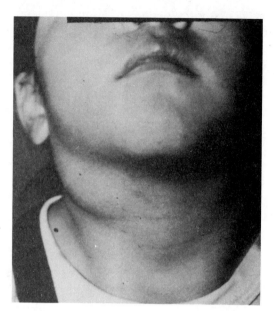

Fig. 11–4.—Clinical picture of lymphadenitis produced by atypical mycobacteria. (From Owens, D. W.: South. Med. J. 67:39, 1974. (By permission of author and journal.)

Group III. Nonphotochromogens

M. intracellulare was so named because of its intracellular growth in tissue culture. It has been reported from chronic pulmonary disease, which in some instances has disseminated to other organs. In one series of 45 cases, 20% of patients died of the active disease within 5 years of onset. The source is apparently soil or house dust. Response to therapy is variable and best results have been obtained by combining antitubercular drugs and surgical resection. The bacillus may cause infections in swine and cattle. Experimentally, it is essentially nonpathogenic for most laboratory animals but has limited pathogenicity for mice and chickens. Initial isolates may require 3–4 weeks to grow.

M. avium produces tuberculosis in chickens and other birds and may also infect cattle, swine and other animals. Pulmonary and cervical lymphadenitis has been infrequently reported in humans. The organism is often resistant to chemotherapeutic agents. Experimentally, it is pathogenic for chickens, mice and rabbits but only to a limited degree for other laboratory animals. It grows well at 37 C and also at 45 C. The growth of most mycobacteria except *M. xenopi, M. phlei, M. smegmatis* and *M. avium*, is inhibited at 45 C.

M. xenopi (isolated from a toad, *Xenopus*) has been reported to cause pulmonary infections more frequently in Europe than in the United States. Favorable response to antibiotics has been reported. It is pathogenic for chickens but it requires a large inocula to demonstrate pathogenicity for other laboratory animals. The source of the organism has not been established. The three species discussed in this group are not always distinguishable and may be referred to as the *M. avium-intracellulare-xenopi* complex. Also, there are three other species in this group, *M. gastri*, *M. terrae* and *M. triviale*, but their pathogenicity for humans has not yet been documented.

Group IV. Rapid Growers

M. fortuitum is also referred to as *M. ranae*. It has been associated with pulmonary infections and localized or "injection" abscesses. There is frequently a minimal response to chemotherapeutic agents. It has limited pathogenicity for laboratory animals, but in mice an ear infection causes a "spinning" disease. It grows in 2 to 4 days at 37 C without pigment production and forms a filamentous microcolony on corn meal agar. It has been isolated from infections in cattle and cold-blooded animals and from soil. Another organism designated as *M. peregrinum* has been described, but it differs only slightly from *M. fortuitum*. Thus, it will not be described separately but considered as part of a complex to include *M. borstelense* and *M. abscessus*. The involvement of these organisms in pulmonary disease is questionable, but they do cause localized abscesses, sometimes after injection of drugs or vaccines. These lesions start as a lump at the injection site and develop into an abscess which may take months to heal. Response to antibiotics is often minimal, and if the lesions do not resolve, excision may be necessary. These organisms are pathogenic for mice but have limited pathogenicity for guinea pigs, rabbits and hamsters. They grow in 3 to 5 days as nonpigmented colonies.

OTHER MYCOBACTERIA

Several other species of mycobacteria are known. These organisms cause disease in animals or are found free in nature. For example: *M. microti* causes tuberculosis in the vole; *M. africanum* causes human tuberculosis in tropical Africa; *M. paratuberculosis* causes a sometimes fatal enteritis of cattle (Johne's disease); *M. lepraemurium* causes chronic rat leprosy of wild rats; *M. phlei* is a nonpathogenic bacillus found on hay. *M. smegmatis* is a nonpathogen present in human smegma – it can be found in urine and in stained smears and may be confused with the tubercle bacillus.

MECHANISM OF PATHOGENICITY

In considering bacterial pathogenicity or virulence factors, one immediately thinks of toxins. However, many disease-producing microorganisms do not elaborate toxins. Thus it is necessary to broaden the concept of mechanisms of pathogenicity to include any substance, product, or method that allows the organism to survive in the tissues of the host. This could include utilization of substrates required for respiration, energy or metabolism which have been obtained at the expense of tissue cells, as well as the products of metabolism or extracellular enzymes that might lyse and kill tissue cells. *M. tuberculosis* is a classic example of a nontoxic yet highly pathogenic organism. Ten cells will eventually cause the death of a guinea pig. To grow in tissue, it requires amino acids, carbohydrates, salts, iron and oxygen, and the source of these substrates is the plasma or cell constituents of the host present in the microenvironment of the tubercle bacillus. Thus the metabolic and respiratory enzymes that successfully compete for these nutrients are basically factors of pathogenicity. A specific example is mycobactin, an iron-chelating growth factor, which makes the iron present in transferrin or in ferritin available to the tubercle bacillus at the expense of the host.

Definitive information is lacking on the effect of the growing tubercle bacilli on the metabolism and nutrition of the human body, although clinically there is frequently weight loss. Studies with avian tuberculosis indicate that in an extensive tuberculous infection, up to 94% of the energy of the chicken is used by the infectious process.

There have been numerous attempts to isolate or demonstrate "virulence factors" from the tubercle bacillus with almost uniformly disappointing results. The cord factor might be an exception as it is toxic to animals, and loss of the cord factor reduces virulence of the organism. However, this relationship is not always direct, as the compound can be isolated from certain nonpathogenic mycobacteria. Nevertheless, the cord factor and sulfatides can alter mitochondrial membranes and disrupt oxidative phosphorylation, which would be deleterious to host cells. Another proposed effect of these lipids is that they rupture the phagosomal membranes within the phagocyte, releasing hydrolases into the cytoplasm thereby causing death of the phagocyte (chap. 1).

Also associated with metabolism and survival in the host is the fact that the tubercle bacillus has adapted itself to an intracellular existence within the macrophages. It grows slowly and in so doing obtains nutrients from the macrophage. Within this protected environment the anionic lipids of the bacillus bind and inactivate macrophage hydrolases, thereby shielding the organism from the effects of antibodies and even from certain chemotherapeutic agents. Thus the continued survival of the organisms contributes to the pathogenicity of the tubercle bacillus.

Delayed hypersensitivity, a key feature of mycobacterial infection, develops in response to the mycobacterial antigens and is both beneficial and detrimental to the tubercle bacillus (see section on Immunity: Beneficial and Harmful Aspects). These effects are not always readily separable. On the beneficial side for the organism is the cytotoxic action of the sensitized lymphocytes, which under appropriate conditions frees the organism from the phagocyte. Cytotoxicity is also a factor in caseation, and liquefaction may facilitate spread of the organism to other areas of the body. On the detrimental side for the bacillus are the properties of the lymphocyte, which, in the presence of the antigen, aggregates macrophages and enhances their microbicidal ability. These macrophages also transform into epithelioid and giant cells which are phagocytic and also confine the tubercle bacillus to one area.

IMMUNITY: BENEFICIAL AND HARMFUL ASPECTS

Mycobacterial cells contain a number of substances which when injected into an experimental animal increase the resistance of that animal to an experimental infection. These substances include cell wall and cytoplasmic components (most of which are not well defined chemically), such as the tuberculoproteins, protein complexes, lipids, lipoproteins, lipopolysaccharides, phospholipids and polysaccharides. The response to these substances, in both the animal and human body, is complex and includes antibody production, hypersensitivity, a granulomatous reaction and cellular immunity. These host responses to the foreign antigens function together with the ultimate purpose of overcoming the invading tubercle bacillus.

Proteins, lipids (particularly phospholipids) and polysaccharides of the tubercle bacillus stimulate the B cells to synthesize humoral antibodies. These are demonstrable by means of the agglutination, gel diffusion or complement fixation tests. Unfortunately, the antibodies are frequently of low or highly variable titer, so the results from such tests have not proven helpful as aids in the diagnosis of tuberculosis. In addition, these antibodies have not been shown to be protective or useful for passive immunization; thus their role, if any, in immunity to tuberculosis has yet to be demonstrated.

Delayed hypersensitivity is an important feature of tuberculosis, as well as of certain fungal, viral and other bacterial diseases. When sensitized T cells come in contact with the antigen, the lymphocyte releases a dozen or more soluble mediators (lymphokines). These are not well defined at the present time, nor is it known whether some have multiple functions, but the mediators affect primarily the monocytes and include migratory inhibitory factor (MIF), chemotactic factor, cytotoxin factor and transfer factor.

MIF is a protein that causes the monocyte to become sticky and adhere to the endothelial wall, which provides a concentration of monocytes in the area of the lymphocytes and the antigen. MIF is demonstrable in vitro (Fig. 11–5). These monocyte-macrophages become more actively phagocytic and have increased killing power

Fig. 11–5.—In vitro demonstration of the migration inhibitory factor (MIF). Peritoneal exudate cells, predominantly macrophages and lymphocytes, are cultured in capillary tubes in the presence or absence of the antigen. The antigen, e.g., tuberculin, causes MIF to be released from specifically sensitized lymphocytes, which in turn blocks the migration of macrophages from the tube. **Left,** control cultured cells from a sensitized guinea pig in the absence of antigen showing cells migrating out from the end of the tube. **Right,** the cells in the presence of antigen showing inhibition of migration. (Courtesy of J. J. Marx, Marshfield Clinic Research Foundation, Marshfield, WI.)

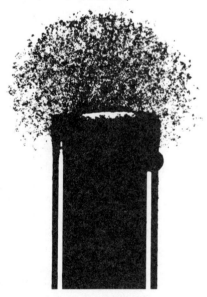
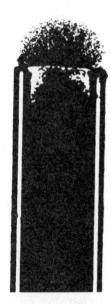

Control   Cells + Antigen

for intracellular parasites. In addition, the chemotactic factor attracts additional macrophages to the site. The lymphocytes also release non-selective cytotoxic factors which can cause death and lysis of a variety of cells, including macrophages, monocytes, lymphocytes or tissue cells. This may be detrimental to the host because of the release of hydrolases from these cells, which in turn can cause additional cell lysis. Also, pharmacologically active substances such as histamine and serotonin are released which promote additional localized tissue and cellular responses.

Transfer factor is a nonantigenic, dialyzable, low molecular weight compound that is not destroyed by RNase, DNase or trypsin. Both lymphocytes and leukocytes release transfer factor. This factor stimulates lymphocytes to undergo blast transformation into sensitized cells, which then initiate a delayed hypersensitivity reaction in the previously nonsensitized host.

With the accumulation of monocytes in the area, these cells are stimulated to undergo transformation into macrophages, and some of these evolve into epithelioid cells which in turn may fuse to form the multinucleated giant cells. All of these cells are phagocytic and play a major role in overcoming the tubercle bacillus. Either before or soon after the bacillus is ingested, the macrophage becomes "activated"; as such it has an enhanced ability to ingest particles, increased mitochondrial content, increased lysosomes and increased killing power for intracellular parasites. The lysosomal membrane fuses with the phagosome, and hydrolases and other enzymes are discharged into the phagocytic vacuole. These enzymes, including lipases and lysozyme, act first on the cell wall and then on other components of the bacterial cell. Such enzymes are also released from the macrophage and they can be deleterious to neighboring tissue cells.

Macrophages are activated by mycobacterial antigens and have increased phagocytic or microbicidal activity for other intracellular parasites such as *Brucella*, *Listeria* and *Salmonella*. However, this increased nonspecific killing power is lost more readily than the specific and is usually not recalled by reintroduction of the mycobacterial antigens.

It has long been appreciated that a state of hypersensitivity is associated with an increased resistance to reinfection with the tubercle bacillus. Several authors have indicated that hypersensitivity and immunity are synonymous. This was challenged with the work of Youmans (1969) and his colleagues when they demonstrated that a mycobacterial ribosomal fraction and RNA stimulated a cellular immunity equal to that obtained with living cells. These fractions did not produce a hypersensitivity, indicating that the response was separate and distinct from delayed hypersensitivity (DH). It is doubtful that the body separates hypersensitivity and this specific cellular response. In all probability they beneficially supplement each other in the overall host response to the invading tubercle bacillus.

TUBERCULINS

There are two types of tuberculins that contain the tuberculo-protein, a nonantigenic, low molecular weight protein of *M. tuberculosis*. These are designated old tuberculin (OT) and purified protein derivative (PPD). Following the original method of Koch, OT is prepared by (1) growing the tubercle bacilli in alkaline 5% glycerine broth, (2) steaming for 1 hour at 100 C, (3) evaporating at 80 C to one tenth of the original volume and (4) filtering to remove the bacilli.

For production of PPD, the tubercle bacilli are grown in a chemically defined medium, killed by autoclaving, then centrifuged. The supernate is precipitated with trichloracetic acid or ammonium sulfate, dialyzed, dried and redissolved in a special buffer. The dosage is calculated on the basis of milligrams of protein per milliliter and expressed as tuberculin units with 0.00002 mg dry weight = 1 tuberculin unit or 1 TU. Three strengths are available:

1 TU = 0.00002 mg PPD in 0.1 ml, or first strength
5 TU = 0.0001 mg PPD in 0.1 ml, or intermediate strength
100 TU = 0.002 mg PPD in 0.1 ml, or second strength

PPD solutions should be kept in the dark and should not be left in the syringe for any length of time as the protein readily absorbs to the glass or plastic, thereby reducing the effective concentration. This loss of potency can be prevented by mixing the PPD with Tween 80; such a stabilized preparation is available and is preferred for use. PPD preparations have been developed for the other mycobacteria, and these are identified by letter designations. The following skin test preparations are used as aids to diagnosis of infections due to mycobacteria: (1) OT, *M. tuberculosis;* (2) PPD-S, Seibert's purified protein derivative from *M. tuberculosis;* (3) PPD-Y, *M. kansasii;* (4) PPD-G, *M. scrofulaceum* and (5) PPD-B, *M. intracellulare.*

Tuberculin Test

Three methods of injection are used: (1) intradermal or Mantoux, (2) injection with a jet gun and (3) Tine or multiple-puncture method. In the Tine method tuberculin is dried on the tips of four stainless steel needles designed to limit skin penetration. Regardless of the method used, the initial injection contains 5 TU of PPD and the area of induration is measured in 48 to 72 hours. If negative, the test can be repeated with the same or increased strength, as the tuberculin will not sensitize the individual. The results are recorded as follows:

Intradermal or jet test induration	Time test induration	Results
10 mm or more	5 mm	Positive
5–9 mm	2–4 mm	Doubtful
0–4 mm	0–2 mm	Negative

Tuberculin Reaction

As presently understood, the sequence of events occurring at a tuberculin skin test site is as follows. After the tuberculin has been injected intradermally, it diffuses slowly into a localized area. The tuberculin combines with the cell-bound antibody on sensitized lymphocytes, which in turn synthesizes and releases the migratory inhibitory factor. MIF makes the cell surface of circulating monocytes sticky, and they adhere to the capillary wall in the vicinity of antigen deposition. These monocytes are transformed into macrophages with increased phagocytic activities. Cytotoxins from the lymphocytes and perhaps other cells are released, causing the death of macrophages, monocytes and tissue cells with consequent release of hydrolases and pharmacologically active substances that provoke an inflammatory response. The accumulation of fluid and cells in the area causes induration. With the degradation of tuberculin (through a combination of enzymatic digestion and phagocytosis), the reaction subsides and the site eventually returns to normal. In some individuals this may take time and occasionally there can be necrosis and scarring. If an excess of tuberculin is injected either subcutaneously or intravenously, a severe systemic reaction can occur which may result in a breakdown of caseous nodules and a reactivation of tuberculosis lesions.

Interpretation of the Tuberculin Test

A positive tuberculin test means that a primary infection, a successful BCG vaccination or an infection with a typical mycobacteria has taken place. The present concept is that viable organisms continue to be present in the host to maintain the antigenic stimulus. Unfortunately, the reaction does not indicate the clinical status of the infection, i.e., whether or not active tuberculosis is present. However, an induration of 15 mm or more often indicates a recent exposure. The possible exception to this is the child who converts from negative to positive or the adult who is known to be negative at least a year before the positive test; these are then considered to be active cases. A doubtful reaction (5-9 mm induration) could indicate (1) the onset of sensitization to *M. tuberculosis*, (2) a response to therapy with a killing of the tubercle bacilli or (3) a cross-reactivity between *M. tuberculosis* and the atypical mycobacteria to determine the etiology. Cross-reactivity with *Nocardia* has also been reported. These individuals can be retested with OT, PPD-S and PPD to the other mycobacteria. A negative reaction means that there are no sensitized lymphocytes and no viable tubercle bacilli. There are some exceptions to this: (1) in miliary tuberculosis there is an overwhelming amount of antigen which blocks the reaction resulting in anergy, and (2) in persons receiving steroids or with lymphoma, the immune response can be altered or suppressed.

Tuberculin Tests for the Atypical Mycobacteria

These tests are done in the same manner as those for *M. tuberculosis*, and the mechanisms of the reaction are the same as described above. There are conflicting reports as to their interpretation and significance, but in general it is indicated that when different PPDs are used, a greater area of induration correlates with the organism causing the infection. There are cross reactions among the atypicals as well as between the atypicals and *M. tuberculosis*.

VACCINES

Living virulent cells, attenuated cells, killed whole cells, cell wall fractions and cytoplasmic constituents have all been shown to increase the resistance of experimental animals to infection with *M. tuberculosis*. The fact that living cells have the highest immunizing capacity led to the studies of Calmette and Guérin in which they maintained a culture of *M. bovis* on artificial media for approximately 12 years. During this time it gradually lost its virulence for guinea pigs but retained immunogenicity. In 1921 this attenuated strain of *M. bovis*, or BCG, was tried in humans. During the subsequent years, this procedure has been involved in controversy with the principal supporter being the World Health Organization, which has sponsored a worldwide vaccination program involving thousands of children.

The principle of BCG vaccination is that skin test-negative persons (primarily children) are injected with living attenuated cells, and as these organisms continue to slowly metabolize, their antigens sensitize T-cells, which in turn activate the macrophages. In this manner the patient acquires a positive skin test and immunity. Booster vaccinations may be given in 4 or 5 years. These children have a decreased incidence of active tuberculosis, and if they do develop an active infection, there is a decreased chance of their developing miliary tuberculosis or tuberculous meningitis. BCG vaccination has been widely used in Europe with some countries requiring children to be vaccinated. Through the efforts of WHO it has also been extensively used in several underdeveloped countries. In the United States, use has been limited to certain high-risk tuberculosis groups or to individuals repeatedly exposed to sputum-positive cases. Use is restricted on the basis that this negates the possible diagnostic value of skin test conversion in individuals and also because available BCG vaccines vary considerably in immunizing capacity. As yet there is no satisfactory method for standardizing this vaccine.

Currently there is a renewed interest in BCG stemming from reports of tumor regression or tumor prevention in animals following vaccination with BCG. There have also been some clinical trials in humans with malignant melanoma, Hodgkin's disease and leukemia with an indication of regression in certain cases. The basis seems to be related to nonspecific increased phagocytic activity of the macrophages and the release of cytotoxic substances which combine to overcome tumor cells.

THERAPY

Chemotherapeutic agents frequently used in the treatment of tuberculosis include streptomycin (SM), para-aminosalicylic acid (PAS), ethambutol and isoniazid (iso-nicotinic acid hydrazide; INH). Rifampicin (rifampin) is now gaining favor because it is bactericidal and is effective against several of the atypicals.

Other agents that have been used include capreomycin, cycloserine, ethionamide, kanamycin, pyrazinamide and viomycin.

The aims of chemotherapy in tuberculosis are to render the patient noninfectious and then to achieve tissue sterilization or cure. The therapy schedules are variable and depend on clinical judgment, but usually for an active case the patient is hospitalized, cultures are taken for sensitivity testing and then a three-drug regimen with concurrent courses of SM, PAS (or ethambutol) and INH is started. This course reduces the probability of selecting drug-resistant mutants of *M. tuberculosis* and provides a latitude for change if drug toxicity or drug hypersensitivity develops in the patient. The effectiveness of the treatment is monitored clinically as well as by smears and cultures of the sputum. As soon as practical, the patient is released from the hospital and his treatment continues on an outpatient basis. Treatment usually extends over a minimum of 2 years with a gradual reduction in the number of drugs, but with INH usually used through the entire period. If the therapy can be maintained through good patient compliance, tuberculosis is almost always successfully treated. Any of the above therapeutic agents may have adverse effects on the patient with varying degrees of severity. These can include nausea, vomiting, diarrhea, eighth nerve damage, optic neuritis, liver damage, renal damage, blood dyscrasias or hypersensitivity. Thus the patient must be monitored with appropriate laboratory tests and clinical observation throughout treatment so that any necessary changes in therapy can be initiated.

The other mycobacteria which cause disease in man (atypicals, unclassified) are frequently resistant to most of the antitubercular drugs with the possible exception of rifampicin. However, resistance is strain-variable, so sensitivity testing should be done as a guide to therapy.

LABORATORY PROCEDURES

MATERIALS. — Sputum, gastric lavage and urine (all early morning specimens) are the usual materials. Other specimens could include cerebrospinal fluid, pleural or peritoneal exudate, swabs from various sources or feces. Where possible, specimens (minimum of three and preferably six) should be collected on successive days. It is important that specimens be taken to the laboratory as soon after collection as possible. Sputum, not saliva or nasal discharge, must be submitted. Sputum is the material brought up from the lungs in conjunction with a productive cough. For the initial work-up, all specimens should be collected before starting chemotherapy.

CONCENTRATION. — Many of the materials to be examined are viscous and often contain vast numbers of normal flora organisms. Procedures are employed to liquefy the specimens, kill most of the other kinds of bacteria (normal flora and contaminants) and sediment the acid-fast bacilli into a small volume. Either the NaOH or the N-acetyl-L-cysteine method is used, with the latter being preferred. Procedural details for concentration, staining, cultivation, and antibiotic sensitivities will not be given but can be found in various laboratory manuals (references, chap. 4).

STAINING.—The sediment from the concentrate is smeared onto slides, heat-fixed and stained by the Ziehl-Neelsen procedure. Acid-fast organisms retain the red basic fuchsin even after decolorization with acid-alcohol. Other more sophisticated techniques can be done, such as fluorochrome staining with auramine or the direct fluorescent antibody technique (chap. 4), which will specifically identify the organism; both will reduce the microscope time required to detect a positive smear. Results from staining can usually be obtained on the same day that the specimen is collected.

CULTIVATION.—Many different media have been devised to grow the tubercle bacillus, with the two most widely used being Löwenstein-Jensen and Middlebrook 7H10. Both are quite complex but yield good growth. Two tubes, one tube each of different kinds of media, are inoculated rather heavily with the sediment from the concentrate and incubated at 37 C in 5% CO_2. It is important to recall that *M. tuberculosis takes 4 to 6 weeks to grow*. Specific identification can be made using the niacin, nitrate and catalase tests (see Table 11–1). Pathogenicity for the guinea pig is also demonstrable.

ANTIBIOTIC SENSITIVITIES.—Susceptibility or resistance to streptomycin, isoniazid, para-aminosalicylic acid or other chemotherapeutic agents can be tested by using dilutions of the chemotherapeutic agent in plates of media. Results are reported on the basis of the culture being susceptible, intermediate or resistant. These may also take 6 weeks or more.

LEPROSY

For 15 centuries or more leprosy has been a most feared disease and has caused people to be ostracized from society. The etiologic agent, *M. leprae*, was described by Hansen in 1874. However, reports of culture of the organism in vitro have provoked continual controversy, and in vitro growth has not been proved; but there is agreement on etiology and that the disease is contracted from a leprous individual.

There are an estimated 10–11 million cases of leprosy or Hansen's disease throughout the world, with the greatest incidence in India, China, Africa, South America and the islands of the South Pacific, although few regions are actually exempt. Between 80 and 150 cases are reported each year in the United States. The Leprosarium in the United States is in Carville, La. Man is the only known source of the disease, with transmission by direct contact with a patient with lepromatous leprosy. It is thought that transmission is via aerosols, but the portal of entry is not established. The incubation period may be from a few months to as long as 30 years. Clinically the disease is divided into three types — lepromatous, tuberculoid and intermediate leprosy — which relate to the level of resistance of the host.

LEPROMATOUS LEPROSY. — This type is progressive and indicates a lack of host resistance. Early in the disease there is conspicuous involvement of the skin with macular or nodular lesions, and as the disease progresses the peripheral nerve trunks become involved as indicated by loss of senses of pain or touch. This nerve involvement tends to be bilateral and relatively symmetric. Loss of eyebrows is common (Fig. 11–6). If untreated, the disease worsens, with bacterial cells usually readily demonstrable in smears from skin lesions or in biopsies. There is a continuous bacteremia approximating 10^5 bacilli per milliliter, as demonstrated by smears of peripheral blood. Histologically, the organisms are found intracellularly in foamy histiocytes; lymphocytes are rarely present. The lepromin test is negative.

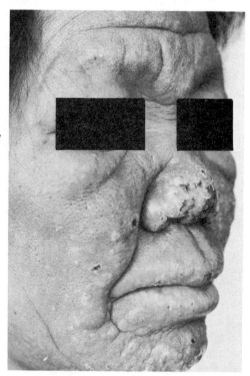

Fig. 11–6. — Lepromatous leprosy. Note the nodular lesions and the loss of eyebrows. (From Arnold, H. L., and Fasal, P.: *Leprosy, Diagnosis and Management* [Springfield, Ill.: Charles C Thomas, Publisher, 1973]. By permission of authors and publisher.)

TUBERCULOID LEPROSY.—This type is usually benign and frequently self-limited because of the cell-mediated immune defenses of the host. In most cases the skin lesions are erythematous, marginally elevated plaques. There is extension to the peripheral nerves causing sensory or motor nerve symptoms, but usually only one or two nerves are involved which may become thickened or nodular and can be palpated. In some instances this nerve damage is rapid and complete, resulting in a disabling deformity. Bacilli are usually not demonstrable in smears or biopsies. Histologically, the lesions are tuberculoid granulomas with epithelioid cells, giant cells and lymphocytes, but usually without organisms. The lepromin test is positive.

INTERMEDIATE LEPROSY.—This is a benign form with flat hypopigmented or erythematous skin lesions. Neuritic manifestations may occur and persist for long periods. These cases may progress to lepromatous or tuberculoid types, or remain unchanged indefinitely. Bacilli are usually not demonstrable in smears or biopsies. The histologic features usually are not definitive and foam cells or a granulomatous reaction is not present. The lepromin test is usually negative or may be weakly positive.

Lepromin Test (Mitsuda test)

This test was introduced by Mitsuda in 1923 when he used a ground-up mixture of autoclaved tissue containing *M. leprae* as a skin test antigen. Such a suspension is injected intracutaneously, and if positive a nodular area of induration 5–10 mm in diameter develops within 3 to 4 weeks. A positive test in conjunction with clinical and histologic evidence is a diagnostic and prognostic aid. The major problems with general use have been difficulties in obtaining standardized suspensions of the bacilli and the occurrence of a false positive reaction in 3% to 75% of noninfected individuals.

Mechanism of Pathogenicity

An understanding of the pathogenetic mechanisms involved in leprosy has been difficult because of inability to grow the bacilli and because of the absence of an experimental model. However, infection of the armadillo results in a model analogous to lepromatous leprosy in man. Skinsnes and co-workers have recently reported isolation and growth of *M. leprae* in vitro. If this work is confirmed, a clearer understanding of pathogenesis should be obtained.

Man is very resistant to the disease as evidenced by difficulty in establishing infections in man and by the long incubation period (average 2–7 years) before signs of the disease. The generation time for M. leprae is about 20 – 30 days, which correlates with slow onset of the disease. M. leprae has a predilection for peripheral body sites, suggesting that the optimum temperature for growth is 30 C. This temperature requirement could explain the absence of lesions in internal organs.

Based on tissue response, the type of clinical disease appears to be dependent on the resistance of the host. For example, in tuberculoid leprosy there is histologic evidence of an immune response, and few organisms are seen in the lesion. However, in lepromatous leprosy, the most severe form of the disease, lymphocytes are rarely seen and numerous organisms are present. The lack of resistance in the lepromatous form of the disease is confirmed by the demonstration of a continuous bacteremia (approximately 10^5/ml of blood) and the presence of large numbers of bacilli in the skin (approximately 10^8/gm) and nasal secretions (10^7/ml). Patients with lepromatous leprosy also do not show hypersensitivity to the lepromin skin test. This correlates with studies which show a decreased number of T cells in peripheral blood, a defective response to mitogens, failure to release MIF and increased survival time of skin homografts. In addition, the presence of chemotactic factor inhibitor (CFI), an inhibitor that acts directly on the C3 and C5 chemotactic factors, correlates with defective skin reactivity.

The bactericidal function of phagocytic cells is the same in patients with lepromatous and tuberculoid leprosy as in normal subjects.

Treatment

Patients with newly diagnosed leprosy should be hospitalized for the initiation of treatment and then, as in tuberculosis, be treated continually on an outpatient basis with dapsone or DDS (4,4′ diamino diphenylsulfone) administered orally. The dosage usually begins at 20 mg/week and slowly progresses to 50 to 100 mg/day for a minimum of 5 years and in some cases for life. Children living with leprous parents should be given dapsone prophylactically for 3 years. More recently rifampicin, either alone or in combination with dapsone, has been shown effective.

Indices for effectiveness of drug treatment include clinical improvement and determination of the morphological index of the bacilli in smears. Smears from skin lesions should be examined at 4- to 6-week intervals, and in cases of favorable response the organisms should show a progressive increase in the numbers of irregularly stained (dead) cells. This irregular staining should begin within 6 months.

Laboratory Aids to Diagnosis

Smears should be made from the edge of the earlobe or from a fold of skin at the margin of a skin lesion. This is done by making a small incision, scraping the edge of the incision, smearing it onto a slide and staining it with an acid-fast procedure. Acid-fast smears of nasal scrapings can also be used. Reports are made in terms of the numbers of bacilli per field and also the morphological index, which is reported on the basis of the number of solidly staining bacilli per 100 organisms. This correlates with the number of living bacilli present and may be used to follow the response to therapy. Punch biopsies of active lesions, taken entirely within the lesion, should also be done. These will determine the type of tissue reaction, as well as the presence or absence of *M. leprae*. Cultures of biopsy tissue or scrapings are negative.

Although cultures are negative, experimental infections can be produced in the footpads of mice and in the armadillo. The footpad technique can be used as an aid to diagnosis or to follow treatment, although it is a time-consuming procedure, taking at least 5 months to establish an infection. The technique is more useful in testing the action of drugs or in evaluating possible vaccines.

PROBLEM SOLVING AND REVIEW

GIVEN: — A 36-year-old man was admitted to the hospital because of low back pain. Two months previously he had had gross hematuria, after which the back pain developed. His physical examination revealed no abnormal findings. Chest roentgenogram showed a rounded calcified area in the right lung and a calcified hilar lymph node. An intravenous pyelogram showed a small calcified area in the left kidney. The right kidney and ureter were normal. There was a marked decrease in function of the left kidney. Acid-fast smears from sputum and urine were negative. The tuberculin test was strongly positive. Surgery was performed and the left kidney was removed. Smears of urine taken at surgery were positive for acid-fast bacilli. Cultures from the urine and kidney were positive for *Mycobacterium tuberculosis* in 6 weeks. The patient finally indicated that in the past he had had spells of severe coughing and night sweats. He was started on isoniazid and ethambutol, which were to be continued for at least 2 years.

PROBLEMS: — 1. How could this type of infection develop? 2. Should additional epidemiologic studies be done? 3. What is the rationale behind multiple drug therapy? 4. How is the tuberculin test read? 5. What is the significance of the positive tuberculin test? 6. How would you identify *M. tuberculosis?* (Ans. p. 237.)

SUPPLEMENTARY READING

Arnold, H. L., and Fasal, P.: *Leprosy. Diagnosis and Management* (2d ed.; Springfield, Ill.: Charles C Thomas, Publisher, 1973).
Barksdale, L., and Kim, K. S.: Mycobacterium, Bacteriol. Rev. 41:217, 1977.
Daniel, T. M., and Janick, B. W.: Mycobacterial antigens: a review of their isolation, chemistry, and immunological properties, Microbiol. Rev. 42:84, 1978.
Dannenberg, A. M.: Macrophages in inflammation and infection, N. Engl. J. Med. 293:489–493, 1975.
Drutz, D. J., Cline, M. J., and Levy, L.: Leukocyte antimicrobial function in patients with leprosy, J. Clin. Invest. 53:380–386, 1974.
Goren, M. B.: Mycobacterial lipids. Selected topics, Bacteriol. Rev. 36:33–64, 1972.
Jopling, W. H.: Leprosy, Practitioner 207:164–172, 1971.
Lederer, E.: The mycobacterial cell wall, Pure Appl. Chem. 25:135–165, 1971.
Rich, A. R.: *The Pathogenesis of Tuberculosis* (2d ed.; Springfield, Ill.: Charles C Thomas, Publisher, 1951).
Riley, R. L., Mills, C. C., O'Grady, F., Sultan, L. U., Wittstadt, F., and Shivpuri, D. N.: Infectiousness of air from a tuberculosis ward, Am. Rev. Respir. Dis. 85:511–525, 1962.
Runyon, E. H., Wayne, L. G., and Kubica, G. P.: Family *Mycobacteriaceae,* in Buchanan, R. E., and Gibbons, N. E. (eds.): *Bergey's Manual of Determinative Bacteriology,* vol. 8 (Baltimore: Williams & Wilkins Co., 1974).
Shan, S. A., and Neff, T. A.: Miliary tuberculosis, Am. J. Med. 56:495–505, 1974.
Skinsnes, O. K., Matsuo, E., Chang, P. H. C., and Andersson, B.: In vitro cultivation of leprosy bacilli on hyaluronic acid bared medium. I. Preliminary report, Int. J. Leprosy 43:193–203, 1975.
Smith, D. T.: Isoniazid prophylaxis and BCG vaccination in the control of tuberculosis, Arch. Environ. Health 23:235–242, 1971.
Storrs, E. E., Walsh, G. P., Burchfield, H. P., and Binford, C. H.: Leprosy in the armadillo. A new model for biomedical research, Science 183:851, 1974.
Ward, P. A., Goralnick, S., and Bullock, W. E.: Defective leukotaxis in patients with lepromatous leprosy, J. Lab. Clin. Med. 87:1025–1032, 1976.
Wolinsky, E.: Bacteriologic standards for the discharge of patients, Am. Rev. Respir. Dis. 102:470–473, 1970.
Youmans, A. S., and Youmans, G. P.: The relationship between sedimentation value and immunogenicity activity of mycobacterial ribonucleic acid, J. Immunol. 110:581–586, 1973.
Youmans, G. P., and Youmans, A. S.: Recent studies on acquired immunity in tuberculosis, Curr. Top. Microbiol. Immunol. 48:129–178, 1969.

ANALYSIS

1. This is uncertain, but it is likely a hematogenous spread from reactivation of his pulmonary infection. 2. Members of the household should be tuberculin tested and have chest roentgenograms. 3. This reduces the chances of selection of resistant strains. 4. The diameter of the area of induration is determined with 10 mm or more being positive; the size or degree of the inflammatory reaction is not significant. 5. It simply means that a hypersensitivity state exists but does not differentiate between active or inactive infection. 6. Acid-fast rod, slow growing, forms buff-colored, rough colonies, niacin positive and pathogenic for laboratory animals.

12 / Actinomyces and Nocardia

Overview

The organisms of this genus produce branching filaments at some stage of their growth, although they more commonly have a diphtheroid morphology. The generic name *Actinomyces* (ray-fungus) was derived from the observation of the fungus-like filaments in specimens from "lumpy jaw" of cattle. The misconception that these organisms were fungi was perpetuated until, on the basis of cell wall composition and sensitivity to antibacterial antibiotics, they were shown to be bacteria. This genus includes five species (*A. bovis, A. israelii, A. naeslundii, A. odontolyticus* and *A. viscosus*) which can be differentiated biochemically and serologically. However, this chapter deals primarily with *A. israelii*, the principal cause of human actinomycosis. The possible role of *A. viscosus* and *A. naeslundii* in causing caries and periodontal disease is also discussed. *A. bovis*, which causes lumpy jaw in cattle, has not been isolated from humans.

Characteristics and Species

The actinomycetes are gram-positive, non-acid-fast, nonmotile and non-spore-forming organisms. They occur as rods or filaments that branch, but most frequently in diphtheroidal arrangements with palisades, Y, V and T forms (Fig. 12–1). They are facultative anaerobes growing best in the presence of CO_2. Except for *A. viscosus*, catalase is not produced. Acids are produced from carbohydrates; the end products of glucose fermentation are acetic, formic, lactic and succinic acids. Propionic acid is not produced. *A. israelii* produces filamentous "spider" microcolonies and "molar-toothed" macrocolonies (Figs. 12–2, 12–3, 12–4). Another organism that morphologically and culturally resembles these actinomycetes is *Arachnia propionica*. It is differentiated on the basis of producing propionic acid from glucose, having diaminopimelic acid in the cell wall and being serologically distinct. It can cause actinomycosis as well as lacrimal canaliculitis.

239

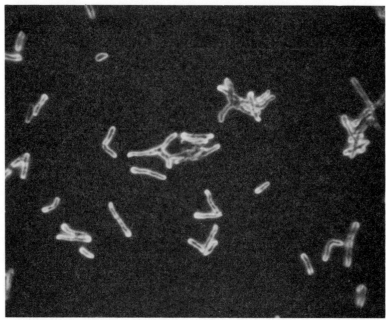

Fig. 12–1.—Darkfield preparation of *Actinomyces israelii*. Note the Y and V forms or diphtheroidal arrangements, which are the typical morphological type of the actinomycetes, particularly when growing in a broth medium. (From Slack, J. M., and Gerencser, M. A.: *Actinomyces, Filamentous Bacteria: Biology and Pathogenicity* [Minneapolis: Burgess Publishing Co., 1975]. Used by permission.)

Fig. 12–2.—Filamentous microcolony or "spider" colony of *A. israelii*. (From Slack, J. M., and Gerencser, M. A.: *Actinomyces, Filamentous Bacteria: Biology and Pathogenicity* [Minneapolis: Burgess Publishing Co., 1975]. Used by permission.)

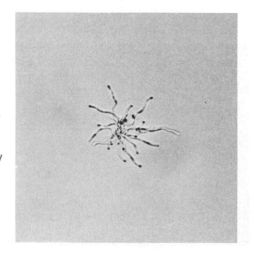

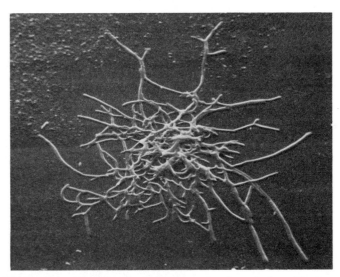

Fig. 12–3.—Scanning electron micrograph of an *A. israelii* microcolony. (From Slack, J. M., and Gerencser, M. A.: *Actinomyces, Filamentous Bacteria: Biology and Pathogenicity* [Minneapolis: Burgess Publishing Co., 1975]. Used by permission.)

Ecology

All species, except *A. bovis*, are inhabitants of the human oral cavity, and thus the source of infection is endogenous. In studies of dental plaque from a series of individuals using the fluorescent antibody technique, *A. israelii* were found in 96% of the specimens with two or more species of actinomycetes in all specimens.

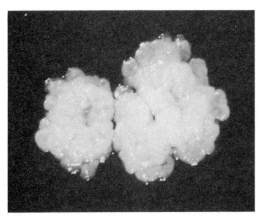

Fig. 12–4.—Mature "molar-toothed" colony of *A. israelii*. (From Slack, J. M., and Gerencser, M. A.: *Actinomyces, Filamentous Bacteria: Biology and Pathogenicity* [Minneapolis: Burgess Publishing Co., 1975]. Used by permission.)

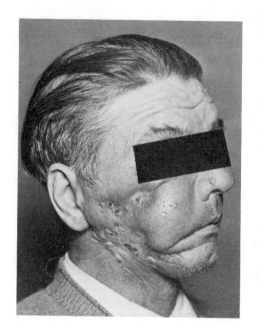

Fig. 12–5.—Cervicofacial actinomycosis. (From Slack, J. M., and Gerencser, M. A.: *Actinomyces, Filamentous Bacteria: Biology and Pathogenicity* [Minneapolis: Burgess Publishing Co., 1975]. Used by permission.)

Actinomycosis

This is a chronic granulomatous disease characterized by suppuration, abscess formation and draining sinuses. Clinically, the disease is usually cervicofacial, thoracic or abdominal, although any organ or area including the central nervous system, bone and skin may be involved. The cervicofacial type of actinomycosis (Fig. 12–5) is the most common. It begins with the organisms entering the tissue from the oral cavity through trauma, such as extraction of a tooth. A persistent swelling develops in the parotid or mandibular region, and the overlying skin often has a reddish purple cast. One or more draining sinuses then develop which discharge a yellowish thick or serous exudate. If the exudate is examined microscopically, the characteristic sulfur granules, which contain branching filaments and peripherally arranged hyaline clubs, can be found.

Mechanisms of Pathogenicity

The actinomycetes produce no toxins or antiphagocytic factors and only a limited number of proteolytic enzymes. Thus they must rely primarily on their ability to grow and successfully compete with cells and tissue for nutrients. In depriving the tissue of nutrients, they cause death of cells and tissue, resulting in necrosis. The filamentous growth could aid survival of the organisms by being a deterrent to phagocytosis. The sulfur granules could be antiphagocytic, and they may interfere with the penetration of antibiotics into the lesion.

As indicated, various species of *Actinomyces* are present in plaque, and thus may be instrumental in plaque formation by two mechanisms: first, by adhering to the pellicle, a protein-salts film which forms on tooth surfaces, and second, by the filaments providing an extensive surface for adherence of numerous other organisms. These two possibilities have experimental support in that both *A. viscosus* and *A. naeslundii* adhere to wire and tooth enamel surfaces forming "in vitro plaque." Actinomycete filaments have been shown to have cocci and rods adhering to the filaments in sections or electron micrographs of plaque. Thus, being a stable member of the plaque microbial population, they contribute to caries formation through acid production from carbohydrates, and to periodontal diseases through complement activation.

The actual factors causing caries are not well established but acidity does play a role. The actinomycetes will lower the pH of glucose broth to pH 4.5 or below, and it is likely that they contribute to the overall acidity of the environment. Less is known about the pathogenesis of periodontal disease, but it has been shown that the polysaccharides of *A. viscosus* will activate complement, resulting in production of chemotactic factors and the migration of phagocytes. Release of lysosomal enzymes from these phagocytes as they lyse may amplify the inflammatory reaction by action of the hydrolases on tissue and on C3 by generation of C3a and C3b.

After trauma to the oral cavity, the cervicofacial infection spreads by direct continuity to the adjacent areas of the face and neck or via the bloodstream to other organs or tissue. Thoracic actinomycosis results from aspiration of material from the oral cavity or by direct extension of a facial or abdominal infection. Abdominal actinomycosis usually develops as the result of an acute perforative gastrointestinal disease (appendicitis or ulcerative diseases). In both of these the development of draining sinuses with sulfur granules is typical.

There is a limited antibody response in actinomycosis, and presumably active immunity does not develop. Treatment is with either antibiotics alone or a combination of antibiotics and surgical drainage. Penicillin is the antibiotic of choice, but massive doses over a prolonged period of time are required for successful therapy.

Laboratory Procedures

In actinomycosis, the materials usually collected are pus or exudates from draining sinuses, or sputum. These should be poured into a Petri dish and examined for the presence of hard yellowish-to-white

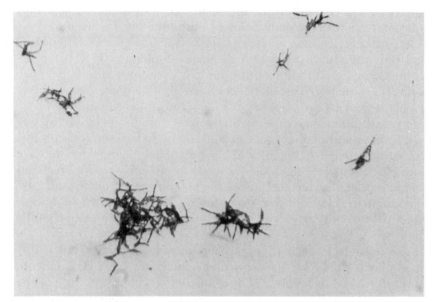

Fig. 12–6.—Gram stain of a broth culture of *Actinomyces israelii.* Note the short filaments with irregular staining and some branching. (From Slack, J. M., and Gerencser, M. A.: *Actinomyces, Filamentous Bacteria: Biology and Pathogenicity* [Minneapolis: Burgess Publishing Co., 1975]. Used by permission.)

granules. Sulfur granules are not always present. One or more of the granules should be transferred to a slide, crushed, smeared and stained by gram's and acid-fast procedures. The presence of gram-positive, non-acid-fast, branching filaments permits a tentative identification as an *Actinomyces* (Fig. 12–6). If conjugated antiserum is available, a specific identification of both genus and species can be made using the direct FA procedure (chap. 4). For cultivation, washed crushed granules or portions of the pus or sputum are inoculated into thioglycolate broth containing rabbit serum and streaked onto Brain Heart Infusion agar and blood agar plates. All cultures are incubated at 37 C but the plates are incubated anaerobically with CO_2. The plates are examined in 12 to 24 hours for filamentous microcolonies which can then be reported as *Actinomyces*. Otherwise, cultures are kept for 5 to 7 days for development of molar-toothed macrocolonies with identification on the basis of morphological features, biochemical reactions, FA findings, and even end products from glucose fermentation or a cell wall analysis.

NOCARDIA

Overview. These are filamentous organisms that are aerobic and acid-fast. The principal pathogen is *Nocardia asteroides*, a pulmonary opportunist with a predilection to cause brain abscesses. As nocardiae are not normal inhabitants of the oropharynx or intestinal tract, a report of their isolation from sputum, exudate or any other material should be considered as indicating an infection.

Characteristics and Species

Three species can cause infections in man: *N. asteroides*, *N. brasiliensis* and *N. caviae*. They are all aerobic, filamentous, acid-fast, non-spore-forming organisms; sometimes the staining is irregular or partial (Fig. 12–7). In cultures, the filaments often fragment into bacillary or coccoid elements. Colonies are variable in appearance and may be buff, orange, red or brown. With age they may turn white due to the formation of white aerial hyphae. Nocardiae produce acid from carbohydrates oxidatively and use a wide variety of compounds, including hydrocarbons, as a source of carbon. They contain diaminopimelic acid, arabinose, galactose and nocardomycolic acid in the cell wall. The hydrolysis of casein, tyrosine and xanthine is used in species differentiation. *N. asteroides* does not hydrolyze any of these substrates, *N. brasiliensis* hydrolyzes both casein and tyrosine and *N. caviae* hydrolyzes only xanthine.

Fig. 12–7.—Acid-fast stain of a smear from a brain abscess showing the acid-fast, filamentous *Nocardia asteroides*.

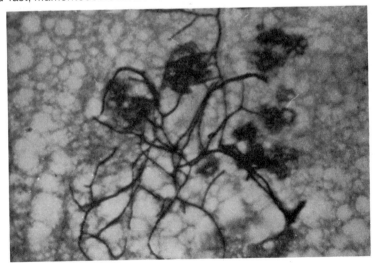

Ecology

Nocardia are inhabitants of the soil and are not normally found in the oral or nasal cavities or in the intestinal tract. Thus if they are isolated, for instance, from sputum, this evidence should be taken as indicating an infection until proven otherwise.

Nocardiosis

The *Nocardia* can cause three clinical manifestations: systemic nocardiosis, mycetoma and a lymphocutaneous syndrome. Systemic involvement is due almost entirely to *N. asteroides. N. brasiliensis* and *N. caviae* cause mycetomas. *N. brasiliensis* causes the lymphocutaneous syndrome which may be transitory, acute or chronic, localized or disseminated. Clinically, it may simulate bronchopneumonia, tuberculosis, lung abscess or neoplasm. Pathologically, it is characterized by acute necrosis with abscess formation. About 30% of the infections remain pulmonary, but they can metastasize to any tissue or organ of the body. There is a predilection for the central nervous system, particularly the brain, where single or multiple abscesses may develop (Figs. 12–7, 12–8). Other organs can be involved including the

Fig. 12–8.—Brain abscess from a case of nocardiosis. Smears and cultures were positive for *N. asteroides.* (From Emmons, C. W., Binford, C. H., and Utz, J. P.: *Medical Mycology* [Philadelphia: Lea & Febiger, 1970]. With permission of author and publisher.)

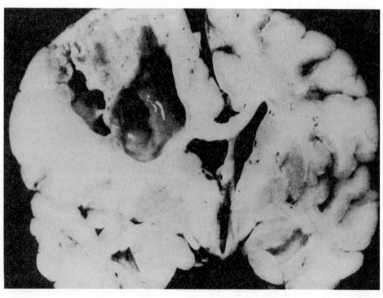

kidney, eye, skin, liver, spleen, adrenals and intestines. Mortality still approximates 45%.

Mycetomas are more common in Africa and India but have been reported from many other countries, including the United States. These are chronic, localized infections of the subcutaneous tissue which form granulomatous masses with the development of abscesses and draining sinuses. The pus may contain granules that can be white, yellow, red, brown or black. Any one of a number of organisms can cause mycetomas, including *Streptomyces, Madurella, Cephalosporium, Phialophora, N. brasiliensis* and *N. caviae*. The organisms are introduced into the skin by thorns, splinters or abrasions, and the infection usually occurs in the lower extremities. The lymphocutaneous syndrome has just recently been described, and it resembles sporotrichosis with inflamed lymphatics and involved lymph nodes. Only *N. brasiliensis* has been reported as a cause of this infection.

The sulfonamides, particularly sulfadiazine, for a prolonged period, are the drugs of choice for treatment. Other antimicrobials have been used with or without sulfonamides, including ampicillin, cycloserine, streptomycin, trimethoprim and minocycline with variable success. Penicillin is of no value. An antibiogram should be done on each isolate to determine antimicrobial sensitivities. Surgical intervention may be necessary. The prognosis is good for patients with pulmonary disease but poor in compromised patients and in those with meningitis.

Mechanisms of Pathogenicity

The *Nocardia* do not produce toxins. The cellular products are not antiphagocytic, although the filamentous growth makes phagocytosis difficult. They can produce a hypersensitivity which could prompt an inflammatory response. Their ability to survive and metabolize in tissue is probably the principal mechanism causing inflammation and necrosis.

Laboratory Procedures

In nocardiosis the specimens collected usually include sputum, bronchial washings, pus, exudate or cerebrospinal fluid; the sputum should not be digested. The material can be spread in a Petri dish and observed for clumps of organisms or granules; *N. asteroides* rarely forms granules, but *N. brasiliensis* and *N. caviae* form white or yellow granules with clubs. Smears are prepared; one is stained by gram's and the other by Kinyoun's acid-fast stain. Filamentous, gram-positive organisms that have variable degrees of acid fastness are identified presumptively as *Nocardia*.

Cultivation is done on plates of Brain Heart Infusion and blood agar aerobically at 37 C. Growth is usually detectable within 4 to 7 days; otherwise, observations are maintained for 3 weeks. The colonies are quite variable in both color and consistency, but most frequently they are buff colored and rather friable. Final identification depends on the results of a battery of tests, including oxidation but not fermentation of sugars, and hydrolysis of casein, tyrosine and xanthine. Animal pathogenicity studies may also be done.

PROBLEM SOLVING AND REVIEW

GIVEN: — A 71-year-old man with a reticulum cell sarcoma involving the root of the mesentery was treated with cyclophosphamide and prednisone, and the patient improved and gained weight. Then he developed a fever with chills and nonproductive cough and was hospitalized. A chest roentgenogram showed a questionable nodular density in the right lower lung and a small infiltrate in the right middle lung. The heart was normal, the liver was slightly enlarged, and the spleen was not palpable. The white blood cell count was 8,100/cu mm, with 2% atypical lymphocytes; enzymes and immunoglobulins were within normal ranges. Tuberculin test was negative. Blood and urine cultures were negative. The 48-hour sputum cultures showed normal flora; in 5 days a few colonies of an aerobic, filamentous acid-fast organism were observed. A needle biopsy of the lesion showed acid-fast organisms. A repeat x-ray film showed definite cavitation of the lesion in the right lower lobe. Intravenous sulfathiazole was begun along with isoniazid; after 5 days isoniazid was replaced by minocycline. The patient improved and within 3 weeks the pulmonary lesion had regressed.

PROBLEMS: — 1. What was the most probable cause of the pulmonary lesion? 2. What would be the source of such an organism? 3. What conditions favored the onset of such an infection? 4. What other organ is this organism likely to infect? 5. Is the disease transmissible from the infected person? 6. How would you culture and identify this organism? 7. What relationship in the cell wall does this organism have with *Mycobacterium* and *Corynebacterium*? (Ans. p. 249.)

SUPPLEMENTARY READING

Berd, D.: Laboratory identification of clinically important anaerobic actinomycetes, Appl. Microbiol. 25:665–681, 1973.
Berd, D.: *Nocardia brasiliensis* infection in the United States, Am. J. Clin. Pathol. 60:254–258, 1973.

ANALYSIS 249

Eastridge, C. E., Prather, J. R., Hughes, F. A., Young, J. M., and McCaughan, J. J.: Actinomycosis: A 24 year experience, South. Med. J. 65:839–843, 1972.
Harvey, J. C., Cantrell, J. R., and Fisher, A. M.: Actinomycosis: Its recognition and treatment, Ann. Intern. Med. 46:868–885, 1957.
Hoeprich, P. D., Brandt, D., and Parker, R. H.: Nocardial brain abscess cured with cycloserine and sulfonamides, Am. J. Med. Sci. 255:208–216, 1968.
Murray, J. F., Finegold, S. M., Froman, S., and Will, D. W.: The changing spectrum of nocardiosis, Am. Rev. Respir. Dis. 83:315–330, 1961.
Slack, J. M., and Gerencser, M. A.: *Actinomyces, Filamentous Bacteria. Biology and Pathogenicity* (Minneapolis: Burgess Publishing Company, 1975).
Slack, J. M., Landfried, S., and Gerencser, M. A.: Morphological, biochemical and serological studies on 64 strains of *Actinomyces israelii*, J. Bacteriol. 97: 873–884, 1969.

ANALYSIS

1. The staining, morphological features and aerobic growth indicate *Nocardia asteroides*. 2. Most likely the soil; human carriers have not been established. 3. The sarcoma and the cytotoxic drugs acted as immunosuppressants, allowing an opportunistic organism to become invasive. 4. The brain. 5. No. 6. Aerobic, filamentous, acid-fast rod which does not hydrolyze casein, tyrosine or xanthine. 7. Nocardomycolic acid in the cell wall.

13 / Enterics, Endotoxins and Enterotoxins

OVERVIEW

The enteric organisms, i.e., the gram-negative bacilli that normally colonize the intestinal tract, have become increasingly important in human disease. This is due to several factors: their presence in man and animals as part of the normal flora, their relative resistance to antibiotics and their ability to survive in the environment. In a patient population whose normal defense mechanisms are impaired by disease or altered via treatment with immunosuppressive drugs or instruments or who have received contaminated drugs, solutions or instruments, gram-negative infection becomes a serious problem. It is estimated that one case of bacteremia due to gram-negative organisms occurs in each 100 hospital admissions. This results in the death of about 100,000 patients each year either directly or indirectly from the infection. This estimate is conservative—the actual number of deaths is probably higher.

Similarities in cultural, physiologic, and serologic properties have made it difficult for the clinical microbiologist and the physician to understand the importance of these organisms. Also, the ability of these organisms to become resistant has created problems in treatment.

In recent years, studies on mode of action of endotoxin, the demonstration and study of enterotoxins and the recognition and importance of R factors have contributed to a partial understanding of this complex group of organisms.

GENERAL CHARACTERISTICS OF ENTERICS

The family Enterobacteriaceae contains the small (0.5×3 μm) aerobic or facultatively anaerobic gram-negative rods (Fig. 13-1). They may be motile by peritrichate flagella or nonmotile. Capsules are present on some; spores are not formed. Indophenol oxidase is not pro-

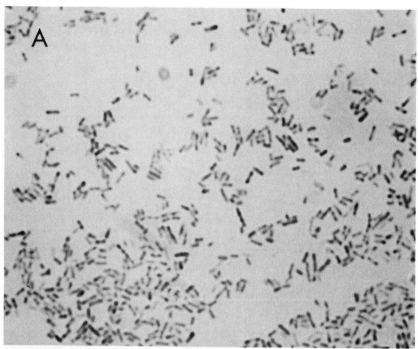

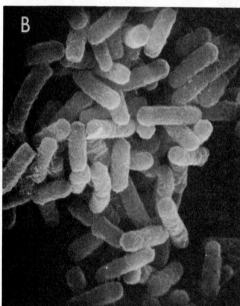

Fig. 13–1. — *E. coli* as observed by conventional light microscopy **(A)** and by scanning electron microscopy **(B)**. (Courtesy of Ruff, R. M., and Allender, P., West Virginia University Medical Center.)

duced. Most grow rapidly on noncomplex media over a wide range of temperatures. Acid is produced from the fermentation of glucose. Usually aerogenic but some anaerogenic strains occur.

CLASSIFICATION AND GENERA

The classification of the family Enterobacteriaceae is complicated because of overlapping serologic, morphological, cultural and biochemical properties. Two classification systems are presently in use and add to this confusion (Table 13–1). The student should be familiar with both systems until there is general acceptance of one or the other.

One of the major differences between the two classification systems is the collapsing of the tribes Escherichieae, Edwardsielleae and Salmonelleae (Ewing classification) into a single tribe Escherichieae. Also, the genus *Arizona* is recognized as a species of *Salmonella (S. arizonae)* in Bergey's classification. The tribe Proteeae remains in both classification systems, but the genus *Providencia* is assigned to the genus *Proteus* as a new species *(Proteus inconstans)* in the classification proposed in the 8th edition of *Bergey's Manual of Determinative Bacteriology.* The genus *Pectobacterium* has been eliminated in Bergey's classification, and these organisms have been assigned to the

TABLE 13–1.—CLASSIFICATION OF
ENTEROBACTERIACEAE

Bergey's Manual —8TH ED.		EWING CLASSIFICATION	
TRIBE	GENUS	TRIBE	GENUS
Escherichieae	*Escherichia* *Edwardsiella* *Citrobacter* *Salmonella* *Shigella*	Escherichieae Edwardsielleae Salmonelleae	*Escherichia* *Shigella* *Edwardsiella* *Salmonella* *Arizona* *Citrobacter*
Klebsielleae	*Klebsiella* *Enterobacter* *Hafnia* *Serratia*	Klebsielleae	*Klebsiella* *Enterobacter* *Serratia*
Proteeae	*Proteus*	Proteeae	*Proteus* *Providencia*
Erwinieae	*Erwinia*	Erwineae	*Erwinia* *Pectobacterium*
Yersinieae	*Yersinia*		

TABLE 13-2.—SEPARATION OF THE ENTERICS
BASED ON LACTOSE FERMENTATION

RAPID LACTOSE FERMENTERS	SLOW OR NON-LACTOSE FERMENTERS	
Escherichia	Proteus	Arizona
Klebsiella	Providencia	Yersinia
Enterobacter	Citrobacter	Salmonella
	Serratia	Shigella

genus *Erwinia*. A significant change in the classification was the addition of a new tribe Yersinieae to the family Enterobacteriaceae.

Differentiation among the "enterics" is based on physiologic characteristics, e.g., fermentation of lactose and other carbohydrates, presence or absence of enzymes such as urease, ability to grow on certain
substrates, end products formed after growth and serologic properties.
The enterics can be divided into two groups based on ability or inability to ferment lactose (Table 13-2). As a general statement, the
frank pathogens are non-lactose fermenters, whereas the opportunists
are both lactose and non-lactose fermenters. For example, the genera
Salmonella, Shigella, certain strains of *Escherichia coli* and *Yersinia*
are frank pathogens and cause serious intestinal diseases. The remaining enterics are opportunists.

The genera *Escherichia, Klebsiella* and *Enterobacter* are commonly
termed coliforms.

ECOLOGY

The enterics are commonly found in and on man. *Escherichia coli* is
the major organism constituting the facultative organisms of the intestinal tract, but it must be stressed that the strict anaerobes (chap. 8) are
the most numerous. *Klebsiella pneumoniae* is found as part of the
normal flora of the upper respiratory tract in a small percentage of the
population. Most of these organisms are also found in animals, on
plants, and in soil and water.

As normal flora, they play a role in the antagonisms that prevent colonization with pathogenic microorganisms. They synthesize important vitamins and have been shown to deconjugate bile acids. Obviously, these organisms do not play a passive role but are important
in the health of man.

CELL WALL

The cell wall of gram-negative bacteria consists of two layers, the
peptidoglycan layer and the outer membrane, and is described in

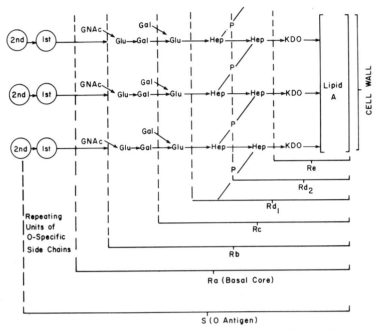

Fig. 13–2.—Chemotypes of lipopolysaccharides isolated from smooth and mutant forms of *Salmonella minnesota*. GNAc, N-acetylglucosamine; Gal, galactose; Glu, glucose; Hep, heptose; KDO, 2-ketodeoxyoctonate.

Chapter 2. The outer membrane contains the endotoxin, a lipopolysaccharide. The lipopolysaccharide is composed of lipid A, which is responsible for toxicity and a terminal polysaccharide responsible for serologic activity (O antigen) (chap. 2; Figs. 2–6, 2–7). Variations in the terminal polysaccharide account for different serologic specificities. S→R dissociation is accompanied by loss of the terminal polysaccharide.

Figure 13–2 shows the basic structure of the various lipopolysaccharide chemotypes. Rough mutants which lack portions of the lipopolysaccharide are designated Ra (contains all components but O-specific terminal polysaccharide) to Re (those which contain only 2-ketodeoxyoctonate and lipid).

OTHER SURFACE COMPONENTS

A number of enterics contain capsules, envelopes or slime layers (K antigens), antigenic substances that may play a role in interfering with phagocytosis and may aid in attachment to tissue. These antigens are polysaccharides and are sometimes useful in serologic differentiation within species and in epidemiologic studies.

Flagella (H antigens) are present in a majority of the enterics. These are protein structures with serologic specificity.

Pili-(fimbriae) are important structures that take part in transfer of genetic material (F pilus) and in attachment to host tissue.

An antigen termed the Kunin antigen or enterobacterial common antigen (ECA) is shared among the members of the enteric group. ECA consists of two amino sugars, D-glucosamine and D-mannosamineuronic acid, and is partly esterified to palmitic acid. Some of the ECA antigen is apparently covalently linked to the endotoxin core, and in this form it is antigenic. A haptenic form of ECA which is not linked to the endotoxin core is also present. Both the haptenic and antigenic forms of ECA bind to erythrocytes and hemagglutination results if anti-ECA serum is added. The biologic significance of ECA is not clear. Antibody to ECA is produced in certain disease states, e.g., chronic pyelonephritis, shigellosis, and peritonitis. The antigen has also been demonstrated by immunofluorescence in patients with pyelonephritis. Tissues (liver, spleen and colon) also contain an antigen which cross-reacts with ECA. It is suggested that the presence of the cross-reacting antigen may increase susceptibility of certain tissues and hosts to infection or that induction of antibody to ECA may result in immunopathology by reaction of anti-ECA with the cross-reacting tissue antigen.

GENETICS

Members of the enterics represent closely related genera that share many characteristics. Evidence for relatedness of the various enteric organisms has been obtained by demonstration that hybridization of chromosomal genes occurs and that episomes can be transferred between various genera. These organisms are similar morphologically, physiologically and biochemically; they share antigens, and immunologic cross reactions are frequently seen. S→R dissociation associated with loss of polysaccharides which confer O-antigen specificity occurs in all species. K antigens and flagellar antigens can also be lost. In addition, antigenic changes such as changes in serotype may result via lysogenic conversion and by recombination after conjugation or transduction. Genetic exchange also results in transfer of physiologic characteristics such as acquisition of ability to ferment lactose by the *Salmonella*, and conversely, loss of lactose fermentation by *Escherichia coli*.

R factors are easily transferred among enterics, and multiple resistance to antibiotics, mediated by these factors, is becoming an increasing problem in treatment of these diseases.

Enterotoxin and hemolysin synthesis in at least one species, E. coli, is controlled by plasmids. Bacteriocin production is also determined by plasmids.

INFECTIONS

The enterics cause diseases of any tissue or organ (chaps. 14 and 15). With the exception of Salmonella, Shigella, and certain strains of E. coli, most infections occur in patients debilitated by preexisting disease or compromised by preexisting disease or treatment. Thus in most cases the enterics are considered provisional pathogens or opportunists. Specific diseases associated with the opportunistic enteric bacilli are discussed in Chapter 14. A common and important aspect of these opportunistic infections is the production of septicemia, frequently in compromised patients, which may be followed by endotoxic shock.

Certain strains of E. coli, the Salmonella, Shigella, Yersinia and a nonenteric genus (Vibrio) are commonly associated with disease of the intestinal tract characterized most commonly by diarrhea. The mechanism for production of diarrhea is not completely understood, but most cases are associated with production of an enterotoxin.

MECHANISMS OF PATHOGENICITY: ENDOTOXINS AND EXOTOXINS

Endotoxins

Clinical Aspects

One of the more dramatic effects of gram-negative septicemia is the development of endotoxin shock. Briefly, there are peripheral and circulatory failure, renal and hepatic failure, and disturbances in ventilation, gas exchange and consciousness. Shock is characterized by a pooling of blood in the pulmonary and splanchnic vasculature, an increase in peripheral vasoconstriction and poor tissue perfusion. The direct myocardial depressant action of LPS, along with decreased venous return due to pooling, results in lowered cardiac output, which causes a drop in blood pressure and peripheral perfusion and resultant release of catecholamines. The catecholamines cause an arteriolar-venular constriction and subsequent acidosis, which initiates capillary congestion and dilation. This in turn accentuates decreased venous return and cardiac output.

Endotoxic shock may not be the result of endotoxin released only

TABLE 13-3.—BIOLOGIC EFFECTS
OF ENDOTOXIN

1. Pyrogenicity
2. Leukopenia and leukocytosis
3. Increased nonspecific resistance
4. Agglutination of platelets
5. Release of interferon
6. Acts as an adjuvant in antibody production
7. Hageman factor activation
8. Complement activation
9. Metabolic changes
10. Endocrine changes
11. Protection against irradiation
12. Necrosis of tumors
13. Shock
14. Disseminated intravascular coagulation (Shwartzman reaction)
15. Tolerance
16. Prevention of gastric emptying
17. Increased rate of peristalsis
18. Labilization of lysosomes

from organisms causing the septicemia. Some work suggests that endotoxin causes the release of additional endotoxin from the normal intestinal flora, and that this latter source of endotoxin is responsible for triggering effects.

Biologic Effects

Many different effects of endotoxin have been described, and some are listed in Table 13-3. The variety and nonspecificity of effects described correlate well with many of the symptoms observed in patients with gram-negative infections.

Mechanisms of Endotoxin Action

The mechanisms by which endotoxin causes its effect on the host are unknown. The affinity of endotoxin for cell membranes suggests that the primary effect may be on the cell surface. The thrombocytopenia and degranulation observed after administration of LPS may result in part from adherence of LPS to platelets. The marked binding of LPS to Kupffer cells has suggested this cell as the target cell. Interaction with polymorphonuclear leukocytes and monocytes results in release of endogenous pyrogen (EP), a low molecular weight, heat-labile protein. The EP causes fever by its effect on the hypothalamus, the thermoregulatory center in the brain; it also causes an increase in some membrane-associated enzymes and alters the flux of cations such as calcium, zinc, iron and also amino acids.

The interaction of endotoxin with leukocytes, platelets and other host systems either directly or indirectly via complement may account for the alteration in the vascular and blood clotting system which results in shock and disseminated intravascular clotting (DIC). The induction of tumor necrosis is probably due to activation of the blood coagulation system or to release of a specific factor, the tumor necrosis factor.

Activation of the prekallikrein-kallikrein system with subsequent release of bradykinin, a potent hypotensive peptide, has also been demonstrated. The release of bradykinin is associated with initial vasodilation and hypotension.

Endotoxin activates the complement sequence, primarily via the alternate pathway, causing (1) contraction of smooth muscle and increased capillary permeability (C3, C5); (2) adherence and degranulation of platelets (C3); (3) coagulation of blood (C6) and (4) release of chemotactic factors (C3a, C5a). It is presumed that many of the effects of endotoxin relate to complement activation.

The mechanisms by which other changes, e.g., metabolic changes, endocrine changes, increased nonspecific resistance, are caused are still unclear. A factor that causes tumor necrosis has been found in mice injected with endotoxin. This suggests that tumor necrosis is due to a specific factor released by endotoxin rather than a direct effect of endotoxin.

LPS is known to cause a marked decrease in liver glycogen. Initially there is a hyperglycemia followed by a hypoglycemia. These changes are accompanied by an increase in activity of certain glycolytic enzymes and by decreases in activity of some glyconeogenic enzymes. Decreases in activity of glyconeogenic enzymes have been associated with decreased synthesis of these enzymes. Studies suggest that macrophages may modulate these changes in enzymes through release of a factor termed glucocorticoid antagonizing factor (GAF). This factor blocks glucocorticoid induction of some enzymes. Macrophages also mediate other biologic effects of endotoxin, e.g., fever via release of endogenous and leukocytic endogenous pyrogen, release of interferon and also substances that modulate responsiveness of lymphocytes to mitogens and antigens.

Endotoxin also selectively affects the hypothalamic-pituitary-adrenal axis resulting in release of adrenocorticotropic hormone and growth hormone but not thyrotropin or luteinizing hormone. The hormonal effect may be brought about by an effect on neuronal elements of the hypothalamus or by direct effect on the pituitary gland. Plasma cortisol is also increased following injection of LPS.

Macrophages, T cells, and B cells are affected directly and indirectly by LPS. Endotoxin causes a proliferation of B cells (mitogenic response). Lymphokine production is also stimulated. The release of chemotactic factors, macrophage inhibiting factor (MIF) and macrophage aggregating factor (MAF), may account for the adjuvant effect of endotoxin. The release of lymphocyte accumulating factor (LAF) from macrophages exposed to LPS may result in T-cell activation.

Disseminated Intravascular Coagulation

The experimental animal correlate to DIC in man is the generalized Shwartzman reaction (GSR). The GSR requires two intravenous injections of endotoxin with resultant production of bilateral renal cortical necrosis. The first injection is the preparative injection and the second injection is the provoking injection. In man, it is assumed that initially a conditioning (preparative injection) occurs which is followed by a provoking reaction.

Disseminated intravascular coagulation is a serious feature of gram-negative bacteremia. Several probable mechanisms for DIC have been suggested. One is that endotoxin causes desquamation of endothelium, which is followed by platelet deposition and subsequent fibrin formation. Endotoxin also causes aggregation of platelets and this facilitates platelet deposition and subsequent fibrin formation. Endotoxin has also been shown to activate factor XII, resulting in thrombin generation and fibrin formation. Finally, complement activation results in granulocyte injury with release of lysosomal cationic proteins and acid mucopolysaccharides, which react with soluble fibrin-monomer complexes and results in clot formation.

Tolerance and Resistance

Injection of sublethal amounts of endotoxin into animals makes them refractory (tolerant) to the biologic effects of endotoxin. Tolerance is a short-lived phenomenon that lasts for only a few days.

The mechanism for tolerance and resistance is unknown. Various studies have suggested that tolerance and resistance are due to (1) increased ability of the reticuloendothelial system (RES) to remove and detoxify endotoxin perhaps by a serum esterase or macrophages, (2) increased stabilization of lysosomes, (3) antibody or (4) loss in ability of cells to release mediators. Recent studies have shown that tolerance may relate to the increased resistance of susceptible RES cells (Kupffer cells), and that increased clearance of the toxin is an ancillary mechanism that efficiently brings the toxin to the resistant cells.

Clinical Correlates

Man is one of the species most reactive to endotoxin. The minimal intradermal inflammatory dose in man is 10^{-3} to 10^{-4} μg. The responses are visible in 1 hour and reach a maximum at 3 hours; infiltrates are mononuclear. With a dose 100 times greater than the minimal inflammatory dose, the inflammatory response increases in intensity and is characterized by a polymorphonuclear response.

Temperature elevation can be evoked in man by intravenous injection of 0.001 μg of endotoxin per kilogram body weight. A latent period of 45 to 90 minutes follows injection with a peak febrile response in about 3 hours. During the phase of ascending temperature, the symptoms are chills, rigor, headache, myalgia, anorexia, nausea and vomiting. Unlike the biphasic fever curve observed in animals, only a monophasic curve is obtained in man. Endogenous pyrogen has been demonstrated in human plasma, monocytes and polymorphonuclear leukocytes.

Leukocytosis, resulting from release of granulocytes from bone marrow reserves, has also been demonstrated. The neutropenia and thrombocytopenia which can be demonstrated in animals have not been shown in man, but this may relate to the low dose of endotoxin employed. Fibrinolysis, hypofibrinogenemia and an increase in factor VIII have also been reported.

Alteration in liver carbohydrate, production of hyperglycemia and hypoglycemia, also occurs in man during infection with gram-negative rods.

Bradykinin is proposed as the cause of the initial drop in blood pressure. This is probably followed by activation of complement and release of additional vasoactive substances.

Tolerance has also been demonstrated in man. Daily intravenous injection of endotoxin does result in pyrogenic tolerance. As in animals, tolerance is relative and not absolute. Tolerance to the intradermal reaction does not develop.

Measurement of Endotoxin

The most common method used for assay of endotoxin is injection of rabbits and determination of pyrogenic response either as maximum fever or as fever over a defined period of time.

Other assays involve determining lethality in mice or in mice sensitized to endotoxin by injection of lead or actinomycin D or by adrenalectomy. An immunoassay for endotoxin and an intracutaneous epinephrine skin sensitivity test have also been used for quantitating endotoxin.

Recently the *Limulus* test has received the attention of many workers interested in detecting and quantitating endotoxin. Amebocytes from *Limulus polyphemus,* the horseshoe crab, are lysed and the lysate is incubated with tissue or other materials containing endotoxin.

The *Limulus* lysate clots in the presence of picogram amounts of endotoxin. A number of clinical investigators have used this test to assay endotoxin in gingival tissue, cerebrospinal fluid, urine and blood with variable results. However, several other substances, including peptidoglycan, also cause clotting of the *Limulus* extract.

Enterotoxins

Several gram-negative bacteria, as well as some gram-positive organisms, cause disease of the intestinal tract evidenced by diarrhea. Mechanistically, diarrhea results either from invasion or penetration of the bowel wall (enteritis) or by a noninvasive mechanism mediated through production of a specific exotoxin. These exotoxins, which affect the intestinal tract (enteron), are referred to as enterotoxins. Some organisms, such as *Shigella dysenteriae*, are invasive and also produce an enterotoxin. Enterotoxins are elaborated by some but not all invasive organisms. The significance of enterotoxin production by the invasive strains is questionable.

The best studied enterotoxins are those produced by *Escherichia coli*, *Vibrio cholerae* and *Staphylococcus aureus*. Mechanistically, the enterotoxin produced by the gram-positive *S. aureus* differs considerably from the enterotoxins produced by the gram-negative organisms (Table 13–4).

Enterotoxic activity has been demonstrated in a number of gram-negative bacterial species, e.g., *E. coli*, *V. cholerae*, *V. parahemolyticus*, *Salmonella*, *Shigella* and *Klebsiella*. Recently, the delta toxin of *S. aureus* has also been reported to show enterotoxic activity.

Except for the gram-positive *S. aureus*, enterotoxin production in food is not the mechanism for production of diarrheal disease. Instead, enterotoxins produced by gram-negative bacteria are synthesized by microorganisms in the intestine.

TABLE 13–4.—PROPERTIES OF ENTEROTOXINS
PRODUCED BY *S. AUREUS* AND *E. COLI*

STAPHYLOCOCCUS	*E. COLI*
1. Preformed in food	1. Produced in intestinal lumen
2. Heat stable	2. Heat labile and heat stable
3. Toxin ingested with food	3. Organism ingested with food
4. Affects CNS	4. Affects intestinal adenyl cyclase or is cytotoxic
5. Produces nausea, vomiting	5. Produces diarrhea
6. Several serotypes	6. One serotype

Classification

Enterotoxins can be classified as cytotonic or cytotoxic. Cytotonic enterotoxins, such as the heat-labile toxins produced by E. coli and V. cholerae, are not toxic for tissue cultures. They cause a change in cellular activity such as increased adenyl cyclase activity, increased intracellular cyclic adenosine monophosphate levels, and increased synthesis of ketosteroids. These changes in activity, at least in certain cell lines, are reflected by a change in cell morphological features, i.e., cell rounding or elongation. Cytotoxic enterotoxins do not affect adenyl cyclase but cause cell destruction in tissue culture. Heat-stable enterotoxins elaborated by some E. coli, Salmonella enteritidis and Klebsiella pneumoniae are examples of cytotoxic enterotoxins.

Mode of Action

V. Cholerae Enterotoxin.—The V. cholerae enterotoxin is referred to as choleragen (cholera-producing). The molecule is a protein (84,000 daltons) that consists of an A region (also referred to as L) and a B region (referred to as H). The A region, the biologically active portion of the molecule, is responsible for activation of adenyl cyclase and the resultant loss of fluids. The B (binding) region is required for attachment of the toxin to the cell surface. Aggregates of the binding protein (choleragenoid) occur normally in culture filtrates of V. cholerae and are nontoxic. The receptor site for choleragenoid and also the B region of choleragen is probably the G_{M1} ganglioside of the cell membrane.

The mechanism by which activation of adenyl cyclase results in increased secretion of water and salts is not known, but it is clear that movement of water and salts from the small intestine lumen to serosa is not affected. In fact, fluids lost by cholera patients can be replaced by oral administration of glucose, water and salts.

The action of choleragen in activating adenyl cyclase is not limited to the enzyme in intestinal mucosa. Choleragen also stimulates steroidogenesis in adrenal cells, inhibits histamine release from lymphocytes by antigen and IgE, and causes morphological changes in melanoma cells among other activities.

E. Coli Enterotoxin.—Two enterotoxins are produced by E. coli: one is heat stable (ST) and one is heat labile (LT). Recent evidence suggests that the heat-stable enterotoxin may be a complex of endotoxin and the heat-labile toxin. Studies on the molecular weight of the heat-labile toxin have given variable results with recent studies indicating a molecular weight of 102,000. The molecular weight of the heat-stable toxin is greater than 10^6. A plasmid that codes for enterotoxin production has been demonstrated.

The mode of action of the heat-labile *E. coli* enterotoxin is identical to that of choleragen, i.e., the enterotoxin activates adenyl cyclase and causes hypersecretion of water and salts. The enterotoxin does not alter absorption. The receptor site is similar but not identical to the receptor necessary for binding of choleragen.

OTHER ENTEROTOXINS.—The mode of action of the cytotoxic enterotoxins is unknown. It appears that these enterotoxins do not directly result in adenyl cyclase activation and increased intracellular cyclic AMP. Some studies suggest that the *Salmonella* enterotoxin may result in increased prostaglandin synthesis, which in turn activates adenyl cyclase.

The role of the cytotoxic enterotoxins in intestinal disease is unclear. Studies with *Shigella dysenteriae*, which produces an enterotoxin, showed that strains which were invasive but did not produce an enterotoxin produced disease in animals as severe as that caused by the invasive and toxinogenic *Shigella*.

Fig. 13–3.—Ileal loop reaction. Four loops of pig small intestine were inoculated with cultures of *E. coli*. The pig was killed after 18 hours. Swelling of the loop indicates an enterotoxigenic *E. coli*. End loops were inoculated with enterotoxinogenic *E. coli*. Organisms injected into middle loops did not produce enterotoxin. (Courtesy of Dr. Harley W. Moon, National Animal Disease Center, Ames, Iowa 50010.)

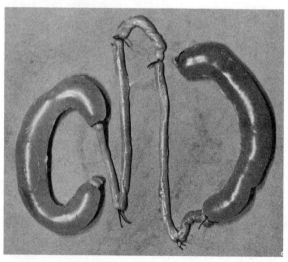

Assays for Enterotoxin
    Enterotoxin can be assayed by several methods. Early studies used ligation of intestinal loops that were inoculated either with enterotoxin-containing filtrates or with enterotoxin-producing bacteria. Fluid accumulation in the loop is evidence of enterotoxin; the method can be quantitated by measuring the amount of fluid accumulation. Other methods include oral feeding of infant rabbits or mice and measurement of intestinal weight as an indicator of fluid accumulation (Fig. 13-3).

Cytotonic Enterotoxins
    More recently, morphological changes (rounding) in adrenal Y-1 cells and synthesis of $\Delta 4,3$-ketosteroids by these cells after exposure to an adenyl cyclase-activating enterotoxin have been used to measure picogram amounts of enterotoxin (Fig. 13-4). Other methods use tissue culture systems, e.g., Chinese hamster ovary. In addition, enterotoxin has been reported to activate adenyl cyclase in solubilized myocardial tissue from cat heart.

Cytotoxic Enterotoxins
    Cytotoxic enterotoxins are assayed using HeLa cells and measuring cell detachment as an indication of toxicity. The heat-stable enterotoxin can be measured by oral feeding of suckling mice. The intestinal tract of the mice is weighed and compared to control mice. The increase in weight is associated quantitatively with the amount of enterotoxin.

IMMUNITY

    Antibody to capsular (K) and O antigens protects animals against infection with homologous organisms. Immunization of animals with rough mutants of *S. minnesota* (see Fig. 13-2) provides immunity against infection with smooth heterologous gram-negative bacilli. The Re mutant, which contains only lipid A and KDO (ketodeoxyoctonate), affords the best protection. In man, high titers of O-specific IgG to the infecting organism correlate with decreased frequency of shock and death in gram-negative bacteremia. Further, high titers of antibody to the Re LPS, i.e., lipid A-KDO, are associated with a reduction in severity and lethality of gram-negative bacteremia.
    In vitro, antibody can neutralize the effects of enterotoxin. Antibody has also been detected in persons who have had diarrhea caused by enterotoxin-producing *E. coli*. Studies in man to evaluate the efficiency of immunizing with toxoid have not been completed.

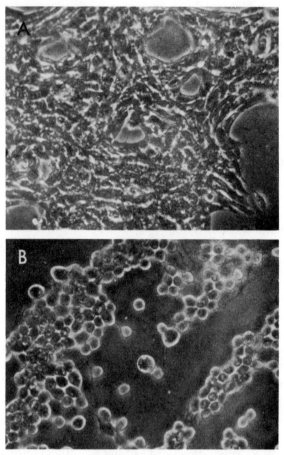

Fig. 13–4.—Detection of *E. coli* enterotoxin. **A,** normal monolayers of Y-1 adrenal tumor cells. **B,** Y-1 adrenal tumor cells after addition of the heat-labile toxin. Note cell rounding. (From Donta, S. T.: Infectious diarrhea, Mod. Med. of Can. 30: 121, 1975. With permission of author and publisher.)

PREVENTION AND TREATMENT

Septic shock is prevented by minimizing the amount of endotoxin or gram-negative organisms in the patient. Thus proper use of catheters, intravenous fluids, and appropriate use of antibiotics minimize risk of infection and therefore induction of endotoxic shock.

Treatment requires use of antibiotics specific for the organism causing sepsis and efforts to maintain adequate tissue perfusion. Generally, this requires stabilization of the cardiopulmonary system.

Diarrhea produced by noninvasive bacteria *(E. coli, V. cholera)* or by those with limited invasiveness *(Salmonella, Shigella)* generally does not require antibiotic therapy. In fact, the carrier state may be prolonged by treatment probably because of antibiotic effects on normal intestinal flora which inhibit the pathogens. Treatment is directed at replacement of water, glucose and salts lost by hypersecretion. Absorption by the small intestine is not affected by the enterotoxin, and therapy by oral administration of water and salts is usually sufficient.

LABORATORY PROCEDURES

The procedures for isolating and identifying enteric organisms are considerably more complex than those required for other organisms. Identification and isolation are expensive and time consuming and require use of many different media and serologic techniques. Considerable expertise is also required for correct identification. Many laboratories cannot handle the large number of specimens associated with an epidemic, and specimens may need to be taken to a laboratory at some distance. Thus transport media, i.e., media designed to prevent pH changes and desiccation, are necessary to protect microbial viability. Several media — Amies transport medium, buffered glycerol-saline and others — are available for this purpose.

Due to the large numbers of normal flora organisms, particularly in stool specimens, and because the pathogens are usually fewer than nonpathogenic organisms, enrichment media are commonly used to facilitate growth of pathogens and inhibit the opportunistic enterics. Three media used for enrichment are tetrathionate, selenite (the medium recommended for general use) and Gram-Negative (GN) broth. Enrichment media, even though designed for isolation of pathogens, are inhibitory for some species or strains; thus it is advisable to use more than one type of medium. In addition to selenite, GN broth is recommended.

The enterics are similar in microscopic and colonial morphological features and usually exist in mixed culture. Thus the primary plating media are differential and to some extent selective. Differential media contain one or more carbohydrates as substrate and an acid-base indicator to detect utilization of these carbohydrates. Some media also permit identification of H_2S production. Bile salts, brilliant green and crystal violet are incorporated into the agar to inhibit other organisms. Eosin methylene blue (EMB) is commonly used as primary plating medium. This medium is differential (lactose fermenters are blue; non-lactose fermenters are uncolored) and shows little selectivity for enteric bacilli. Salmonella-Shigella (S-S), Hektoen-Enteric (HE) and deoxycholate citrate are differential and moderately selective. As an example of differential and selective properties, the *Salmonella* spp. and *Shigella* spp. grow as yellow colonies on S-S agar whereas the lactose fermenters are red. Growth of organisms other than *Salmonella* and *Shigella* is markedly inhibited. Use of appropriate differential and selective media enables one to select colonies of non-lactose fermenters (probable pathogens) and lactose fermenters (probable opportunists).

Colonies isolated from the primary plating media are then inoculated into primary differential media, e.g., Triple Sugar Iron (TSI), Russell's Double Sugar (RDS) or Kligler's Iron (KI) agar slants. These media contain two to three carbohydrates (glucose and lactose, sometimes sucrose) as indicators of acid production, and in some cases an indicator for H_2S production (RDS, KI). As an example of their use, TSI slants contain glucose, lactose and sucrose. If only glucose is fermented, the butt of the tube becomes yellow or acid because of glu-

TABLE 13-5.—DIFFERENTIAL CHARACTERISTICS
OF TRIBES OF ENTEROBACTERIACEAE[*]

TEST OR SUBSTRATE	TRIBES[†]				
	ESCHERICHIEAE	EDWARDSIELLEAE	SALMONELLEAE	KLEBSIELLEAE	PROTEEAE
Hydrogen sulfide (TSI)	−	+	+	−	+ or −
Urease	−	−	−	− or (+)	+ or −
Indole	+ or −	+	−	−	+ or −
Methyl red	+	+	+	−	+
Voges-Proskauer	−	−	−	+	−
Citrate (Simmons')	−	−	+	+	d
KCN	−	−	− or +	+	+
Phenylalanine deaminase	−	−	−	−	+
Jordan's tartrate	+ or −	−	d	+ or −	+ or −
Mucate	d	−	d	+ or −	−
Mannitol	+ or −	−	+	+	− or +

[*]Adapted from Ewing, W. H., and Martin, W. J.: Enterobacteriaceae, in Lennette, E. H., Spaulding, E. H., and Truant, J. P. (eds.): *Manual of Clinical Microbiology* (2d ed.; Washington, D.C.: American Society for Microbiology, 1974).

[†]Symbols: +, 90% in 1-2 days; −, 90% or more do not give the reaction; (+), delayed reaction, positive in 3 days or more; d, different biochemical reactions; + or −, most cultures positive; − or +, most cultures negative.

cose fermentation while the top slanted portion of the medium becomes red or alkaline. If lactose, sucrose, or both are fermented, both the slant portion and the butt are yellow, indicating acid production. Bubbles indicate gas production and a black precipitate is evidence of H_2S production. This permits further differentiation of the organisms into groups that ferment one or more carbohydrates with or without production of gas and with or without H_2S.

Final identification of the enterics requires inoculation into other media for further biochemical characterization. This may include detection of (1) specific enzymes (urease, decarboxylases, deaminases); (2) utilization of certain substrates (citrate, acetate); (3) specific products of metabolism (acids, indole, acetylmethylcarbinol) and (4) specific types of metabolism (oxidation or fermentation of selected substrates). Table 13–5 lists some reactions that can be used to differentiate this diverse group. The interested student is encouraged to consult the Manual of Clinical Microbiology and Identification of the Enterobacteriaceae for more specific identification schemes. Serologic identification of the O, K and H antigens may also be required for complete identification and for epidemiologic studies. Colicin typing and phage typing can be used for epidemiologic studies. The overall procedure used for identification of the enterics is diagrammed in Figure 13–5.

Fig. 13–5.—Laboratory approach to identification of enterics.

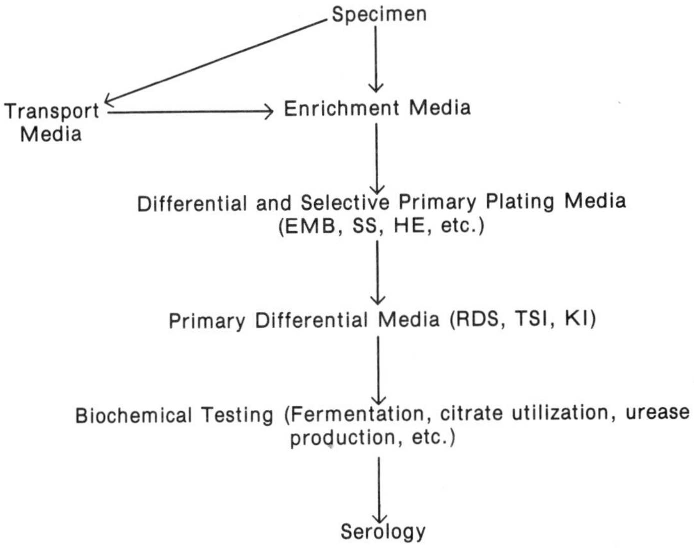

PROBLEM SOLVING AND REVIEW

No. 1. GIVEN: — A 60-year-old man was hospitalized because of prostatic hypertrophy. Several hours after surgery, he appeared alert but restless. He had some fever; his skin was warm and flushed and he was hypotensive. Cultures of blood and urine were collected and sent to the laboratory. A few hours later his condition markedly deteriorated. He was mentally confused, his temperature was subnormal; urine output was low (oliguria) and he was markedly hypotensive. Blood analysis showed he had hypoglycemia; he had low platelet and leukocyte counts, a decrease in fibrinogen and an increase in fibrin split products.

PROBLEMS: — 1. What is your clinical diagnosis? 2. What is the probable cause? 3. What is the bacterial component which causes the signs and symptoms? 4. What are the basic physiologic problems? 5. How do you explain the temperature increase and the hypoglycemia? 6. How would you explain the DIC? 7. What causes the hypotension? (Ans. p. 271.)

No. 2. GIVEN: — An epidemic of diarrhea occurred in several adults who had just returned from a vacation in Mexico. The patients had no fever; they had some abdominal cramping. Gram stain of the stool showed only gram-negative rods characteristic of those found normally in the intestinal tract. Leukocytes were not observed. The bacteriologic report indicated only *E. coli* present. The diarrhea and other symptoms subsided without treatment.

PROBLEMS: — 1. What is the probable cause of the diarrhea? 2. What is the mechanism? 3. How could you determine if the organism produced an enterotoxin? 4. Assume that gram stain of the stool showed many polymorphonuclear leukocytes. What is the significance of leukocytes in the feces? (Ans. p. 271).

SUPPLEMENTARY READING

Berry, L. J.: Bacterial toxins, CRC Crit. Rev. Toxicol. 5:239–318, 1977.
Donta, S. T., and Smith, D. M.: Stimulation of steroidogenesis in tissue culture by enterotoxigenic *Escherichia coli* and its neutralization by specific antiserum, Infect. Immunol. 9:500–505, 1974.
Edwards, P. M., and Ewing, W. H.: *Identification of the Enterobacteriaceae* (3d ed.; Minneapolis: Burgess Publishing Co., 1972).
Elin, R. J., and Wolff, S. M.: Biology of endotoxin, Annu. Rev. Med. 27: 127–141, 1976.
Ewing, W. H., and Martin, W. J.: Enterobacteriaceae, in Lennette, E. H.,

Spaulding, E. H., and Truant, J. P. (eds.): *Manual of Clinical Microbiology* (2d ed.; Washington, D.C.: American Society for Microbiology, 1974).

Finkelstein, R. A.: Cholera Enterotoxin, in Schlessinger, D. (ed.): *Microbiology, 1975* (Washington, D.C.: American Society for Microbiology, 1975).

Giannella, R. A.: Suckling mouse model for detection of heat-stable *Escherichia coli* enterotoxin: Characteristics of the model, Infect. Immunol. 14:95–99, 1976.

Gots, R. F., Formal, S. B., and Gianella, R. A.: Indomethacin inhibition of *Salmonella typhimurium, Shigella flexneri* and cholera-mediated rabbit ileal secretion, J. Infect. Dis. 130:280–284, 1974.

Keusch, G. T., and Donta, S. T.: Classification of enterotoxins on the basis of activity in cell culture, J. Infect. Dis. 131:58–63, 1974.

Makela, P. H., and Mayer, H.: Enterobacterial common antigen, Bacteriol. Rev. 40:591–632, 1976.

McCabe, W. R.: Immunization with R mutants of *S. minnesota*. I. Protection against challenge with heterologous gram-negative bacilli, J. Immunol. 108:601–610, 1972.

McCabe, W. R., Carling, P. C., Bruins, S., and Grealy, A.: The relation of K-antigen to virulence of *Escherichia coli*, J. Infect. Dis. 131:6–10, 1975.

Muller-Berghous, G., Bohn, E., and Hobel, W.: Activation of intravascular coagulation by endotoxin: The significance of granulocytes and platelets, Br. J. Haematol. 33:213, 1976.

Zinner, S. H., and McCabe, W. R.: Effects of IgM and IgG antibody in patients with bacteremia due to gram negative bacilli. J. Infect. Dis. 133:37–45, 1976.

ANALYSIS

No. 1.—1. Gram-negative shock; endotoxic shock. 2. Gram-negative bacteremia or septicemia caused by *E. coli*. 3. Endotoxin. 4. Underperfusion of tissue. DIC. 5. Endogenous pyrogens from tissue cells (Kupffer cells) affect the hypothalamus causing temperature increase. Increased enzyme activity causes depletion of liver glycogen. 6. Activation of complement with injury to the granulocytes. Endothelial damage and platelet deposition. Activation of Hageman factor XII. 7. Release of bradykinin and activation of complement resulting in release of vasoactive substances.

No. 2.—1. Enterotoxin probably produced by *E. coli*. 2. The enterotoxin activates adenyl cyclase and causes hypersecretion of water and salts. 3. (*a*) Inject organism into ligated intestinal loops and observe for fluid accumulation. (*b*) With tissue cultures, determine if a cytotonic or cytotoxic effect is produced with culture filtrates in an appropriate tissue culture system. (*c*) Determine if adenyl cyclase is activated. 4. Presence of leukocytes indicates that the organism is invasive.

14 /Opportunistic Enteric Bacteria

OVERVIEW

Of the *Enterobacteriaceae,* the *Salmonella, Shigella* and certain *E. coli* are considered frank pathogens. The remaining genera, which are part of the normal intestinal flora, cause disease in persons whose resistance to infection has been altered. These infections are difficult to diagnose because the types of diseases and the signs and symptoms are not characteristic for a given genus or species. Also, in some cases the same or related organisms can be isolated from patients without evidence of disease, and the physician must interpret the significance of the isolated organisms. In other cases the patient may show little, if any, evidence of disease but may quickly become bacteremic and develop shock. Treatment poses another problem in that susceptibility to the various chemotherapeutic agents varies and resistant forms emerge rather quickly.

ESCHERICHIA COLI

General Characteristics

Escherichia coli is a gram-negative rod (0.4–0.7×1–3 μm) (Fig. 14–1). It is a facultative anaerobe and grows on simple nutrient media. Some isolates may be motile, others are nonmotile. They usually ferment lactose and produce gas from glucose. Indole is produced and acetate but not citrate is used as the sole carbon source. Some strains produce a β-hemolysin.

Species

Escherichia coli is the single species within this genus. Other species which formerly were in the genus *Escherichia (E. freundii)* are now classified in the genus *Citrobacter (C. freundii* and *C. diversus).* Diseases produced by *Citrobacter* are similar to those produced by *E. coli.*

273

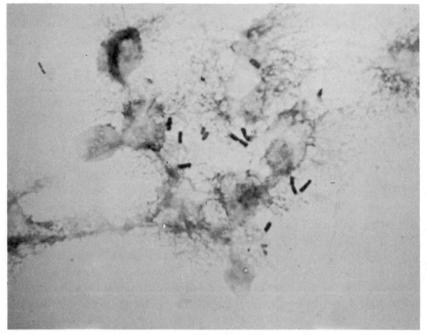

Fig. 14–1.—*E. coli* in urine (unspun).

Ecology

Escherichia coli is found as part of the normal flora of the intestinal tract of man and animals. It is the predominant facultatively anaerobic rod in the colon and is found in concentrations approaching 10^8/gm feces.

Antigens

Escherichia coli is antigenically complex and contains antigens that cross-react with other enterics. There are 157 somatic (O) antigens, 52 flagellar (H) antigens and 93 capsular or envelope (K) antigens. These antigens have been well studied, and serotyping based on these antigens is used in understanding the epidemiology of infections caused by this organism.

The K antigens can be subdivided into three types: L, A and B. These antigens can be differentiated by heating and determining loss of antibody binding power or temperature required for loss of antigenicity. Because the K antigens cover the O antigens, they may prevent agglutination by O-antiserum. Some K antigens may play a role in adherence of the microorganisms to tissue cells.

The O antigens are cell wall polysaccharides and are not inactivated by heat. The flagellar antigens are protein and are inactivated by heat.

With the use of specific antiserums, *E. coli* can be serotyped and designated as, for example, O26: K60 (B6): H11. This designation indicates that the given strain contains O antigen 26, a K antigen designated as K 60. The K antigen is of the B type and specifically B6. The H or flagella antigen is designated as H11.

Pili are also present. These antigens are also important in adherence.

Toxins and Hemolysins

ENTEROTOXIN: — Two enterotoxins, a heat-labile and a heat-stable toxin, have been described. Both of these toxins cause fluid accumulation in ligated ileal loops. The heat-stable enterotoxin is cytotoxic for tissue culture cells; it does not activate adenyl cyclase. The heat-labile toxin is an activator of adenyl cyclase, and the resultant increased concentration of cyclic AMP is responsible for hypersecretion of fluids into the bowel lumen and diarrhea (chap. 13).

HEMOLYSIN: — Two hemolysins have been described. One is cell bound and living organisms are needed to demonstrate lysis of erythrocytes. The other hemolysin is cell-free and filterable. Both hemolysins produce a beta-hemolysis. Their role in disease is not completely understood.

ENDOTOXIN: — Endotoxin is described in Chapter 13. Much of the work with endotoxin has been done with the endotoxic lipopolysaccharide from *E. coli.*

Infections

Escherichia coli can cause disease in any organ or tissue. It is frequently associated with urinary tract infections (pyelonephritis, cystitis) and with diarrhea, particularly in children and in travelers. However, it can also cause meningitis, pneumonia, septicemia, endocarditis, wound infection and abscesses in various organs. *E. coli* is a major cause of meningitis in newborns. This organism is responsible for 80–90% of urinary tract infections and is the most important agent in nosocomial (hospital-acquired) infections.

Urinary Tract Infections

Acute infections of the kidney (pyelonephritis) are characterized by chills, fever, flank pain and tenderness (Fig. 14–2). Dysuria (pain on voiding), which is symptomatic of cystitis, may also be noted. Frequent urination (polyuria) and nocturia (frequent urination at night) are also symptoms of pyelonephritis. The white blood cell count is

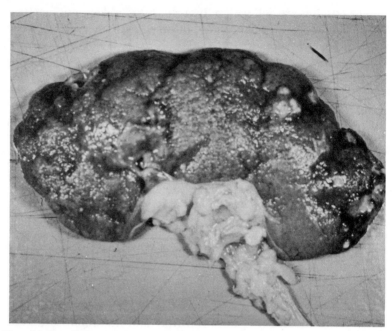

Fig. 14–2.—Outer surface of kidney shows pyelonephritis (irregular depressions and multiple abscesses). (Courtesy of Dr. Winfield Morgan, Department of Pathology, West Virginia University Medical Center.)

elevated with an increase in the number of polymorphonuclear leukocytes and there is proteinuria, pyuria and bacteriuria. Pyelonephritis is classified as uncomplicated if there is no history of prior urinary tract infection or structural or neurologic lesions. *E. coli* isolated from patients with uncomplicated pyelonephritis responds favorably to chemotherapy. Complicated pyelonephritis is associated with an alteration of the urinary tract (residual changes due to recurrent infection, obstruction due to stones, neurologic lesions) that predisposes the patient to infection and reinfection. Patients with complicated pyelonephritis are difficult to treat because the causative organisms are resistant to chemotherapy or because the obstruction interferes with antibiotic activity. In some patients, particularly the elderly, chronic infection, characterized by repeated episodes of infection, can occur.

Asymptomatic bacteriuria is the most common form of urinary tract infection. The symptoms are mild and frequently are unrecognized. About 5% of pregnant women have asymptomatic bacteriuria early in pregnancy and, if untreated, about 40% later develop acute symptomatic bacteriuria.

Intestinal Tract Disease

Certain strains of *E. coli* (enteropathogenic *E. coli*) are associated with intestinal tract disease. Two different forms of the disease have been described, a cholera-like disease and a dysentery or *Shigella*-like disease. The cholera-like form of the disease is caused by enterotoxin-producing strains, whereas the dysentery-like disease is caused by invasive organisms.

Epidemics of infantile diarrhea caused by *E. coli* can be a major problem in nurseries. Until recently, certain serotypes of *E. coli* were believed to be implicated in infantile diarrhea, and serotyping was used to identify these enteropathogenic strains. Newer data indicate that a correlation between serotype and enteropathogenicity does not exist and that serotyping is an epidemiologic tool.

The diarrhea of travelers may have several microbial and parasitological causes. An important agent in this disease is the enterotoxin-producing *Escherichia coli*.

Mechanisms of Pathogenicity

The mechanism of pathogenicity of *E. coli* and other enteric bacteria is only beginning to be understood. The K antigen apparently acts as an adherence factor; it is also antiphagocytic and may inhibit the complement-dependent bactericidal action of serum. *E. coli* isolated from patients with urinary tract infection contain more K antigen than strains isolated from feces or from patients with bacteremia. Pili also play a role in attachment and adherence of the cells to tissue. The O antigen is antiphagocytic and permits survival of the organism in the absence of anti-O antibody. If the organism survives and a bacteremia develops, the endotoxin is released and either directly or indirectly causes septic shock.

In persons who ingest enteropathogenic strains of *E. coli*, two different interactions and processes may occur. In both cases the organisms attach to the intestinal mucosa. If the *E. coli* contains a plasmid coding for enterotoxin production, enterotoxin is produced. The heat-labile enterotoxin reacts with the mucosal cells of the small intestine and activates adenyl cyclase. The increase in adenyl cyclase activity causes increased levels of intracellular cyclic AMP and hypersecretion of water and salts. However, water resorption is not affected, permitting replacement of fluids and salts by the oral route. The mechanism of action and the precise role of the heat-stable toxin are not known but it also causes hypersecretion of water and salts. The heat-stable toxin apparently does not activate adenyl cyclase.

E. coli which do not produce enterotoxin but which are invasive produce a dysentery or Shigella-like disease. The organisms invade the ileum and colon. The mechanism for production of diarrhea is unknown but is probably the result of an inflammatory response.

The role of the hemolysin in disease is unknown. Hemolytic strains are frequently isolated from patients with urinary tract infections, and some experimental data suggest that hemolytic strains may be associated with more kidney disease than nonhemolytic strains. Hemolysis is not a feature of disease caused by *E. coli*.

Immunity

Innate or natural immunity to *E. coli* and other enteric bacteria is probably the most important facet of immunity. Infection with *E. coli* and similar organisms occurs in neonates compromised by lack of placental transfer of antibody (neonatal meningitis), and in others whose normal defense mechanisms are altered by disease or cytotoxic drugs or bypassed by one method or another (urinary tract catheterization, intravenous catheters). Anatomic alterations due to prior or existing disease or natural processes such as pregnancy also increase susceptibility.

Antibodies to the O, K and H antigens are produced as a result of infection and are important in opsonization. Antibody to the capsular and O antigens protects animals against experimental infection with homologous organisms. In man, high titers of IgG antibody are associated with a reduction in frequency of shock and death. It is suggested that IgM antibody may function to prevent infection with serum-sensitive strains of *E. coli*. Serum-resistant strains that cause bacteremia are probably not affected by IgM but will be opsonized if IgG antibody is produced. IgA antibodies are found in urine but their importance is not known. Antibody to the heat-labile enterotoxin is produced during natural disease due to enterotoxin-producing strains and after experimental challenge with enterotoxin-producing strains.

Prevention

Since most serious infections are hospital-acquired, control is difficult. Most infections are associated with inappropriate use of antibiotics and with use of cytotoxic drugs or contaminated materials. Infection can be minimized by good hospital care, i.e., proper use of antibiotics, aseptic techniques and proper use of urinary catheters.

Treatment

The antibiotic resistance patterns of *E. coli* are variable, and antibiotic sensitivity testing must be done. Most *E. coli* are sensitive to one of the following: tetracyclines, chloramphenicol, sulfonamides, ampicillin, or cephalexin.

Treatment must be approached with an understanding of the reason for infection. The underlying conditions that predispose or the site of infection that served as a focus for bacteremia must be identified and corrected. The patient must be carefully monitored with antibiotics and supportive therapy promptly given to patients with septicemia and signs of endotoxic shock.

Intestinal tract disease caused by the enterotoxin-producing strains does not require treatment with antibiotics. The water and salts lost should be replaced to correct dehydration.

Laboratory Procedures

All specimens should be gram stained and checked for gram-negative rods and for presence of pus cells (see Fig. 14–1). Stools may also be gram stained for detecting pus cells, which helps in differentiating invasive from noninvasive disease. Gram stain of stools from patients with enterotoxin-producing *E. coli* will not contain polymorphonuclear leukocytes.

Appropriate specimens (cerebrospinal fluid, pus, sputum, urine, and stool) are inoculated onto selective and differential media (chap. 13).

Blood cultures are processed in the usual manner and periodically subcultured to selective and differential media.

In diagnosis of urinary tract disease, it is important to identify patients with bacteriuria, particularly those who are asymptomatic, and also to distinguish between upper and lower urinary tract infections. Bacteriuria is detected by quantitative bacterial counts of the urine (quantitative urine culture) (chap. 4). Bacterial counts of 1,000 cells per milliliter in a clean catch specimen are not significant and reflect contamination of the specimen by urethral flora. Counts of 10^5 or more are significant and indicate bacteriuria. Intermediate counts are of questionable significance.

Infection of the kidney results in local production of immunoglobulins that react specifically with the infecting organisms. Antibody is not produced in lower urinary tract infections, and thus the organisms are not coated with immunoglobulins. This allows differentiation of upper and lower tract infections. Immunofluorescence with fluorescein-labeled anti-IgG is used to detect immunoglobulins on the bacterial surface.

KLEBSIELLA-ENTEROBACTER-SERRATIA

General Characteristics

Organisms of this group are gram-negative, facultatively anaerobic, non-spore-forming rods (Fig. 14–3). The *Klebsiella* are not motile and

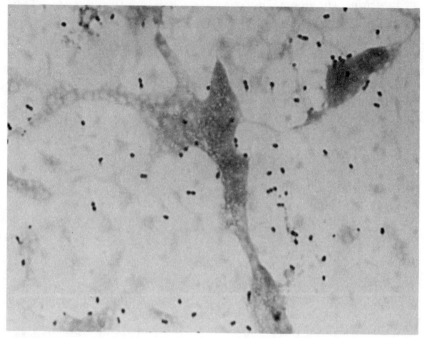

Fig. 14–3.—*Klebsiella pneumoniae* in cerebrospinal fluid from a patient with meningitis.

do not decarboxylate ornithine; the *Enterobacter* and *Serratia* are motile by peritrichous flagella and decarboxylate ornithine. The *Serratia* produce an extracellular DNase and many strains produce prodigiosin, a red pigment. None of the organisms in this group has special requirements for growth. Lactose is fermented.

Species
There are three species of *Klebsiella*, each of which can cause disease: *K. pneumoniae, K. rhinoscleromatis* and *K. ozaenae*. Four species of *Enterobacter*—*E. cloacae, E. aerogenes, E. hafniae* and *E. agglomerans*—have also been isolated from man. Three species of *Serratia* are recognized: *S. marcescens, S. rubidaea* and *S. liquefaciens*.

Ecology
The *Klebsiella* are found in the upper respiratory tract and the intestinal tract of about 5% of the population. The *Enterobacter* can be isolated from the intestinal tract of man, but they also exist as free-living saprophytes. The *Serratia* are found in water, soil and food.

Antigens and Toxins

The *Klebsiella* contain acidic polysaccharide capsules (K antigen). There are 80 serologically distinct capsules, some of which cross-react with the capsular polysaccharide of *Streptococcus pneumoniae* and other organisms. Eleven different O types have been described. Serologic classification is based on differentiation of the capsular polysaccharide. The *Enterobacter* spp. contain O and H antigens and some contain K antigens. For the *Serratia*, 15 O and 13 H antigens have been described.

Broth filtrates of *K. pneumoniae* cause fluid accumulation in ileal loops. The mechanism for this enterotoxic activity is unknown. The *Klebsiella, Enterobacter* and *Serratia* all contain endotoxin.

Infections

The urinary tract is a common site of nosocomial infections caused by *Klebsiella pneumoniae*. Bacteremia, meningitis, pneumonia and necrotizing enterocolitis also have been reported. *K. pneumoniae* is frequently found in persons who have a systemic disease such as diabetes or an underlying bronchopulmonary disease or viral infection of the respiratory tract. Chronic alcoholics are susceptible to pneumonia caused by *K. pneumoniae*. Other infections — sinusitis, endocarditis, liver abscess, enteritis and salpingitis — also have been reported.

Klebsiella pneumoniae along with other organisms, e.g., other enterics and *Pseudomonas aeruginosa,* cause a necrotizing pneumonia. The disease is acute with fever, malaise, dry cough and often pleuritic pain. The cough later becomes productive with copious amounts of thick, bloody, purulent sputum. The onset may also be insidious with weeks to months of malaise, low-grade fever, cough and loss of weight. Abscess formation and necrosis are common with cavity formation, bronchiectasis and pulmonary fibrosis. A septicemia occurs in about 25% of the cases of pneumonia caused by *K. pneumoniae*. The case fatality rate is 40–60%.

Differentiation of pneumonia caused by *K. pneumoniae* and other gram-negative rods from that caused by *S. pneumoniae* is important because *K. pneumoniae,* unlike *S. pneumoniae,* is resistant to penicillin. Secondly, the infectious process associated with gram-negative organisms frequently leads to necrosis and abscess formation with irreversible lung changes.

The *Enterobacter* and *Serratia* both produce diseases identical to those described for *K. pneumoniae*.

282   OPPORTUNISTIC ENTERIC BACTERIA

Klebsiella ozaenae causes a progressive fetid atrophic rhinitis. *Klebsiella rhinoscleromatis* causes a slow-growing, granulomatous, tumor-like mass in the external nares or the mucosa of the nose, throat, pharynx or larynx. Biopsy of the tumor-like mass shows large, swollen mononuclear cells with many encapsulated gram-negative cells in the cytoplasm. These cells are termed *Mikulicz's cells.*

Mechanisms of Pathogenicity

The normal, healthy individual does not become infected by *Klebsiella, Enterobacter* or *Serratia.* Colonization without tissue invasion usually results. However, if the organisms lodge in the alveoli either (1) because of aspiration from the upper respiratory tract or of aerosols produced during inhalation therapy or (2) because of functional alteration of the mucociliary blanket, they proliferate and an inflammatory response leading to disease occurs. Patients with anatomical alterations of the urinary tract due to preexisting disease or mechanical means (catheterization) also are susceptible to infection with these organisms. Frequently, catheterization results in deposition of the organisms into the urinary tract and the patient develops cystitis or pyelonephritis. In some patients the organisms disseminate from the primary infected area, resulting in bacteremia and endotoxic shock.

Immunity

The capsule of *K. pneumoniae* is antiphagocytic, and antibody to the capsule facilitates phagocytosis. Because they produce a capsule, the *Klebsiella* are better equipped to cause disease. The *Enterobacter* and *Serratia* spp. are readily phagocytosed and killed by polymorphonuclear leukocytes in the presence of fresh serum. Immunization of animals results in production of IgM and IgG antibody and complement-independent opsonins. Immunity is serotype-specific and directed against the O antigen.

Treatment

The *Klebsiella* are sensitive to kanamycin, gentamicin, polymyxins, chloramphenicol, cephalothin and streptomycin and are usually resistant to carbenicillin and ampicillin. Except for resistance to the cephalosporins, the *Enterobacter* are sensitive to the same antibiotics as the *Klebsiella.* Both the *Enterobacter* and *Serratia* produce a cephalosporinase.

The *Serratia* are generally more resistant to antibiotics than *Klebsiella* or *Enterobacter.* They are resistant to polymyxin B and colistin in addition to the cephalosporins as mentioned above. Most isolates are, however, sensitive to gentamicin, kanamycin, chloramphenicol and carbenicillin.

Laboratory Procedures

Gram stain of specimens from wounds, cerebrospinal fluid and sputum should be done (see Fig. 14–3).

Specimens are inoculated onto differential and selective media (chap. 13). The *Klebsiella* are nonmotile and do not decarboxylate ornithine, which is useful in differentiating these organisms from the *Enterobacter* and *Serratia*. Usually, the *Klebsiella* colonies are large and mucoid (due to capsule), which helps in differentiating them from other enterics. *Serratia marcescens* produces an extracellular DNase, which differentiates them from the *Enterobacter*. Also, many but not all isolates of *Serratia* produce the red pigment prodigiosin. Detection of prodigiosin may require incubation at room temperature.

PROTEUS

General Characteristics

These organisms are gram-negative, facultatively anaerobic, non-spore-forming rods ($0.4–0.6 \times 1.0–3.0 \ \mu m$). They may appear as coccobacilli or filaments or in pairs or chains. They are motile by peritrichous flagella and do not ferment lactose. Phenylalanine is deaminated to phenylpyruvic acid, which differentiates these organisms from other enterics. All species, except *P. inconstans,* rapidly decompose urea.

Species

The genus Proteus contains five species: *P. vulgaris, P. mirabilis, P. rettgeri, P. morganii* and *P. inconstans. P. inconstans* includes those organisms previously assigned to the genus *Providencia: P. alcalifaciens* and *P. stuartii.*

Ecology

These organisms are found in the intestinal tracts of man and animals and are free-living in nature, soil, water, sewage and decaying animal matter.

Antigens and Toxins

O, H, and K antigens are present, and schemes have been developed for serologic grouping. Patients with rickettsial infections develop antibodies that agglutinate certain strains of *Proteus* (OX-2, OX-19 and OX-K). These strains of *Proteus* share antigens with the *Rickett-sia*. Agglutination of these *Proteus* strains by serum from patients with rickettsial infections is called the Weil-Felix test and is useful in differentiating among infections caused by the various rickettsia (chap. 21).

Toxins other than endotoxin have not been described.

Infections

Proteus most frequently causes urinary tract infections. Septicemia and infection of other organs and tissues have also been reported on occasion. These organisms have been isolated from wounds and from patients with gastroenteritis. *Proteus mirabilis* is the most commonly isolated species. Nosocomial outbreaks with *P. rettgeri* and *P. incon-stans* have been reported.

Mechanisms of Pathogenicity

Like the other enterics, organisms of the genus *Proteus* are opportunists and cause disease only in debilitated persons or when inoculated into susceptible tissues via urinary or intravenous catheters. All

Fig. 14–4.—Bisected kidney showing renal calculi and hydronephrosis. (Courtesy of Dr. Winfield Morgan, Department of Pathology, West Virginia University Medical Center.)

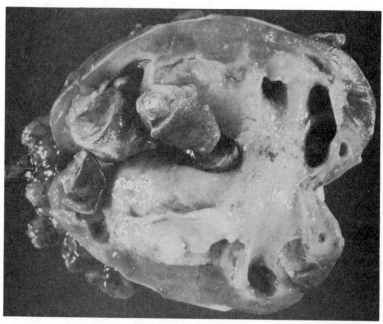

the *Proteus*, except *P. inconstans (Providencia)*, produce urease. The urease splits urea into CO_2 and NH_4^+. The ammonia released by the bacterial enzyme alkalinizes the urine (normal pH = 6.5) and lowers resistance of the tissue by inactivating C4. Alkalinization disrupts the urothelium and allows the organism to penetrate the renal parenchyma and cause tissue damage. Magnesium and calcium salts are precipitated at alkaline pH, and thus infection may contribute to production of renal calculi (stones) (Fig. 14–4). Experimentally, killed *Proteus*, which retain urease activity, cause kidney damage. Conversely, inhibitors of urease activity decrease renal damage.

Treatment

The antibiotic susceptibility is variable and laboratory testing for sensitivity is necessary as a guide to therapy. The organisms are frequently sensitive to gentamicin. Of the *Proteus* species, only *P. mirabilis*, the *Proteus* spp. most frequently isolated from urinary tract infections, is sensitive to penicillin G and ampicillin. *P. vulgaris*, often referred to as indole-positive *Proteus*, is resistant to penicillin. It should be pointed out that all *Proteus* spp. except *P. mirabilis* produce indole, thus indole-positive *Proteus* is not synonymous with *P. vulgaris*.

Laboratory Procedures

All specimens, especially urine, should be gram stained and observed for presence of gram-negative rods and leukocytes.

Cultures from appropriate sources (dependent on disease process) should be inoculated on selective and differential media. The ability to deaminate phenylalanine differentiates *Proteus* from other non-lactose fermenters. *P. inconstans* can be differentiated from other *Proteus* by absence of urease activity.

P. vulgaris and *P. mirabilis* both show "swarming" on noninhibitory agar medium. "Swarming" is the ability to migrate and cover part or all of the surface of the agar plate with a sheet of bacterial growth (Fig. 14–5). This creates a problem in clinical microbiology because it may result in overgrowth of other pathogenic organisms. Agars with sodium azide, phenylethyl alcohol or chloral hydrate are used to suppress growth of *Proteus* and inhibit spreading.

YERSINIA PSEUDOTUBERCULOSIS AND Y. ENTEROCOLITICA

General Characteristics

Y. pseudotuberculosis and *Y. enterocolitica* are non-lactose fermenting, gram-negative rods (0.5–0.8×1.5–2.0 μm). They are non-

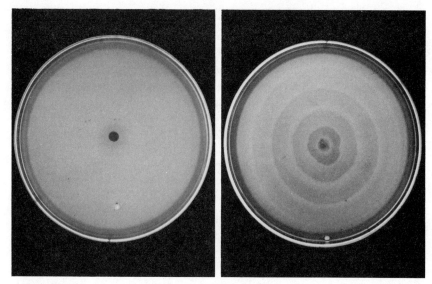

Fig. 14–5.—Growth of *Proteus* on agar. Note swarming **(right)** evidenced by waves of growth on surface. Nonswarming strain is on left.

spore-forming, facultative anaerobes that are motile at 22–25 C but nonmotile at 35 to 37 C. *Y. enterocolitica* grows best at 25 C. *Y. pseudotuberculosis* grows best at 37 C. *Y. pestis* causes a different disease and is described in Chapter 18.

Ecology

Both species of *Yersinia* are found in various domestic and wild animals (pigs, dogs, birds, chinchilla, cattle) and are transmitted to man through water and food contaminated with feces. In animals, *Y. pseudotuberculosis* causes an infection associated with mesenteric glands; the lesions grossly resemble tubercles. *Y. enterocolitica* has been isolated from the feces and lymph nodes of sick and healthy animals and from humans without evidence of the disease.

Antigens

Y. enterocolitica is divided into 17 serotypes based on the O antigens. Six serotypes have been described for *Y. pseudotuberculosis*. Cross reactions with *Brucella, Vibrio* and *Salmonella* have been reported. No toxins other than endotoxins have been demonstrated.

Infections

Both *Y. pseudotuberculosis* and *Y. enterocolitica* cause similar diseases. They have been isolated from patients with gastroenteritis, acute terminal ileitis, mesenteric lymphadenitis and septicemia. The septicemic form is associated with underlying disease, for example, cirrhosis of the liver, diabetes, leukemia, blood dyscrasias such as sickle cell anemia, and immunosuppressive treatment.

Infants usually develop fever, diarrhea and vomiting, whereas older children have an appendicitis-like syndrome. Many cases of infection with Y. enterocolitica are misdiagnosed as appendicitis. Adults develop fever and abdominal pain. Some cases are associated with arthritis or erythema nodosum. In addition, several other diseases, e.g., Reiter's syndrome, meningitis, panophthalmitis, have been associated with Y. enterocolitica infections.

Fever, malaise, hepatosplenomegaly, abdominal pain, diarrhea and vomiting are common features of diseases produced by both organisms. Abscesses of the liver, spleen and bone are associated with a subacute localizing form.

Both hospital-acquired and intrafamily outbreaks of Y. enterocolitica infections have been reported.

Mechanisms of Pathogenicity

These organisms are ingested with contaminated food and water. They penetrate the intestinal mucosa primarily in the ileocecal area. The lymph nodes in the intestinal wall and mesenteries become inflamed and focal areas of necrosis result. Ulceration of the intestinal mucosa can result and a septicemia may follow. The mechanism by which these changes occur is unknown. The only important bacterial factor that has been described is endotoxin.

Immunity

Serologic responses to the type antigens can be used to determine infection, but studies on the role of humoral or cellular immunity in these infections have not been done. Hypersensitivity to Y. pseudotuberculosis is produced and persists for years.

Treatment

Streptomycin, kanamycin and tetracycline have been used to treat Y. pseudotuberculosis. Y. enterocolitica infections have been treated with gentamicin, kanamycin, colistin, chloramphenicol, streptomycin, tetracycline and sulfamethoxazole-trimethoprim.

Laboratory Procedures

Blood cultures should be collected on patients with septicemia. Fecal specimens, lymph nodes and other tissues are inoculated onto blood agar, Eosin Methylene Blue agar or MacConkey's agar for isolation. The Yersinia do not ferment lactose. Cultures should be incubated at 25 C and 37 C. *Y. enterocolitica* grows best at 25 C, and incubation at this temperature offers a selective advantage in isolation. Both *Y. enterocolitica* and *Y. pseudotuberculosis* are motile at 25 C but not at 37 C. *Y. pseudotuberculosis* and *Y. enterocolitica* are urease producers and do not ferment lactose. *Y. enterocolitica* decarboxylates ornithine and ferments sucrose, whereas *Y. pseudotuberculosis* does not.

The serologic response may also be measured and be of value in diagnosis and epidemiology.

PROBLEM SOLVING AND REVIEW

No. 1. GIVEN: — A 45-year-old man was admitted to the hospital with complaints of pleuritic chest pain for several days. He reported that he was "sweating" and had had several shaking chills. His temperature was 39.5 C. His pulse was 132 beats per minute and his respiration rate was increased. He had a productive cough. A bloody (currant jelly) sputum was obtained. His white blood cell count was 25,000/cu mm with polymorphonuclear leukocytes predominant. The patient's family reported that he was a heavy drinker and had returned from a long drinking binge.

PROBLEMS: — 1. What is the presumptive diagnosis? 2. How would you try to establish a bacterial diagnosis? 3. If gram-negative encapsulated rods were observed in the gram stain, what might be the etiologic agent? 4. What are the characteristics of this organism? 5. What is the source of the organism? 6. How do the pathologic features of *K. pneumoniae* differ from those of *S. pneumoniae*? (Ans. p. 290.)

No. 2. GIVEN: — A 21-year-old woman was approximately 24 weeks pregnant with her second pregnancy. This pregnancy had been entirely uncomplicated until 1 week prior to admission, when the patient noted some increased frequency of urination but no dysuria, nocturia or hematuria. This progressed until 2 days prior to admission when she noted an increased feeling of malaise and felt febrile. She also complained of a low back and right flank pain. She appeared to be quite ill with marked flank and costovertebral tenderness and a temperature of 39.6 C. She had malaise and actually appeared somnolent. Her urinary output had decreased somewhat, but she had taken no fluids.

PROBLEMS: — 1. What is your provisional diagnosis? 2. What could you do to obtain data to support the clinical diagnosis? 3. The cultures showed a non-lactose fermenting, gram-negative rod that exhibited swarming on an agar plate. What organism would you suspect? 4. What property of the organism described in (3) do you associate with the ability of this organism to produce disease? 5. What other gram-negative organisms are associated with pyelonephritis? (Ans. p. 291.)

No. 3. GIVEN: — A 10-year-old boy had a 2-day history of fever, vomiting, diarrhea and intermittent abdominal pain. Physical examination showed a temperature of 39.4 C and generalized abdominal tenderness to deep palpation. Hemoglobin was 15.3 gm/100 ml and the white blood cell count was 35,100/cu mm, with 75% neutrophils, 10% bands, 9% lymphocytes and 6% monocytes. He was treated with penicillin G benzathine and discharged. Two days later he returned with the previous symptoms, pain in the lower right quadrant of the abdomen and temperature of 39 C. The patient was then diagnosed as having acute appendicitis and an appendectomy was done. Blood, stool, urine and a swab of the peritoneal cavity were submitted for culture.

Cultures were reported as negative for *Salmonella* and *Shigella*. A gram-negative non-lactose-fermenting organism that was motile at 25 and 37 C was isolated.

PROBLEMS: — 1. What is the probable cause of the boy's illness? Why? 2. How might a diagnosis other than appendicitis have been obtained? 3. What is the probable source of the organism? (Ans. p. 291.)

SUPPLEMENTARY READING

Battone, E. J.: *Yersinia enterocolitica:* A panoramic view of a charismatic microorganism, CRC Crit. Rev. Microbiol. 5:211–241, 1977.

Buffenmyer, C. L., Rycheck, R. R., and Yee, R. B.: Bacteriocin (Klebocin) sensitivity typing of *Klebsiella,* J. Clin. Microbiol. 4:239–244, 1976.

Dans, P. E., Barrett, F. E., Casey, J. I., and Finland, M.: *Klebsiella-Enterobacter* at Boston City Hospital. 1967, Arch. Intern. Med. 125:94–101, 1970.

Donta, S. T.: Tissue culture assay of antibodies to heat-labile *Escherichia coli* enterotoxins, N. Engl. J. Med. 291:117–212, 1974.

DuPont, H. L., Formal, S. B., Hornick, R. B., Snyder, M. J., Libonati, J. P., Sheahan, D. G., LaBrec, E. H., and Kalas, J. P.: Pathogenesis of *Escherichia coli* diarrhea, J. Med. (Basel) 285:1–9, 1971. ·

Evans, D. G., Evans, D. J., Jr., and Deupont, H. L.: Virulence factors of enterotoxigenic *Escherichia coli,* J. Infect. Dis. 136 (Supp.):S118, 1977.

Gangarosa, E. J., and Merson, M. H.: Epidemiological assessment of the relevance of the so-called enteropathogenic serogroups of *Escherichia coli* in diarrhea, N. Engl. J. Med. 296:1210–1213, 1977.

Gorbach, S. L., Kean, B. H., Evans, D. G., Evans, D. J., and Bessudo, D.: Travelers' diarrhea and toxigenic *Escherichia coli,* N. Engl. J. Med. 292: 933–936, 1975.

Griffith, D. P., and Musker, D. M.: Prevention of infected urinary stones by urease inhibition, Invest. Urol. 11:234, 1973.
Guerrant, R. L., Moore, R. A., Kirschenfeld, P. M., and Sande, M. A.: Role of toxigenic and invasive bacteria in acute diarrhea of childhood, N. Engl. J. Med. 293:567–573, 1975.
Hill, H. R., Hunt, C. E., and Matsen, J. M.: Nosocomial colonization with *Klebsiella*, type 26, in a neonatal intensive care unit associated with an outbreak of sepsis, meningitis, and necrotizing enterocolitis, J. Pediatr. 85: 415– 419, 1974.
Johnson, E., and Ellner, P. D.: Distribution of *Serratia* species in clinical specimens, Appl. Microbiol. 28:513–514, 1974.
Jones, S. R., Smith, J. W., and Sanford, J. P.: Localization of urinary tract infections by detection of antibody-coated bacteria in urine sediment, N. Engl. J. Med. 290:591–593, 1974.
Kaslow, R. A., Lindsey, J. O., Bisno, A. L., and Price, A.: Nosocomial infection with highly resistant *Proteus rettgeri*, Am. J. Epidemiol. 140:278–286, 1976.
Kayser, B., Holmgren, J., and Hanson, L. A.: The protective effect against *E. coli* of O and K antibodies of different immunoglobulin classes, Scand. J. Immunol. 1:27– 32, 1972.
Klipstein, F. A., and Engert, R. F.: Enterotoxinogenic intestinal bacteria in tropical sprue. III. Preliminary characterization of *Klebsiella pneumoniae* enterotoxin, J. Infect. Dis. 132:200– 203, 1975.
Maki, D. G., Hennekens, C. G., Phillips, C. W., Shaw, W. V., and Bennett, J. V.: Nosocomial urinary tract infection with *Serratia marcescens:* An epidemiologic study, J. Infect. Dis. 128:579–587, 1973.
Rose, H. D., and Babcock, J. B.: Colonization of intensive care unit patients with gram negative bacilli, Am. J. Epidemiol. 101:495–501, 1975.
Rubin, S. J., Brock, S., Chamberland, M., and Lyons, R. W.: Combined serotyping and biotyping of *Serratia marcescens*, J. Clin. Microbiol. 3:582–585, 1976.
Rudoy, R. C., and Nelson, J. D.: Enteroinvasive and enterotoxigenic *Escherichia coli*, Am. J. Dis. Child. 129:668–672, 1975.
Smith, J. W., Jones, S. R., and Kajser, B.: Significance of antibody-coated bacteria in urinary sediment in experimental pyelonephritis, J. Infect. Dis. 135: 577–581, 1977.
Somberkoff, M. S., Moldaves, N. H., and Rahal, J. J., Jr.: Specific and nonspecific immunity to *Serratia marcescens* infection, J. Infect. Dis. 134: 348–353, 1976.
Windblad, S. (ed.): *Yersinia, Pasteurella* and *Francisella*. Contributions to Microbiology and Immunology, vol. 2 (Basel: S. Karger, 1973).

ANALYSIS

No. 1.– 1. Bacterial pneumonia. 2. Perform gram stain and capsule stain of the sputum and send sputum and blood to the laboratory for culture. 3. *Klebsiella pneumoniae*. 4. Gram-negative, encapsulated rod. It is a lactose fermenter and is nonmotile. 5. Probably the upper respiratory tract of the patient. The organism entered the lower tract by aspiration of saliva or because of alteration of the mucociliary action. 6. Pneumonia caused by gram-negative rods results in extensive, irreversible tissue damage that heals by fibrosis.

No. 2. – 1. Urinary tract infection, probably pyelonephritis. 2. Gram stain of uncentrifuged urine. Presence of bacteria is significant. A midstream urine should be submitted for culture. 3. *Proteus vulgaris* or *Proteus mirabilis*. Probably *Proteus mirabilis* since it is associated with urinary tract infection more frequently than *Proteus vulgaris*. 4. Urease production which alkalinizes the urine and disrupts the urothelium. Ammonia produced by urease activity may also inactivate C4 and lower tissue resistance. 5. *E. coli, Klebsiella, Serratia*, etc.

No. 3. – 1. *Yersinia enterocolitica*. The characteristics of the organism suggest *Y. enterocolitica* and also because infections with this organism mimic acute appendicitis. 2. Cultures should have been obtained on the first visit. The laboratory should have been alerted to the possibility of *Y. enterocolitica*. 3. Animals, food, water, human carriers.

15 / Salmonella and Shigella

OVERVIEW

The *Salmonella* and *Shigella* are very important organisms in disease production. The organism that causes the most serious disease is *Salmonella typhi*. Improved methods of sanitation and immunization have resulted in control of typhoid fever, and, in fact, routine immunization is no longer recommended. Still, in 1976, there were 419 cases of typhoid fever reported to the Center for Disease Control. The potential for limited outbreaks, however, remains, as evidenced by an outbreak in 1973 associated with a contaminated water supply that involved 210 persons.

Gastroenteritis, caused by the *Salmonella* sp., is a major cause of food-borne disease and affects more than 2×10^6 persons each year. The widespread distribution of these organisms in pets and in animals used for food makes control of this disease very difficult.

The *Shigella* also continue to be important agents of disease. Outbreaks still occur in the United States, but the *Shigella* species endemic in the United States (*S. flexneri* and *S. sonnei*) usually do not cause serious disease or high mortality. Outbreaks associated with contaminated water and ice on a passenger cruise ship, food served at a county fair, a school water supply and swimming in the Mississippi River attest to the presence and public nuisance created by these organisms. An epidemic of dysentery caused by the more virulent *S. dysenteriae* recently occurred in Central America.

SALMONELLA

General Characteristics

The *Salmonella* are gram-negative, facultative anaerobic rods $(0.6 \times 2-3 \ \mu\text{m})$ that do not ferment lactose or sucrose. They produce H_2S and are motile except for *S. enteritidis* bioserotype *Pullorum*. Special growth factors are not required. All species except *S. typhi* and

293

TABLE 15-1.—ANTIGENIC ANALYSIS OF SALMONELLAE

		ANTIGENIC FORMULA			
			H		
SPECIES	SEROGROUP*	0	PHASE 1	PHASE 2	Vi
*S. enteritidis** bioserotype *Paratyphi* A or *S. paratyphi* A†	A	1, 2, 12	a	–	–
S. enteritidis serotype *Typhimurium** or *S. typhimurium*†	B	1, 4, 5, 12	i	1, 2	–
S. choleraesuis	C	6, 7	c	1, 5	–
S. enteritidis serotype *Enteritidis** or *S. enteritidis*†	D	1, 9, 12	g,m	–	–
S. typhi	D	9, 12	d	–	Vi

*Edwards-Ewing classification scheme.
†Kauffmann-White classification scheme.

some serotypes of *S. enteritidis* produce gas. As a group, they are biochemically complex and are speciated primarily by serologic analysis.

Species

Two classification systems are in use. One system (Kauffmann-White) recognizes each serotype as a species. About 1,800 species have been identified by serologic analysis. The second system (Edwards-Ewing) recognizes three species: *S. choleraesuis, S. typhi* and *S. enteritidis*. The remaining species in the Edwards-Ewing system are bioserotypes, or serotypes, of *S. enteritidis* (Table 15-1). For example, *S. typhimurium* (Kauffmann-White system) is recognized as *S. enteritidis* serotype *Typhimurium* and *S. paratyphi* A is identified as *S. enteritidis* bioserotype *Paratyphi* A in the Edwards-Ewing system.

Arizona hinshawii is considered by some to be a species of *Salmonella (S. arizonae)*.

Ecology

The *Salmonella* consist of a large and diverse group of organisms with different ecological associations. One species, *S. typhi,* shows a strict host preference and is found primarily in man and only on occasion in nonhumans. A second species, *S. choleraesuis,* is found primarily in animals and rarely infects man, but when it does, the disease

is serious. The third species, S. enteritidis, shows little host preference. These organisms are found in animals and readily infect man
and animals. The Arizona sp. (Salmonella arizonae) causes diseases
similar to those of the Salmonella.

Salmonella are found in rats, mice, insects and also in poultry, eggs,
egg products, cattle, sheep, swine, horses, dogs, cats and turtles. The
high incidence of gastroenteritis caused by the Salmonella spp. is not
difficult to understand because of the ease of contamination of food
products by rodents, the use of animals for food, which may be infected or contaminated during processing, and the use of extracts of animal tissues and insects as food additives and in pharmaceutical products. Many infections of man result from association with household
pets (dogs, cats, snakes, turtles, etc.). Infected dogs and turtles represent a major source of Salmonella.

Antigens

The Salmonella contain three different antigens, the O, H, and Vi
antigens. The O antigens, like O antigens for other bacteria, are located in the cell wall. The serologic specificity of the O antigen is determined by the terminal polysaccharide portion of the lipopolysaccharide. Each Salmonella may contain two or more heat-stable O antigens, some of which are shared with other Salmonella spp (see
Table 15–1).

The H antigens are heat-labile flagellar antigens, and each species
or bioserotype may produce one or more sets of flagellar antigens.
Species or serotypes containing one set of antigens are termed monophasic; those with two sets are termed diphasic. The bacteria synthesize only one set of antigens at a given time and are said to be in a certain phase (phase 1 or phase 2) when expressing a certain antigenic
set. Each phase may contain one or more antigens. For example, S.
choleraesuis (Fig. 15–1) are diphasic, i.e., they may produce flagellar
antigen C (phase 1) or flagellar antigens 1, 5 (phase 2). The phase 1
antigens are specific and are shared by only a few species or serotypes
and are designated by lower-case letters. The phase 2 antigens are

Fig. 15–1.—Phase variation in S. choleraesuis.

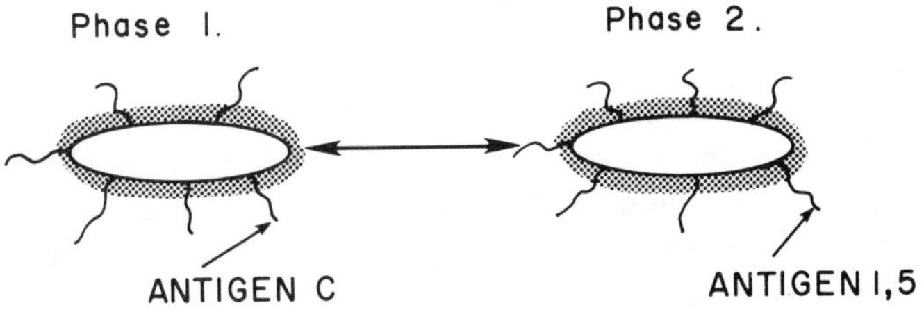

Phase I.   Phase 2.

ANTIGEN C   ANTIGEN I,5

shared among several species; they are less specific than the phase 1 antigens and are designated by Arabic numerals (see Table 15–1).

A third antigen, the Vi antigen, is a K-like or capsular antigen. It is termed Vi because this antigen relates to virulence. The Vi antigen is a polymer of N-acetyl-D-galactosamine uronic acid. Only two species of *Salmonella, S. typhi* and *S. choleraesuis*, contain the Vi antigen, but other enteric bacteria, e.g., *Citrobacter* and *Escherichia*, may also contain the Vi antigen.

Specific antisera are used for determining the antigenic formula of the *Salmonella*. Knowing the antigenic formula, one can designate the species, serotype, or both. An abbreviated example of this scheme is shown in Table 15–1.

Note that several antigens (example, O antigens 1, 12) are shared among several serogroups. Among the phase 2 flagellar antigens, antigen 1 is also found in more than a single species. Identification is based on the total antigenic formula with the differences in antigenic formula being the basis for species or serotypes.

Detection of antibody response in man to O, H and Vi antigens can be used in the serologic diagnosis of infections caused by the *Salmonella*.

Genetics

The *Salmonella*, like other bacteria, undergo an S→R dissociation. Loss of ability to synthesize O, H and Vi antigens and acquisition of new O antigens by lysogenic conversion have been documented. Acquisition of ability to ferment lactose has also been described. Antibiotic resistance mediated by R factor transfer has been demonstrated in the laboratory and in clinical isolates and represents a problem in using antibiotics to treat these infections.

Phage typing is useful in epidemiologic characterization of some species of *Salmonella*, notably *S. typhi*.

Toxins

Two substances important in the pathogenesis of *Salmonella* infection have been described. One is endotoxin; the other is an enterotoxin. The enterotoxin is a cell wall-associated factor that causes diarrhea when fed orally to mice.

Infections

Several types of disease occur after infection with *Salmonella*. The type of disease is in general related to the infecting species and is a measure of virulence and invasiveness of the organisms. Figure 15–2 outlines the pathogenesis of the diseases (salmonelloses) caused by the *Salmonella*.

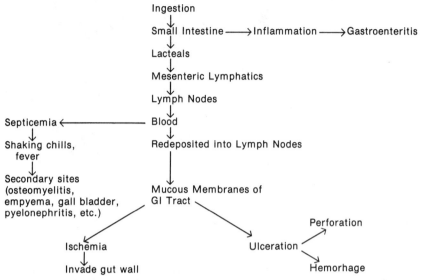

Fig. 15–2. – Pathogenesis of the salmonelloses.

Enteric Fever (Typhoid Fever)

The etiologic agent of typhoid fever, *S. typhi,* is acquired by ingestion of bacilli obtained either directly from an infected person or carrier or indirectly through food or water contaminated by a patient or carrier.

The incubation period is 7–14 days. The initial symptoms may be mild. Initially there is fever which rises in a stepwise manner to 40 C; the fever may continue through the second and third week of the disease. Onset of symptoms is gradual with anorexia, lethargy, malaise, general aches and pains. The patient complains of a dull, continuous headache which is frontal. Most have a nonproductive cough and there may be nosebleed. Although some patients have diarrhea, constipation is the most common intestinal complaint.

The patient is severely ill during the second and third weeks of the disease. Small maculopapular lesions (2–5 mm in diameter) called rose spots may occur on the trunk. The rose spots result from intracapillary agglutination of the organism. The patient is weak and may be confused; the face is dull and expressionless. Delirium is common. The abdomen may be tender on palpation and distended. Convalescence is slow – the patient may fully recover only after a month or more. Secondary foci of infection may lead to serious complications with hemorrhage or perforation of the intestine and

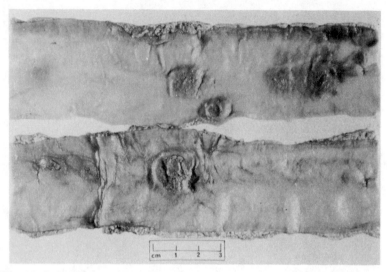

Fig. 15–3.—Ulcerated Peyer's patches in small intestine from a patient with typhoid fever. (From Emond, R. T. D. (ed.): *Color Atlas of Infectious Diseases* [Chicago: Year Book Medical Publishers, Inc., 1974]. Courtesy of editor and publisher.)

peritonitis (Fig. 15–3); thrombophlebitis, cerebral thrombosis, cholecystitis, encephalopathy, pneumonia, osteomyelitis, meningitis and endocarditis may also occur.

Similar signs and symptoms may occur after infection with other *Salmonella*.

Septicemia

A septicemia, without evidence of intestinal disease, may follow ingestion of the *Salmonella*. This syndrome is characterized by a prolonged and intermittent febrile state, chills, anorexia, and weight loss. There is a marked anemia, hepatosplenomegaly and persistent bacteremia. In the noncomplicated septicemia, the leukocyte count is usually normal. Localized infection with a polymorphonuclear leukocytosis may occur. Foci of infection may form in any organ or tissue. *S. choleraesuis* is commonly associated with the septicemic form of *Salmonella* infection.

Gastroenteritis

This is the most common form of *Salmonella* infection. The incubation period is 8–24 hours. Nausea and vomiting may occur initially and are followed by abdominal pain and mild or severe diarrhea. The patient's temperature ranges from 38 to 39 C; the leukocyte count is usually normal. Leukocytes are found in the stool. The patient usually recovers with or without treatment within 5 days. Dehydration and electrolyte loss may be quite marked, particularly in the young and elderly. *S. enteritidis* bioserotype *Typhimurium* is the major cause of gastroenteritis in the United States, although almost any species or serotype can be involved.

Mechanisms of Pathogenicity

Many host factors relate to the ability of the *Salmonella* to survive in man. First, the organisms must be able to survive the acidity of the stomach and enter the intestinal lumen. This may be facilitated by ingestion of *Salmonella* in food, which may buffer the gastric acid, or with water, which may dilute the gastric acid and facilitate survival of the organism. Any surgical procedure or disease that affects gastric acidity predisposes to infection. *S. typhi* possesses the Vi antigen, which may afford protection against gastric acidity. Persons with diseases such as liver cirrhosis, lupus, neoplastic processes, sickle cell anemia or malaria are susceptible to *Salmonella* infection. Whether or not infection occurs clearly depends on the number of organisms, virulence and resistance of the host.

In the intestinal lumen the organisms must survive the antagonistic effects of the normal flora and their products. About 1 million *Salmonella* must be ingested to cause disease in man. Treatment with antibiotics, which alters the oral flora, markedly reduces the number of bacilli required to initiate disease in man. In fact, antibiotic therapy in patients with *Salmonella* gastroenteritis prolongs survival of organisms as indicated by the prolonged carrier state.

In gastroenteritis, the mechanism for diarrhea is unknown but is probably related to production of an enterotoxin. It is clear that invasiveness of epithelial cells and growth in the lamina propria are prerequisites for production of enteritis but other factors are also required for disease production. Penetration of the mucosa and submucosa results in an inflammatory response in the colon and ileum and then diarrhea. Despite the alteration in histologic features, increased transmucosal permeability is unchanged and is apparently not the mechanism for production of diarrhea. Enterotoxic activity, associated with activation of adenyl cyclase, has been demonstrated but the activation of adenyl cyclase by *Salmonella*, unlike that caused by *V. cholerae*, is inhibited by indomethacin. Indomethacin, an inhibitor of prostaglandin synthesis, prevents the increase in adenyl cyclase, suggesting that the *Salmonella*, as a result of inflammation, increase prostaglandin synthesis, which causes the loss of salts and diarrhea.

If the *Salmonella* species is of sufficient virulence, it penetrates the intestinal wall, enters the lymphatic system and then disseminates throughout the host and establishes infection in other organs. After penetration, the organisms are phagocytized by macrophages and transported to other tissue. Survival in the macrophage is probably due to the O antigen or Vi antigen. With some organisms, e.g., S. *choleraesuis*, the intestinal lesions may not be evident.

Organisms associated with enteric fever penetrate the intestinal wall, multiply in the lymph nodes and submucosa, and then disseminate throughout the body. Continued growth in the intestinal wall may result in perforation.

Many of the signs and symptoms of enteric fever and septicemia can be related to endotoxin (chap. 13). Other factors that might relate to signs and symptoms have not been described.

Immunity

Immunity to *Salmonella* gastroenteritis apparently is not produced. Immunization with killed preparations of S. *typhi* results in production of circulating antibodies and low-level immunity to S. *typhi*. However, infection can occur in patients with high levels of anti-O, H and Vi antibodies. The mechanism of immunity is not clear. The experimental data suggest that opsonin, the enhanced activity of macrophages containing cytophilic antibody, and an accelerated inflammation due to hypersensitivity constitute acquired immunity. Humoral antibody is apparently important in clearing organisms from the blood, but cellular immunity is necessary to prevent bacterial multiplication in tissues.

Prevention and Control

Salmonella infection is prevented by maintenance of good methods of sanitation, control of vectors such as flies which may transmit the bacilli, immunization of those at risk because of travel or occupation and detection and control of carriers. Acetone-killed S. *typhi* vaccines are available but are not recommended for routine immunization. Present methods of sanitation, the low incidence of typhoid fever and low efficacy of the vaccine no longer make routine immunization practical unless one is working with the organism or traveling in an endemic area. Vaccines are available for S. *typhi* and S. *enteritidis* bioserotype *Paratyphi* A and serotype *Paratyphi* B but not for other *Salmonella*.

Animals and man are the sources of *Salmonella*. After infection, humans may continue to excrete organisms in the absence of disease for weeks to years. About 3% of patients recovering from typhoid fever become chronic carriers and thus a source for future outbreaks unless adequately treated or placed under surveillance so as not to be a source for infection. Women become carriers of S. *typhi* more frequently than men. Three types of carriers are recognized: (1) convalescent carriers who excrete bacilli for 1 to 2 months, (2) chronic carriers who may excrete organisms for years and (3) intermittent carriers who excrete periodically.

Nosocomial outbreaks of salmonellosis also occur. The source may be infected patients or staff with transmission to other patients either directly or indirectly via environmental contamination. Hospitalized patients, because of depressed host resistance due to preexisting disease, are markedly susceptible to infection.

Treatment

It must be stressed that patients with *Salmonella* gastroenteritis should not be treated with antibiotics because of the prolonged carrier state that results and the risk of inducing resistance to the antibiotic. Therapy to replace the fluid and electrolyte loss should be instituted.

Patients with bacteremia, enteric fever or secondary infection must receive chemotherapy. Chloramphenicol is the antibiotic of choice, but chloramphenicol-resistant strains due to a chloramphenicol-resistance plasmid have caused epidemics. Ampicillin is also used but resistance may occur. Trimethoprim-sulfamethoxazole can be used for treatment of infections caused by resistant strains.

Cholecystectomy may be necessary to eliminate the chronic carrier state and is effective in 85% of the cases. Ampicillin is used for treatment of chronic carriers without gallbladder disease.

Laboratory Procedures

Stool

Gram stain of feces from patients with gastroenteritis should be done. The presence of inflammatory cells helps in differentiating intestinal disease caused by invasive bacteria from that due to noninvasive bacteria, viruses and parasites. Feces should be inoculated onto differential, selective, and enrichment media (chap. 13). After 18 to 24 hours' incubation, non-lactose-fermenting colonies should be inoculated into other media for final identification and then serogrouped and typed. Agglutination testing using polyvalent serum should also be done on the initial isolates of non-lactose fermenters.

Blood

Blood cultures should be obtained on patients with septicemia and enteric fever. Blood cultures are usually positive during the first 2 weeks of the disease in patients with enteric fever. About 50% of blood cultures are positive during the 3d week. Rose spots and bone marrow can also be cultured.

Blood for serologic testing may also be helpful in diagnosis of typhoid fever. A fourfold increase in agglutination titer is significant. Determination of serum agglutinins is referred to as the Widal test.

Other Cultures

Urine, sputum and synovial fluid may also be cultured during the latter phases of typhoid fever. Urine cultures are positive in about 25% of patients with enteric fever during the 3d and 4th weeks of disease.

SHIGELLA

General Characteristics

The *Shigella* are gram-negative, facultatively anaerobic, non-spore-forming rods ($0.5-0.7\times2-3\ \mu m$). They are non-motile and do not produce H_2S, which helps differentiate them from most of the *Salmonella*. They grow well on most media and have no special growth requirements. They are non-lactose fermenters and produce acid but usually not gas from glucose and other carbohydrates. *Shigella sonnei* may show delayed fermentation of lactose.

Species

All members of the genus *Shigella* cause bacillary dysentery. Four species constitute the genus: *S. dysenteriae*, *S. flexneri*, *S. boydii* and *S. sonnei*. *Shigella dysenteriae* causes the most serious disease.

Ecology

The *Shigella* are parasites of man and are found only rarely in other primates. In the United States, *S. flexneri* and *S. sonnei* are the predominant isolates with *S. sonnei* most frequently isolated.

Genetics

Both S and R colony types of *Shigella* have been described. Colicins and phages are produced, and attempts have been made to classify *Shigella* by phage and colicin susceptibility. R factors are readily acquired and the transfer of these factors along with antibiotic resistance, both single and multiple, has created a problem in treatment.

Multiple-antibiotic resistance in *Shigella* was first noted in Japan in the 1950s, and by the end of the 1960s the majority of *Shigella* (about 80%) isolated in Japan were resistant to most antibiotics. Multiply resistant *Shigella* have been isolated in the United States. Reports from

TABLE 15-2.—SEROGROUPS AND SEROTYPES OF *SHIGELLA*

GROUP	NO. OF SEROTYPES	SCIENTIFIC NAME	COMMON NAME
A	10	S. dysenteriae	Shiga's bacillus
B	6	S. flexneri	Flexner's bacillus
C	15	S. boydii	Boyd's bacillus
D	1	S. sonnei	Sonne-Duval bacillus

different geographic areas and even from different institutions in a geographic area are variable, but a recent report on *Shigella* isolated in New York City indicates resistance to one or more antibiotics for 66% of the isolates.

The *Shigella* are susceptible to bacteriophage but phage typing is not useful for epidemiologic studies.

Antigens

The *Shigella* can be divided into four groups based on major O antigens and into from one *(S. sonnei)* to many serotypes based on other O antigens (Table 15-2).

Some strains of *Shigella* contain an envelope (K) antigen which prevents agglutination with anti-O serum. The K antigen can be removed by boiling.

An interesting relationship exists between the *Shigella* serogroups' ability to ferment mannitol and virulence. Group A *(S. dysenteriae)*, the most virulent species, usually does not ferment mannitol, whereas organisms in groups B, C and D usually ferment mannitol.

Toxins and Virulence Factors

The *Shigella* contain endotoxins. Exotoxins with neurotoxic, enterotoxic and cytotoxic activity have been described. In rabbits, the neurotoxic activity results in hindlimb paralysis after parenteral injection. Cytotoxicity for tissue culture cells, fluid accumulation in ileal loops and activation of adenyl cyclase have also been reported. Whether these activities are due to a single toxin is as yet unclear but probable.

Virulent strains of *Shigella* are able to penetrate epithelial cells. The mechanism is not known but it is unrelated to exotoxin production.

Infections

The incubation period for shigellosis is 2-3 days. The onset of disease is abrupt with fever and abdominal cramping and then diarrhea. The abdomen is tender but not rigid. The stools are watery and con-

TABLE 15-3.—DIFFERENTIATION OF BACILLARY AND
AMEBIC DYSENTERY

	BACILLARY DYSENTERY	AMEBIC DYSENTERY
Etiology:	*Shigella* sp.	*Entamoeba histolytica*
Type of disease:	Usually acute	Chronic, not acute
Tissue localization:	Limited to intestinal tract	Cause hepatic and brain abscesses
Lesion:	Superficial mucosal ulcer	Shallow, undermining ulcer
Cellular infiltrate:	Polymorphonuclear leukocytes	Mononuclear cells

tain mucus, blood and polymorphonuclear leukocytes. Tenesmus also occurs. In the usual case, the fever lasts about 3 days. Some patients may not have fever, the diarrhea may not be severe and the stool may not contain blood and mucus. Usually the disease subsides within a week. The infection is confined to the intestine, primarily the colon. Penetration of the intestinal mucosa results in inflammation and formation of a superficial ulcer. The fluid and electrolyte loss may be quite large and shock may result. In some cases a pseudomembrane composed of fibrin, polymorphonuclear leukocytes, cell debris and bacteria may cover the ulcer. Only rarely is there a bacteremia. Excretion of *Shigella* usually continues for about 1 month with a small number of patients excreting bacilli for 3 months or more.

In some cases, particularly in those countries where *Entamoeba histolytica* is prevalent, differentiation between dysentery produced by this protozoan and the *Shigella* sp. may be necessary (Table 15-3).

Mechanisms of Pathogenicity

In man infection can occur after ingestion of as few as 200 organisms. Whether infection occurs depends on factors such as ability of the organisms to survive the acidity of the stomach and the antagonistic effects of the normal bowel flora. Sodium bicarbonate administered along with *Shigella* to human volunteers or animals increases the ability to cause infection. The organisms must penetrate intestinal epithelial cells and multiply in the intestinal wall of the terminal ileum and colon. Unlike the *Salmonella*, the *Shigella* have only limited invasiveness and penetrate only into the submucosa or lamina propria. Infection results in inflammation which progresses to a shallow ulcer sometimes covered with a pseudomembrane. Because of the pseudomembrane, the ulcers are referred to as diphtheritic.

Infections with *S. dysenteriae* have a higher mortality than infections with other *Shigella*. This has been associated with production of an exotoxin that has both neurotoxic and enterotoxic activities. Neurologic symptoms (meningismus) are associated with S. *dysenteriae* infection and it is suggested that these may be due to the neurotoxin. The heat-labile enterotoxin is cytotoxic for HeLa cells, causes accumulation of fluid in intestinal loops and thus is associated with diarrhea. Some reports indicate that the enterotoxin is only cytotoxic, whereas others state that it activates adenyl cyclase. Studies in man on the role of the enterotoxin in human disease showed that epithelial penetration (invasiveness) is the primary virulence property. Shigellosis can be produced with strains that do not elaborate enterotoxin, but the disease is milder than that produced with strains that are both invasive and enterotoxin producers. Strains that produce enterotoxin but are not invasive do not cause disease. An enterotoxin with similar biologic and immunologic properties has been isolated also from S. *flexneri*, but it is produced in lower amounts by S. *flexneri* than by S. *dysenteriae*.

It is clear that enterotoxin alone is not required for production of disease. Indomethacin administered prior to or during infection results in inhibition of fluid production, suggesting that prostaglandins may also be important in causing diarrhea.

Immunity

Low levels of circulating antibodies to the *Shigella* are produced after infection, but these antibodies are not effective because the infection is localized to the large intestine. Secretory immunoglobulins may be important in recovery from the disease. Repeated episodes of bacillary dysentery occur; however, the symptoms are less severe in patients reinfected with the same serotype, suggesting partial but not complete immunity.

Experimentally, immunity after infection with a live *E. coli–Shigella* hybrid has been demonstrated.

Prevention

The *Shigella* cause disease only in man and primates. Man is the reservoir for the organism, which is transmitted by carriers through food or water contaminated by feces, or by mechanical vectors such as flies. Young children (<5 years), debilitated persons and malnourished persons are most susceptible to the disease. About 60% of isolations are from children under 10 years of age. Population groups with substandard sanitation due to conditions of crowding and those who are unable to maintain personal hygiene have a high incidence of shigellosis. After infection, carriers may excrete organisms for 3 to 5 weeks with about 3–6% becoming intermittent carriers.

Prevention requires good sanitation and personal hygiene. Vaccines are not available.

Treatment

Except for serious cases of the disease, antibiotic usage is discouraged because of the ability of the organism to acquire antibiotic resistance factors. The disease is usually self-limiting and only supportive therapy (fluid replacement) is necessary. Generally, antidiarrheal drugs are not recommended because they prolong fever, diarrhea and excretion of organisms.

In serious cases ampicillin is the antibiotic of choice. Chloramphenicol and tetracycline also may be used. Patients with organisms resistant to ampicillin and chloramphenicol have been successfully treated with trimethoprim-sulfamethoxazole.

Laboratory Procedures

Stool specimens or rectal swabs obtained by sigmoidoscopy should be obtained. Gram stains of mucus will show clumps of neutrophils, macrophages and erythrocytes. Mucus from the stool specimens should be plated immediately. If a delay between obtaining the specimen and culture occurs, the specimen should be placed in a transport medium such as glycerol saline (1 gm feces per 10 ml solution).

Specimens are cultured in an enrichment broth and also on differential and selective medias. After incubation, non-lactose-fermenting organisms are selected, tested by agglutination with specific serogroup antisera and then inoculated into media for determining motility, gas production and other characteristics. The *Shigella* are nonmotile, non-lactose fermenters (except for *S. sonnei*) and do not produce gas or hydrogen sulfide.

PROBLEM SOLVING AND REVIEW

No. 1. Given: — A 28-year-old man was seen at the outpatient clinic with complaints of anorexia, malaise, sore muscles and a headache that had persisted for several days. He also had a sore throat and a nonproductive cough. He had a fever of 37.8 C. The patient was unsure of his immunization history but thought he had been immunized against everything during military service 10 years previously. The patient was employed as a laborer on a road construction project. He had returned from a fishing trip to Mexico 3 days before he came to the clinic. He had not felt well during the last 2 days of his trip and for that reason had returned early. The patient's disease was diagnosed as infectious mononucleosis. He was given penicillin and aspirin and sent home.

A week later the patient returned to the hospital. He was acutely ill;

he still had a fever of 39.5 C, and he complained of constipation. He was mentally confused and did not respond well to questioning. Physical examination showed a few maculopapular lesions scattered over the abdomen and chest and hepatosplenomegaly. The white blood cell count was 6,500/cu mm with normal differential; hemoglobin was 14.1 gm/100 ml and there was a slight anemia and proteinuria.

PROBLEMS: — 1. What is the probable diagnosis? 2. What specimens should you send for laboratory diagnosis? 3. The organism isolated from blood and stool cultures was a gram-negative, motile, non-lactose fermenter. Serologic studies reported a 1:100 *Salmonella* titer. What is the probable genus of the organism? 4. How would you determine species of the organism? 5. What is the mechanism for production of the maculopapular rash? 6. What microbial or host factor is responsible for fever and other symptoms? 7. What is the source of the organism? 8. What antibiotics would be used in treatment? 9. What is a possible complication of this disease? (Ans. p. 309.)

NO. 2. GIVEN: — An outbreak of diarrhea in a retirement home was reported to the local department of health. The patients had a low-grade fever, approximately 37.6 C, and complained of cramping followed by numerous watery stools. Several patients were severely dehydrated.

Gram stain of mucus from the stool showed gram-positive cocci, gram-negative rods and numerous polymorphonuclear leukocytes. Stool specimens were sent to the laboratory for culture. A non-lactose-fermenting, nonmotile, non-gas-producing organism was isolated.

PROBLEMS: — 1. What is the most likely causative organism (genus and species)? 2. What is the probable source? 3. What is the location of the organism in man? 4. What is the likelihood of a septicemia? 5. What other specimens should be sent to the laboratory? 6. What is the appropriate approach to treatment? (Ans. p. 309.)

SUPPLEMENTARY READING

Askeroff, B., and Bennett, J. V.: Effect of antibiotic therapy in acute salmonellosis on the fecal excretion of salmonellae, N. Engl. J. Med. 281:636–640, 1969.
Baine, W. B., Herron, C. A., Bridson, K., Barker, W. H., Jr., Lindell, S., Mallison, G. F., Wells, J. G., Martin, W. T., Kosuri, M. R., Carr, F., and Voelker, E., Sr.: Waterborne shigellosis at a public school, Am. J. Epidemiol. 101:323–332, 1975.
Charney, A. N., Gots, R. E., Formal, S. B., and Giannella, R. A.: Activation of intestinal mucosal adenylate cyclase by *Shigella dysenteriae* I enterotoxin, Gastroenterology 70:1085–1090, 1976.

308   SALMONELLA AND SHIGELLA

Hoffman, T. A., Ruiz, C. J., Counts, G. W., Sachs, J. M., and Nitzkin, J. L.: Waterborne typhoid fever in Dade County, Florida. Clinical and therapeutic evaluation of 105 bacteremic patients, Am. J. Med. 59:481–487, 1975.

Farmer, J. J., III, Hickman, F. W., and Sikes, J. V.: Automation of *Salmonella typhi* phage typing, Lancet 2:787–790, 1975.

Feldman, R. E., Baine, W. B., Nitzkin, J. L., Saslaw, M. S., and Pollard, R. A., Jr.: Epidemiology of *Salmonella typhi* infection in a migrant labor camp in Dade County, Florida, J. Infect. Dis. 130:334–342, 1974.

Giannella, R. A., Formal, S. B., Dammin, G. J., and Collins, H.: Pathogenesis of salmonellosis. Studies of fluid secretion, mucosal invasion, and morphologic reaction in the rabbit ileum, J. Clin. Invest. 52:441–453, 1973.

Giannella, R. A., Gots, R. E., Charney, A. N., Greenough, W. B., III, and Formal, S. B.: Pathogenesis of *Salmonella*-mediated intestinal fluid secretion. Activation of adenylate cyclase and inhibition by indomethacin, Gastroenterology 69:1238–1245, 1975.

Giannella, R. A., Washington, O., Gemski, P., and Formal, S. B.: Invasion of HeLa cells by *Salmonella typhimurium*: A model for study of invasiveness of *Salmonella*, J. Infect. Dis. 128:69–75, 1973.

Johnson, R. H., Lutwick, L. I., Huntley, G. A., and Vosti, K. L.: *Arizona hinshawii* infections. New cases, antimicrobial sensitivities, and literature review, Ann. Intern. Med. 85:587–592, 1976.

Kinsey, M. D., Dammin, G. J., Formal, S. B., and Giannella, R. A.: The role of altered intestinal permeability in the pathogenesis of *Salmonella* diarrhea in the Rhesus monkey, Gastroenterology 71:429–434, 1976.

Koupal, L. R., and Deibel, B. H.: Assay, characterization and localization of an enterotoxin produced by *Salmonella*, Infect. Immun. 11:14–22, 1975.

Levine, M. M., DuPont, H. L., Formal, S. B., Hornick, R. B., Takeuchi, A., Gangarosa, E. J., Snyder, M. J., and Libonati, J. P.: Pathogenesis of *Shigella dysenteriae* I (Shiga) dysentery, J. Infect. Dis. 127:261–270, 1973.

Levine, M., Gangarosa, E., Barrow, W., and Weiss, C.: Shigellosis in custodial institutions. V. Effect of intervention with streptomycin-dependent *Shigella sonnei*, Am. J. Epidemiol. 104:88–92, 1976.

Marecki, N. M., Hsu, H. S., and Mayo, D. R.: Cellular and humoral aspects of host resistance in murine salmonellosis, Br. J. Exp. Pathol. 56:231–243, 1975.

McIver, J., Grady, G. F., and Keusch, G. T.: Production and characterization of exotoxin(s) of *Shigella dysenteriae* type I, J. Infect. Dis. 131:559–566, 1975.

Merson, M. H., Tenney, J. H., Meyers, J. D., Wood, B. T., Wells, J. G., Rymzo, W., Cline, B., DeWitt, W. E., Skaliy, P., and Mallison, G. F.: Shigellosis at sea: An outbreak aboard a passenger cruise ship, Am. J. Epidemiol. 101:165–175, 1975.

Neu, H. C., Cherubin, C. E., Longo, E. D., and Winter, J.: Antimicrobial resistance of *Shigella* isolated in New York City in 1973, Antimicrob. Agents Chemother. 7:833–835, 1975.

Rosenberg, M. L., Weissman, J. B., Gangarosa, E. J., Reller, L. B., and Beasley, R. P.: Shigellosis in the United States: Ten-year review of nationwide surveillance. 1964–1973, Am. J. Epidemiol. 104:543–551, 1976.

Rout, W. R., Formal, S. B., Dammin, G. J., and Giannella, R. A.: Pathophysiology of *Salmonella* diarrhea in the Rhesus monkey. Intestinal transport, morphological and bacteriological studies, Gastroenterology 67:59–70, 1974.

Weissman, J. B., Williams, S. V., Hinman, A. R., Haughie, G. R., and Gangarosa, E. J.: Foodborne shigellosis at a country fair, Am. J. Epidemiol. 100: 178–185, 1974.

ANALYSIS

No. 1.– 1. Enteric fever, malaria, brucellosis, Rocky Mountain spotted fever. 2. (*a*) Blood for culture and serologic study; (*b*) Stool for culture. 3. *Salmonella* sp. 4. Determine O, H and Vi antigens. Identify by Kauffmann-White scheme. 5. Intracapillary agglutination of *Salmonella* sp. 6. Endotoxin. 7. Food or water contaminated by a carrier. 8. Chloramphenicol or ampicillin. 9. Perforation of intestine, spread to other organs.

No. 2.– 1. *S. sonnei.* 2. Carrier, contaminated food and water. 3. Terminal ileum and colon. 4. Organism is limited to mucosal and submucosal tissue. A septicemia is unlikely. 5. None. 6. Supportive therapy – antibiotics only in severe cases.

16 / Pseudomonas

OVERVIEW

Infection with *Pseudomonas* spp. commonly occurs in hospitalized patients and represents an important cause of morbidity and mortality in patients compromised by other diseases, e.g., cystic fibrosis, leukemia, or burns. The widespread distribution of these organisms in man and his environment requires development of methods for identifying their source and for controlling them. Studies using pyocin production and sensitivity, bacteriophage sensitivity, and serologic typing are now leading to a partial understanding of the epidemiology and importance of these organisms.

A large number of enzymes, hemolysins and toxins produced by *P. aeruginosa* have been studied, and some understanding of the mechanism of pathogenicity has been obtained. Some studies suggest it may be possible to immunize certain population groups, and hopefully an approach will develop that will minimize the role of these organisms in diseases of debilitated patients.

GENERAL CHARACTERISTICS

The family Pseudomonadaceae contains straight or curved, gram-negative, non-spore-forming, aerobic rods ($0.5-1.0 \times 1.5-4.0$ μm). They are motile by polar flagella. Many species produce phenazine pigments. They are oxidase positive (except for *P. maltophila*), non-fermentative and grow readily on usual bacteriologic mediums. Optimal growth occurs at 35 C (except for *P. fluorescens*) but some species grow at 42 C.

SPECIES

Several species of *Pseudomonas* have been described. Those of importance to man include *P. aeruginosa, P. cepacia, P. putida, P. fluorescens, P. stutzeri, P. maltophila, P. alcaligenes, P. pseudomallei* and *P. mallei*. A partial list of the characteristics of this group is in Table 16-1.

TABLE 16-1.—CHARACTERISTICS OF
MEDICALLY IMPORTANT *PSEUDOMONAS* SPECIES

SPECIES OF *PSEUDOMONAS*

TEST OR SUBSTRATE	AERUGINOSA	FLUORESCENS	PUTIDA	PSEUDOMALLEI	MALLEI	CEPACIA	STUTZERI	ALCALIGENES	MALTOPHILA
Glucose oxidation	100°	100	100	100	100	100	100	(100)	56 (44)
Maltose oxidation	0	70	35	100	100	100	100	31	100
Indophenol oxidase	100	100	100	100	67	90	100	100	0
Growth at 42 C	100	0	0	100	0	71	100	100	10
Lysine decarboxylase	0	0	0	0	0	93	0	0	20 (43)
Arginine dihydrolase	96 (3)	98	07	100	83 (17)	0	0	0	0
Ornithine decarboxylase	0	0	0	0	0	29	0	100	0
Nitrate reduced to gas	94	2	0	85	0	0	100	0	0
Pyocyanin	58	0	0	0	0	0	0	0	0
Motility	93	100	100	100	0	100	100	100	100

°Percent of strains giving positive reaction. Numbers in parentheses indicate that reactions are positive but delayed.
Adapted from Hugh, R., and Gilardi, G. L.: Pseudomonas, in Lennette, E. H., Spaulding, E. H., and Truant, J. P. (eds.): *Manual of Clinical Microbiology* (2d ed., Washington, D.C.: American Society for Microbiology, 1974).

ECOLOGY

The pseudomonads are ubiquitous and are found in soil, fresh water, marine environments, the intestinal tract of man, and on plants and vegetables. One species, *P. mallei*, causes a disease in horses (glanders) which is transmissible to man. *P. aeruginosa* is the most common species causing disease in humans. Acquisition of *Pseudomonas* spp. by hospitalized patients is via food and water (including contaminated ice machines), common bathtubs, sinks, nebulizer reservoirs, contaminated catheters, drugs, disinfectants, intravenous fluids and soap. The organisms are more resistant than other agents to commonly used disinfectants and survive readily in moist environments.

PSEUDOMONAS AERUGINOSA

Cell Wall and Other Structures

A polysaccharide slime layer covers the cell wall and is found in largest amounts on isolates from patients with cystic fibrosis. The composition has not been characterized with certainty, but studies suggest the presence of uronic acids containing O-acetyl groups. Purified preparations are toxic and cause death in animals. Active and passive immunization protects against the toxic effect of the slime and against challenge with live organisms. The cell wall lipopolysaccharide has a specific pyocin-receptor activity and has associated endotoxin activity but it is not as toxic as endotoxins from other gram-negative organisms. Unlike other enterics, lipid A of *P. aeruginosa* lacks β-hydroxymyristic acid. Polar flagella and pili have been demonstrated. The pili function in attachment of the organism to the cell surfaces or in enabling the organism to resist phagocytosis is unknown. The cell wall and outer structures are similar to those of other gram-negative rods.

Antigens

Serologic studies by agglutination and agglutination-absorption, show that *P. aeruginosa* can be divided into 10 to 16 serogroups based on O antigens and on heat-labile antigens (presumed to be flagellar antigens). Antisera against the slime layer can also be used to immunotype *P. aeruginosa* in a mouse infection-protection system. Seven serotypes or immunotypes based on antigenicity of the slime layer have been described. Serotyping can also be done by slide agglutination using the seven lipopolysaccharide antisera or antisera derived from immunization with boiled whole cell antigen.

Genetics, Phages and Pyocins

The pseudomonads are quite complex. They produce pyocins (bacteriocins) and are susceptible to pyocins produced by other strains of *Pseudomonas*. Production of phage and susceptibility to phage are variable. R factor transfer of antibiotic resistance has also been demonstrated.

Enzymes, Hemolysins and Toxins

A number of bacterial products of potential significance in infections have been recognized. Among these are a heat-stable (a glycolipid) and a heat-labile (phospholipase C) hemolysin. Several enzymes, e.g., proteases, collagenase and elastase, have been isolated and associated with tissue destruction.

A leukocidin, active on human leukocytes, probably functions by altering selective permeability of the leukocyte membrane.

P. aeruginosa contains an endotoxin and an exotoxin. The heat-labile protein exotoxin has a molecular weight of 66,000 and is lethal to animals in microgram amounts. It is an inhibitor of protein synthesis with a mode of action similar to that described for the *Corynebacterium diphtheriae* exotoxin (Chap. 10). It specifically catalyzes the transfer of the ADP-ribosyl moiety from NAD to elongation factor 2, resulting in inactivation of EF2 and cessation of protein synthesis. Like diphtheria toxin, it is composed of two fragments, A and B, and requires reduction and denaturation for full activity. Intact toxin is inactive. The slime layer is also toxic but the mechanism is unknown. An enterotoxin has also been described but its mechanism of action is unknown.

Two pigments, fluorescein (water soluble) and pyocyanin (chloroform soluble), are produced both in vitro and in vivo. These two pigments are responsible for the blue-green diffusible color associated with cultures of *P. aeruginosa* and with pus produced during infection.

Infections

The pseudomonads are frequently associated with wound and urinary tract infections, although the organisms can cause pneumonia, meningitis, endocarditis, otitis media, septic arthritis and necrotizing lesions of skin (Fig. 16–1), cornea and intestinal tract. Corneal infec-

Fig. 16–1.—Necrosis of skin in patient with *Pseudomonas* septicemia. (Courtesy of Dr. Edmund Flink, Department of Medicine, West Virginia University Medical Center.)

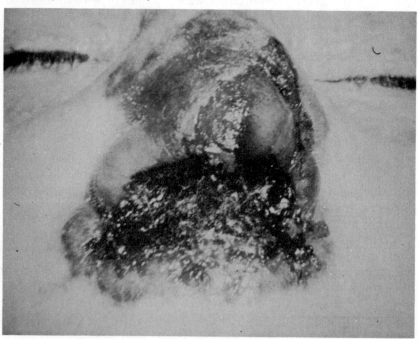

tions are destructive and can result in loss of sight. Mortality in pulmonary infections is high because of necrosis and abscess formation. Infections with these organisms are frequently found in patients with burns, cystic fibrosis or cardiopulmonary disease. Also, patients with neoplasms or granulocytopenia associated with chemotherapy, heroin addicts, postoperative patients on respirators and patients with urinary catheters have increased risk of developing *Pseudomonas* infections. Septicemia as a result of dissemination from the primary site of infection may cause death due to septic shock. In one study, 2.5% of the patients admitted with burns developed *Pseudomonas* septicemia; mortality was 76%.

Mechanisms of Pathogenicity

The pseudomonads are opportunistic organisms that readily colonize and infect the body surfaces of humans predisposed because of immunologic defects or alterations in body surfaces or host resistance.

A large number of possible virulence factors may singly or in combination play a role in human diseases caused by these organisms. The surface components of the organism (slime layer and endotoxic lipopolysaccharide) have antiphagocytic functions and probably help in establishment and survival of the organisms. The slime produced by these organisms may interfere with the function of the mucociliary blanket in removal of organisms from the respiratory tract. A leukocidin may also prevent phagocytosis and contribute to establishment and survival of these organisms in the host.

Two bacterial components or products may relate to the shock frequently associated with *Pseudomonas* infection. One factor is the endotoxin, but a second factor, a heat-labile exotoxin (PA toxin; exotoxin A) may be more important in pathogenesis of *Pseudomonas* infections. In mice this heat-labile protein toxin causes a drop in circulating leukocytes and death in 24–48 hours. In dogs, hypotensive shock follows injection of the exotoxin. Dermonecrotic lesions are also produced in animals. The PA toxin inhibits protein synthesis in a manner similar to that described for *C. diphtheriae*. Increasing amounts of antibody (IgG) to the exotoxin have been demonstrated in patients with *Pseudomonas* infection and indicate in vivo production of toxin. Lower levels of antibodies are found in the serums of controls and may reflect antibody formed as a result of normal colonization. Antibody to the exotoxin protects against infection with live heterologous *P. aeruginosa*, and may be significant in preventing disease. The exotoxin has been demonstrated in culture filtrates of approximately 90% of clinical isolates.

Hemorrhagic necrotic lesions are associated with infections of the skin, eyes and internal organs. Similar lesions are produced in experimental animals injected with the proteases, elastase, collagenase and with the exotoxin.

The role of the hemolysin in disease is not clear. The phospholipase C hemolysin may be important in pneumonia by destroying lung surfactant, thereby resulting in atelectasis and necrosis. The glycolipid hemolysin may also contribute to destruction of lung surfactant and be important in pulmonary disease.

A heat-labile substance, probably an enterotoxin, in conjunction with other enzymes and toxins may be responsible for the necrosis and fluid loss associated with a necrotizing enteritis which occurs in humans.

The blue-green color of pus obtained from *Pseudomonas* infections is due to the production of two pigments, pyocyanin and fluorescein, by organisms growing in tissue. Determining fluorescein in tissue with Wood's light is useful in detecting severe infections of burned surfaces. One other substance that apparently is not involved in pathogenesis but is a hallmark associated with *P. aeruginosa* is trimethylamine. This aromatic compound, which gives off a fruity, grape-like odor, can be a key to recognizing *P. aeruginosa* in infectious processes and in culture.

Immunity

Susceptibility to infection is associated with humoral and cellular deficiencies of the immune system. IgM and IgG antibodies develop after infection and correlate with increased opsonization and protection. IgA antibodies are also produced. Active immunization with a heptavalent lipopolysaccharide preparation has been used and shows promising results in protecting patients. Elevated antibody titers are obtained by immunization but are of short duration. Killing of *P. aeruginosa* requires neutrophils, which are often deficient in patients with *Pseudomonas* infection, and granulocyte transfusions may be necessary.

Treatment

Antibiotic therapy is not too successful with up to 80% mortality in patients with pulmonary disease and septicemia. Resistance to antibiotics frequently occurs. Aminoglycoside antibiotics, e.g., gentamicin, tobramycin, amikacin, as well as colistin and carbenecillin, are used, but antibiotic sensitivity tests must be used as a guide to therapy. Gentamicin and carbenicillin act synergistically in vivo and are used in combination in serious infections. Sulfamylon is useful in patients with infected burns. Recently, silver sulfadiazine and povidone-iodine have been used with good results.

OTHER PSEUDOMONAS SPECIES

Pseudomonas cepacia (formerly recognized as EO-1, *P. kingii* and *P. multivorans*) have been isolated from water, saline solutions, and disinfectants in a hospital. These organisms have been associated with infections in patients with granulomatous disease and have been isolated from several clinical sources, e.g., blood, cerebrospinal fluid, joint fluid and abscesses. *P. cepacia* bacteremia after open heart surgery has been associated with pressure transducers that were cleaned with quaternary ammonium disinfectant contaminated with *P. cepacia*.

Several other species of *Pseudomonas* (*P. fluorescens, P. maltophilia, P. stutzeri, P. putida* and *P. alcaligenes*) have been isolated from clinical specimens and may cause wound, urinary tract and other infections.

P. pseudomallei is found in soil and causes disease in rodents and domestic animals. Humans may acquire the disease through the skin via abrasions or by ingestion or inhalation. Inapparent infection, as determined by serologic evidence, also occurs. Acute or subacute pneumonitis or pneumonia, as well as a rapidly fatal fulminating septicemia, may result. The pulmonary disease can be confused with tuberculosis or respiratory fungal disease. The disease is found in Southeast Asia and in Central and South America.

P. mallei causes a disease of equines called glanders, which is characterized by focal involvement of the lungs with suppuration. The organism can be transmitted to man through skin abrasions or inhalation. Glanders is rarely seen in the United States, although infections acquired elsewhere have been seen here.

LABORATORY PROCEDURES

The type of specimen depends on the disease and localization in the host. The specimen is plated on blood agar, selective-differential media such as MacConkey, eosin methylene blue or deoxycholate. Non-lactose fermenters that do not cause a change in triple sugar iron or Russell's double sugar agar should be tested for motility, pigment production, ability to oxidatively use glucose, and for indophenol oxidase. *P. aeruginosa* is generally characterized by the production of the pyocyanin pigment. However, only about half of the strains produce this pigment (see Table 16–1). Some other differential characteristics of the *Pseudomonas* species are listed in Table 16–1. Identification and differentiation among the species are difficult, and a reference source such as the *Manual of Clinical Microbiology* should be consulted.

Investigators attempting to understand the epidemiologic characteristics by distinguishing among isolates of *P. aeruginosa* have used serology, pyocin typing, phage typing, and determination of antibiogram. Differences in amount of pyocins produced, the ability to change pyocin types, changes in the bacteriophage lytic pattern and the complexity of serotyping have made epidemiologic studies difficult. It is generally agreed that serotyping should be done but that it should be augmented by other methodologies.

PROBLEM SOLVING AND REVIEW

GIVEN: – A patient was admitted to the burn ward after an industrial accident. Four days later the nurse noticed blue-green pus on the burn dressings. The patient then became toxic, developed shock and died.

PROBLEMS: – 1. What organisms do you suspect as the etiologic agent? 2. What caused the blue-green pus? 3. Would you expect to see fluorescence if you exposed the patient to Wood's light? Why? 4. What activities of the organism do you associate with *(a)* establishment of the infection, *(b)* destruction of skin and *(c)* development of shock? 5. What is the source of the organism? 6. If this were an epidemic, how would you identify the point source? 7. How might one have prevented infection and death in this patient? (Ans. p. 319.)

SUPPLEMENTARY READING

Artenstein, M. S., and Stanford, J. P. (eds.): Symposium on *Pseudomonas aeruginosa*, J. Infect. Dis. [Suppl.] 130:1–166, 1974.
Baltch, A. L., and Griffin, P. E.: *Pseudomonas aeruginosa* bacteremia: a clinical study of 75 patients, Am. J. Med. Sci. 274:119, 1977.
Duncan, N. H., Hinton, N. A., Penner, J. L., and Duncan, I. B. R.: Preparation of typing antisera specific for O antigens of *Pseudomonas aeruginosa*, J. Clin. Microbiol. 4:124–128, 1976.
Howe, C., Sampath, A., and Spotnitz, M.: The pseudomallei group: A review, J. Infect. Dis. 124:598–606, 1971.
Hugh, R., and Gilardi, G. L.: Pseudomonas, in Lennette, E. H., Spaulding, E. H., and Truant, J. P. (eds.): *Manual of Clinical Microbiology* (2d ed.; Washington, D. C.: American Society for Microbiology, 1974).
Iglewski, B. H., and Kabat, D.: NAD-dependent inhibition of protein synthe-

sis by *Pseudomonas aeruginosa* toxin, Proc. Natl. Acad. Sci. U.S.A. 72: 2284–2288, 1975.

Matsumato, H., and Tazaki, T.: Relationships of O antigens of *Pseudomonas aeruginosa* between Hungarian types of Lanyi and Hab's type or Verder and Evans type, Jap. J. Microbiol. 13:209–211, 1969.

Pollock, M., Callahan, L. T., III, and Taylor, N. S.: Neutralizing antibody to *Pseudomonas aeruginosa* exotoxin in human sera: Evidence for *in vivo* toxin production during infections, Infect. Immunol. 14:942–947, 1976.

Pollock, M., Taylor, N. S., and Callahan, L. T., III: Exotoxin production by clinical isolates of *Pseudomonas aeruginosa*, Infect. Immunol. 15:776–780, 1977.

Reynolds, H. Y., Levine, A. S., Wood, R. E., Zierdt, C. H., Dole, D. C., and Pennington, J. E.: *Pseudomonas aeruginosa* infections. Persisting problems and current research to find new therapies, Ann. Intern. Med. 82:819–831, 1975.

Scharmann, W., Jacob, F., and Porstendörfer, I.: The cytotoxic action of leucocidin from *Pseudomonas aeruginosa* on human polymorphonuclear leucocytes, J. Gen. Microbiol. 93:303–308, 1976.

ANALYSIS

1. *Pseudomonas aeruginosa*. 2. Pyocyanin production. 3. Yes, because of production of fluorescein. 4. *(a)* Slime layer, endotoxin, leukocidin; *(b)* elastase, protease; *(c)* endotoxin and PA exotoxin. 5. Other patients, staff, environment. 6. Serologic tests, phage typing, colicin typing. 7. Immunize patients predisposed to infection with the heptavalent lipopolysaccharide vaccine.

17 / Vibrios

OVERVIEW

With two exceptions, cholera has not appeared in the United States since 1911. However, in 1973 a single case of cholera due to *V. cholerae* serotype Inaba, biotype *eltor* occurred in Texas, and more recently another case has been reported from Alabama. These patients had not been in an endemic area and the source of the infection has not been uncovered. Recently, *V. cholerae* and *V. parahaemolyticus* have been isolated from the Chesapeake Bay. Worldwide, cholera is still an important disease. In 1961 the seventh pandemic of cholera began in Indonesia and spread to Asia, Africa and Eastern Europe. It is estimated that 100,000–200,000 cases of cholera appear each year.

Cholera is an important and interesting disease because it is an example whereby the signs and symptoms of the disease result from an altered host physiologic response (intestinal secretion) without penetration of host tissue by the organism. Cholera can be treated successfully largely by replacing fluids and salts lost as a result of the physiologic alteration.

A second species, *Vibrio parahaemolyticus*, has been recognized as a pathogen of increasing importance. It was first isolated in Japan from patients with food-borne disease in the 1950s, and it now accounts for several hundred cases each year. After the Japanese experience *V. parahaemolyticus* was recognized in many other countries, and in 1971 laboratory documentation of food-borne disease caused by this organism was reported in the United States.

GENERAL CHARACTERISTICS

The vibrios are gram-negative, non-spore-forming, facultatively anaerobic rods (0.5×1.5–3.0 μm) that are slightly curved (Fig. 17–1). Capsules are not produced. They are motile by a single polar flagellum and grow at 37 C. Indophenol oxidase is produced, which differ-

321

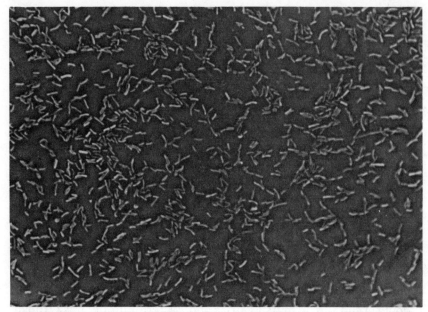

Fig. 17–1.—*Vibrio cholerae*. Note slightly curved rods. (Courtesy of Dr. R. Ganguly, Departments of Medicine and Microbiology, West Virginia University Medical Center.)

entiates *Vibrio* from the enteric bacteria. The organisms ferment lactose slowly. *V. cholerae* grows best at pH 7.0 but will grow profusely at pH 7.6 to 8.6. Growth is obtained on nutrient media.

SPECIES

Vibrio cholerae causes a disease of man characterized by a profuse diarrhea. Four biotypes—*cholerae, eltor, proteus* and *albensis*—are recognized and can be differentiated by a number of characteristics (Table 17–1). *Vibrio parahaemolyticus* is a halophilic organism found in coastal and estuarine water; the requirement for high salt concentration for growth enables differentiation of *V. cholerae* from *V. parahaemolyticus*. These are two biotypes of *V. parahaemolyticus* (Table 17–2). Both *V. parahaemolyticus* biotype *parahaemolyticus* and biotype *alginolyticus* are associated with disease; organisms of the former biotype cause an acute enteritis in man after ingestion of contaminated seafood. Both biotypes cause nonintestinal infections. Other species of *Vibrio*, referred to as nonagglutinable cholera-like *Vibrio* (NAG) or non-cholera *Vibrio* (NCV) also produce a cholera-like dis-

VIBRIO CHOLERAE 323

TABLE 17-1.—DIFFERENTIAL CHARACTERISTICS OF
BIOTYPES OF *V. CHOLERAE*

| | BIOTYPE | | | |
	CHOLERAE	ELTOR	PROTEUS	ALBENSIS
Tube hemolysis	−	d°	+	−
Sucrose fermentation	+	+	+	+
Mannose fermentation	+	+	+	−
Voges-Proskauer at 22 C	−	+	d	+
Nitrates reduced to				
nitrites	+	+	−	+
Lysine decarboxylation	+	+	−	+
Agglutination by				
O 1 antiserum	+	+	−	−

°d, delayed reaction.
Adapted from Buchanan, R. E. and Gibbons, N. E. (eds.): *Bergey's Manual of Determinative Bacteriology* (8th ed.; Baltimore: Williams & Wilkins Co., 1974).

TABLE 17-2.—SOME DIFFERENTIAL
CHARACTERISTICS OF *V. PARAHAEMOLYTICUS*
BIOTYPES

| | BIOTYPES | |
TEST OR SUBSTRATE	PARAHAEMOLYTICUS	ALGINOLYTICUS
Triple sugar iron	Alkaline/acid	Acid/acid
Voges-Proskauer	−	+
Sucrose fermentation	−	+
Methyl red	+	−

ease in man. *Campylobacter fetus* (formerly *Vibrio fetus*) is a microaerophilic organism that causes diseases in animals and man.

CELL WALL AND ASSOCIATED STRUCTURES

The cell wall of the vibrios is typical of a gram-negative bacterium. Flagella and pili have also been demonstrated.

VIBRIO CHOLERAE

Antigens

Agglutinating and bactericidal antibodies are produced in response to lipopolysaccharide (O) antigens. Based on O antigens, the vibrios can be divided into six serogroups. *V. cholerae* biotypes *cholerae* and *eltor* are in O group I. Vibrios belonging to other serogroups are com-

TABLE 17–3.–DIFFERENTIATION OF *V. CHOLERAE* BIOTYPES *CHOLERAE* AND *ELTOR*

TEST	BIOTYPES	
	CHOLERAE	ELTOR
Group IV cholerae phage susceptibility	+	−
Voges-Proskauer test at 22 C	−	+
Polymyxin B sensitivity	+	−
Chicken erythrocyte agglutination	−	+

monly referred to as NCV or as NAG (nonagglutinable in O group I antiserums) vibrios. For example, *V. cholerae* biotypes *proteus* and *albensis* are often referred to as NAG vibrios. *Vibrio cholerae* can be further differentiated into two serotypes, Ogawa and Inaba. A third serotype (Hikojima) has been described, but it may be a variant of the Ogawa type. A protein antigen isolated from the cell wall induces vibriocidal antibody. A single flagellar (H) antigen is shared among the vibrios. The enterotoxin (choleragen) responsible for the acute diarrhea is antigenic, and enterotoxins from different strains are immunologically identical.

Genetics

Phages have been isolated and used for development of phage typing schemes. Susceptibility of the *cholerae* biotype to specific phage (Mukerjee's type IV) is used to separate it from the *eltor* biotype (Table 17–3). Lysogeny has also been demonstrated. Bacteriocins (vibriocins) are produced and there have been attempts to use vibriocin typing as an epidemiologic tool. Conjugation, sex pili and R factor transfer have also been shown.

Toxins, Hemolysins and Enzymes

An endotoxin similar in structure and function to that of other gram-negative organisms is produced, but it is of doubtful importance in disease. A filterable antigenic hemolysin causes a beta-hemolysis, but its role in disease, if any, is unknown. Hemolysin production is associated with the *eltor* biotype. A mucinase and neuramidinase are also produced but their role in infection is not clear. An enterotoxin (choleragen) is produced both in vitro and in vivo. It consists of two major regions or subunits designated A and B. The A (active) portion binds to the cell surface and activates adenyl cyclase. The enterotoxin is antigenic and antibody neutralizes the toxin by binding to the B region and preventing attachment to the cell surface receptor. The nature of the mucosal cell receptor is unclear. Some work suggests that it is a G_{M_1} ganglioside, but other data suggest that it is not the receptor even though it binds to the B region of the toxin.

Infections

V. cholerae is a parasite solely of man. The organism enters the host who ingests food or water contaminated by a carrier. It attaches to the mucosal cell surface of the small intestine but does not invade the intestinal mucosa. After an incubation period of 8 to 72 hours, there is an acute onset of nausea, vomiting, diarrhea and abdominal cramping. There may be only a slight fever or slight hypothermia. The patient rapidly becomes dehydrated because of profuse diarrhea (may lose 10-12 liters of fluid per day). Tachycardia, tachypnea and low or ab-

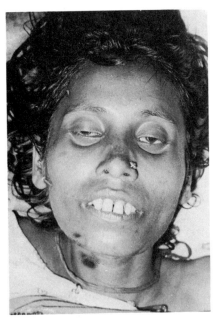

Fig. 17-2.—Note sunken eyes *(left)* and wrinkled skin on hands *(right)* typical of cholera. Both result from acute loss of fluid. (Courtesy of Dr. S. Pal, Director, Cholera Research Center, Indian Council of Medical Research, Calcutta, India.)

sent blood pressure are common signs. The pulse is thready or absent. The patient has sunken eyes and cheeks and may be cyanotic (Fig. 17–2). The patient becomes acidotic, hypokalemic and may develop hypovolemic shock with death occurring in a few hours to a few days. A similar disease picture, but usually milder, can be produced by the NCV or NAG vibrios.

Mechanisms of Pathogenicity

The organism is not invasive and therefore there is neither damage to the intestinal tract nor secondary sites of infection. About 10^8 organisms are required to establish infection. The importance of gastric acidity as a barrier to infection is shown by the fact that persons who have undergone gastrectomy are especially sensitive to infection. Also, in experimental infections, $NaHCO_3$, administered to lower the gastric pH, reduces the infective dose from 10^8 to 10^4 organisms. In the small intestine, the organisms adhere to villi where they multiply and produce choleragen, which binds to the mucosal cell. The enterotoxin activates adenyl cyclase, resulting in an increase in intracellular cyclic AMP and hypersecretion of chloride, bicarbonate ions and water from the mucosa to the lumen. Sodium and water readsorption from the intestinal lumen is not affected, and oral replacement of fluid and salts often reverses the physiologic effect of the enterotoxin.

Immunity

The nature of immunity in cholera is not clear, but it may result from antibody which either prevents adherence of the organism to the small intestine or which neutralizes the enterotoxin.

Infection results in short-lived immunity lasting 4–12 months. Homologous immunity, but not heterologous immunity, is produced after infection. Vibriocidal, agglutinating, secretory IgA and antienterotoxin antibodies are produced after infection. There is poor correlation between serum antibody titer and immunity. IgA antibody is present in the intestinal contents of immunized persons after infection and correlates with immunity.

Vaccines composed of killed V. *cholerae* are available. The protection afforded is short (3–6 months) and the host response is variable.

Prevention

Since cholera is spread by contaminated food and water, prevention of this disease rests with education, sanitation, and detection and treatment of carriers. Convalescent carriers can harbor organisms up to 11 months, but usually the carrier state is less than 20 days. The organisms are sequestered in the gallbladder in these chronic carriers and are detected only in purged stools. However, small-bowel cultures of asymptomatic carriers are negative and repeated rectal swabs are required to isolate the organism. The ratio of asymptomatic carriers to clinical cases due to the *cholerae* biotype is 4:1, whereas the ratio in outbreaks caused by *eltor* is 10:1.

Vaccines in current use are not effective, particularly against large doses of organisms. Cholera immunization is not required for U.S. travelers.

Treatment

Treatment requires replacement of water and electrolytes, either orally or intravenously, to correct the acidosis, hypokalemia and dehydration. Since intestinal absorption is unaffected by the cholera toxin, oral replacement is possible in mild cases. In severe cases intravenous administration is necessary to rapidly correct the fluid-electrolyte changes with oral administration used to maintain fluid-electrolyte balance. Tetracycline may be used to reduce the bacterial load and thereby interrupt toxin production. It also reduces the period of excretion of organisms.

Laboratory Procedures

Fecal specimens, rectal swabs or vomitus should be obtained within the first 24 hours of illness. The specimen can be examined by dark-field microscopy and observed for motile vibrios. If motile organisms resembling *V. cholerae* are observed, antisera is added to the specimen to determine if motility is inhibited, thereby confirming the identification serologically. Examination of direct smears by fluorescent antibody is also useful in patients with disease. Specimens should be promptly inoculated into an enrichment medium such as alkaline peptone water and inoculated directly onto agar plants, or placed in a transport medium. Both selective (thiosulfate-citrate bile salts agar) and nonselective media (nutrient agar or taurocholate gelatin agar) should be inoculated. Because these bacteria can grow at a high pH (7.8), isolation is not difficult. Growth usually is obtained in 18 to 24 hours. The vibrios produce indophenol oxidase, which differentiates them from the enterics. The "string" test helps in presumptive identification of *V. cholerae*. In this test the organisms are emulsified in 0.5% sodium deoxycholate. A mucus-like string is observed as the inoculating loop is lifted away from the slide. Serologic tests should be done with isolated colonies to determine the serogroup. Final identification of *V. cholerae* requires inoculation into media for determination of biochemical properties (see Table 17–1).

V. cholerae biotypes *cholerae* and *eltor* can be differentiated by phage susceptibility, hemolysin production, susceptibility to polymyxin B and production of acetylmethyl carbinol (Table 17–3).

Acute phase serum taken as early as possible and convalescent serum (10–21 days after onset) may be used to obtain serologic evidence of infection.

VIBRIO PARAHAEMOLYTICUS

Antigens

The cell wall is covered by a capsular polysaccharide antigen (K). Like the K antigens of other bacteria, it prevents agglutination with anti-O serum but can be removed by heating.

All *V. parahaemolyticus* share a common H antigen. Using both O and K antigens, one can divide *V. parahaemolyticus* serologically into 12 serogroups (O antigens) and 52 serotypes (K antigens).

Toxins

HEMOLYSINS. — Four different hemolysins have been demonstrated. Two are cell bound and have phospholipase A and lysophospholipase activity. The other two hemolysins, one heat labile and one heat stable, are found in culture filtrates. The heat-stable hemolysin, the Kanagawa hemolysin, lyses human and rabbit erythrocytes and is produced by those strains which infect humans. The Kanagawa hemolysin is a protein that is cardiotoxic in vitro and in vivo and has also been reported to have enterotoxic activity. Antibody to the Kanagawa hemolysin is found in the serums of infected patients.

ENTEROTOXIN. — Fluid accumulation in ligated ileal loops and a rounding of Chinese hamster ovary cells, both indicators of enterotoxin, have been reported. However, the mode of action is still not clear.

ENDOTOXIN. — Endotoxin is produced but its importance in disease is not clear.

Infections

V. parahaemolyticus is a halophilic organism found in coastal waters which is acquired by injection of raw fish or shellfish contaminated with *V. parahaemolyticus* biotype *parahaemolyticus*. The average incubation period for the gastroenteritis produced by these organisms is 15–24 hours. The symptoms resemble those of cholera and are primarily nausea, abdominal cramping, and a watery diarrhea. Blood and mucus are not usually found in the stool. Headache, fever and chills are present in a small percentage of the patients. The disease may last from several hours to several days (average 3 days).

Localized infections may also occur with biotypes *parahaemolyticus* and *alginolyticus*.

Mechanisms of Pathogenicity

The means by which the diarrhea occurs is unclear. The symptoms (fever, chills, headache) suggest invasion of the intestinal tract. However, in vitro studies report that *V. parahaemolyticus* is cytotoxic for tissue culture (HeLa) cells but does not invade the cells. The profuse, watery diarrhea indicates an enterotoxin as being responsible. Enterotoxic activity as demonstrated by accumulation of fluid in ileal loops inoculated with either live organisms, culture filtrates, or the thermostable Kanagawa hemolysin has been reported. Only strains that produce the Kanagawa hemolysin cause gastroenteritis.

Prevention

Infection with *V. parahaemolyticus* biotype *parahaemolyticus* is acquired by eating uncooked fish or shellfish that have been improperly refrigerated. Steaming or cooking kills the microorganisms, but the food is often recontaminated by use of common containers and utensils. Localized infections are acquired by direct contact with the marine environment. Vaccines are not available.

Treatment

The enteritis is usually self-limiting but death can occur. Treatment is largely supportive and includes replacing fluid and electrolytes lost and controlling electrolyte balance. Antimicrobial agents are not recommended except in severe cases. The organism is sensitive to chloramphenicol, tetracycline, erythromycin, kanamycin and cephalothin.

Laboratory Procedures

Fecal specimens, rectal swabs and vomitus are cultured in enrichment media, such as 1% alkaline peptone water containing 3% NaCl, and are also plated directly on a selective medium such as thiosulfate-citrate bile salts (TCBS). Incubation is at 35 to 37 C. After the organisms have been isolated, they are identified by determining cultural, biochemical, and serologic characteristics (see Table 17–2). Strains of *V. parahaemolyticus* that cause food-associated gastroenteritis produce a β-hemolysin under defined conditions and in a special medium and are termed Kanagawa positive. Preliminary identification can be obtained in 24 to 48 hours.

CAMPYLOBACTER (VIBRIO) FETUS

General Characteristics

This organism was previously classified as a *Vibrio* because of similarity in morphological and other characteristics but is now assigned to the genus *Campylobacter*. It is found in animals and causes abortions in sheep and cattle and has been reported to cause septicemia, endocarditis, enteritis and abortion in humans. Transmission is probably by direct contact with infected animals or by ingestion of contaminated food. It is sensitive to most antimicrobial agents.

Laboratory Procedures

Fecal specimens, rectal swabs and blood cultures are inoculated into *Brucella* medium containing 10% blood. The organisms are gram-negative, slender, curved bacilli that are motile by a single flagellum. They are microaerophilic, do not ferment carbohydrates and grow at 25 C.

PROBLEM SOLVING AND REVIEW

NO. 1. GIVEN: — Twenty-four hours after returning from a business trip to India, several bankers developed a severe diarrhea. They were acutely ill; their skin was dry and shriveled. They complained of nausea, mild abdominal pain and severe cramping. Hematocrit reading was 60%. The diarrhea was characterized as brown to clear in color. Pulse rate was 145 beats per minute, respirations were 29 and blood pressure was unobtainable. Hemoglobin was 18.0 gm/100 ml; white blood cell count was 13,000/cu mm. Blood chemistry values were sodium 136 mEq/liter, potassium 3.1 mEq/liter, and BUN 40 mg/100 ml. Gram stain of isolated colonies from a stool culture showed a gram-negative, slightly curved, motile bacillus. The patients were hydrated with intravenous glucose and salts, and recovery was uncomplicated.

PROBLEMS: — 1. What is the probable causative organism? 2. How was it acquired? 3. Is there invasion of intestinal tissue? 4. What is the mechanism for production of diarrhea? 5. What is the site of tissue invasion? (Ans. p. 331.)

NO. 2. GIVEN: — Several fraternity brothers reported to the student health service with complaints of headache, abdominal cramping, vomiting, and a profuse, watery diarrhea. Questioning revealed that the patients had eaten steamed crabs and drunk large amounts of beer at a picnic on the previous day. They were treated with intravenous fluids and recovered without complications. The culture report indicated the organism was Kanagawa positive.

PROBLEMS: — 1. What is the most likely etiologic agent? 2. What is the probable source and why? 3. If a gram stain on the stools had been done, what most likely would have been seen? 4. What cultures should be taken? 5. What is the significance of the culture report? (Ans. p. 332.)

SUPPLEMENTARY READING

Barker, W. H., Jr.: *Vibrio parahaemolyticus* outbreaks in the United States, Lancet 1:551–554, 1974.

Barua, D., and Burrows, W.: *Cholera* (Philadelphia: W. B. Saunders Co., 1974).

Carruthers, M. M.: Cytotoxicity of *Vibrio parahaemolyticus* in HeLa cell culture, J. Infect. Dis. 132:555–560, 1975.

Cash, R. A., Music, S. I., Libonati, J. P., Craig, J. P., Pierce, N. F., and Hornick, R. B.: Response of man to infection with *Vibrio cholerae*. II. Protection from illness afforded by previous disease and vaccine, J. Infect. Dis. 130: 325–333, 1974.

Cash, R. A., Music, S. I., Libonati, J. P., Snyder, M. J., Wenzel, R. P., and Hornick, R. B.: Response of man to infection with *Vibrio cholerae*. I. Clinical, serologic, and bacteriologic responses to a known inoculum, J. Infect. Dis. 129:45–52, 1974.

Colwell, R. R., Kaper, J., and Joseph, S. W.: *Vibrio cholerae, V. parahaemolyticus*, and other vibrios: Occurrence and distribution in Chesapeake Bay, Science 198:394–396, 1977.

Finkelstein, R. A.: Cholera, CRC Crit. Rev. Microbiol. 2:553–623, 1973.

Ganguly, R., Clem, L. W., Bencic, Z., Sinha, R., Sakazaki, R., and Waldman, R. H.: Antibody response in the intestinal secretion of volunteers immunized with various cholera vaccines, Bull. W.H.O. 52:323–330, 1975.

Hallett, A. F., Botha, P. L., and Logan, A.: Isolation of *Campylobacter fetus* from recent cases of human vibriosis. J. Hyg. (Camb.) 79:381, 1977.

Honda, T., Goshima, K., Takeda, Y., Sugino, Y., and Minwatani, T.: Demonstration of the cardiotoxicity of the thermostable direct hemolysin (lethal toxin produced by *Vibrio parahaemolyticus*, Infect. Immunol. 13:163–171, 1976.

Honda, T., Shimizu, M., Takeda, Y., and Miwatani, T.: Isolation of a factor causing morphological changes of Chinese hamsters ovary cells from the culture filtrate of *Vibrio parahaemolyticus*. Infect. Immunol. 14:1028–1033, 1976.

Pierce, N. F., Banwell, J. G., Gorbach, S. L., Mitra, R. C., and Mondal, A.: Convalescent carriers of *Vibrio cholerae*. Ann. Intern. Med. 72:357–364, 1970.

Van Heyningen, S.: Cholera toxin, Biol. Rev. 52:509, 1977.

ANALYSIS

NO. 1. — 1. *Vibrio cholerae* or the non-cholera vibrios. 2. Ingestion of water or food contaminated by a carrier. 3. No. 4. Organisms produce an enterotoxin that activates adenyl cyclase and results in hypersecretion. 5. Small intestine.

No. 2. – 1. *V. parahaemolyticus* or the non-cholera vibrios. 2. Steamed crabs improperly cooked or recontaminated after cooking and improper refrigeration. 3. Gram-negative rods. 4. Stool culture only. 5. Kanagawa positive means that a thermostable hemolysin was produced. This is characteristic of *V. parahaemolyticus* strains associated with food-borne disease.

18 / Brucella, Francisella, Yersinia and Pasteurella

OVERVIEW

The *Brucella, Francisella, Yersinia* and *Pasteurella* cause diseases referred to as zoonoses, i.e., diseases of animals. Man becomes infected when he comes in contact with the animal reservoir or vector. The diseases caused by these genera differ considerably in epidemiologic characteristics. For example, the *Brucella* are found primarily in domestic animals and represent a hazard primarily to those involved in animal husbandry and working in abattoirs. Transmission is usually by direct contact. The *Yersinia* and *Francisella* are found in wild animals and are maintained in these animals via feeding of infected arthropods. These organisms are transmitted to man through contact either with the arthropod vector (bubonic plague and tularemia) or infected animals (tularemia) or with aerosols from persons with pulmonary plague (pneumonic plague). The *Pasteurella* are part of the normal flora of animals and are transmitted to man by direct contact and usually cause disease in a host with impaired defense mechanisms.

The plague bacillus has played an important role in the history of man. It was responsible for over 200 million deaths and caused the death of as much as 50% of the population of the Roman Empire during the reign of Justinian. It has been suggested that during the epidemic of "black death" in Europe in the 14th century, 25 million people, one fourth of the population, were killed. Plague still exists in several parts of the world and sporadic outbreaks occur in the western and southern United States.

BRUCELLA

General Characteristics

The *Brucella* are gram-negative, coccobacillary $(0.5-0.7 \times 0.6-1.5$ μm), non-motile, non-spore-forming bacteria (Fig. 18–1). Upon primary isolation they are generally encapsulated, but propagation in the

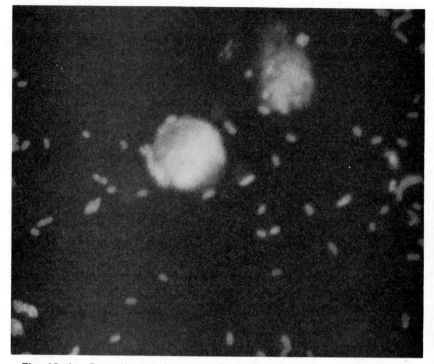

Fig. 18–1.—*Brucella suis* in tissue. Fluorescent antibody stain. (Courtesy of Dr. William Hausler, State Hygiene Laboratory, University of Iowa.)

laboratory results in loss of the capsule. Optimal temperature for growth is 37 C, and they are strict aerobes. A medium consisting of a protein digest, vitamins, salts and glucose is needed for growth. One species, *Brucella abortus*, requires an elevated CO_2 atmosphere for initial isolation but loses the CO_2 requirement after laboratory propagation.

Species

Four species of *Brucella* are pathogenic for man: *B. abortus, B. suis, B. melitensis* and *B. canis*. These species can be differentiated on the basis of CO_2 requirement, urease production, H_2S production, inhibition by certain dyes, and by agglutination tests (Table 18–1). *B. abortus, B. suis* and *B. melitensis* contain several strains or biotypes.

Ecology

The *Brucella* cause disease primarily in animals but also disease in persons in contact with infected animals or their products. The organ-

TABLE 18-1.—CHARACTERISTICS OF THE *BRUCELLA*

SPECIES	NO. OF BIOTYPES	CO$_2$ REQUIREMENT	H$_2$S PRODUCTION	HYDROLYSIS OF UREA	GROWTH ON MEDIA CONTAINING: THIONINE	BASIC FUCHSIN
B. melitensis	3	–	–	Slow	+	+
B. abortus	9	+	+	Slow	–	+
B. suis	4	–	+	Rapid	+	–
B. canis	1	–	–	Rapid	+	–

isms are excreted in milk, vaginal secretions, urine and are found in the infected fetus and fetal membranes of infected animals. The organisms survive for long periods in damp soil and water, and this represents a reservoir for infection of other animals. They can survive for 21 days in the refrigerated carcass of infected animals.

Antigens and Toxins

Capsules are found on cells from smooth and mucoid colonies.

Two carbohydrate antigens, designated A and M, are found in the cell wall of *B. abortus*, *B. melitensis* and *B. suis*. These antigens are found in all three species but in different amounts. The A antigen is the major antigen in *B. abortus* and *B. suis*, and the M antigen is the major antigen in *B. melitensis*. Monospecific sera to the A and the M antigen, prepared by absorption, are used to differentiate these organisms. Immunologic cross-reactivity occurs between the *Brucella*, *Yersinia*, *Francisella* and *Vibrio*.

Toxins other than endotoxin have not been demonstrated.

Genetics

The brucellae undergo the classic smooth to rough dissociation, with an accompanying loss in virulence and antigens. An attenuated strain (*B. abortus* 19) can be used for vaccination of animals. Other avirulent strains are under investigation as immunizing agents for man.

Infections

The primary effect of *Brucella* on animal hosts other than man is abortion. In cattle this is called Bang's disease, and is primarily caused by *Brucella abortus*. The other three species of *Brucella* also have preferred hosts: *B. suis* (swine), *B. melitensis* (goats) and *B. canis* (dogs). However, these species can infect other animal species. For example, *B. melitensis* can also cause disease in cattle, sheep and horses. Humans acquire infection through direct animal contact or by ingestion of contaminated foods.

Animals

In domestic animals the organs infected with *Brucella* are the mammary glands and the genital tract. The *Brucella* localize in the supramammary nodes and are shed in the milk of lactating females. They have a predilection for placental tissue because of its high concentration of erythritol. Infected animals can harbor and shed *Brucella* for years. The disease is transmitted to other animals by contact with a contaminated fetus, placental tissues or milk. The *Brucella* enter the host via ingestion, through the skin and mucous membranes or through abrasions of the skin. The organisms travel to regional lymph nodes, and after an ensuing septicemia the *Brucella* localize in the genital tract, where they multiply extensively. This results in necrosis of placental cotyledons and an infected fetus that may be aborted. Except for abortion, the animals are asymptomatic.

Humans

B. suis is the most frequent cause of disease in man. The disease occurs chiefly in abattoir workers but also in veterinarians and in those employed in dairy farming. The organisms enter a human host through the mucous membranes of the oropharynx, abraded skin, or conjunctiva. In most cases the infection is obtained by direct contact. Infection by inhalation occurs in slaughterhouse workers. Also, organisms can be ingested in unpasteurized milk or products made from unpasteurized milk. In the host, the organisms are engulfed by neutrophils and monocytes and localize in the lymph nodes. They proliferate intracellularly and are then released from the lymph nodes and infect phagocytic cells in the sinusoids of the reticuloendothelial system. If the host mounts a sufficient cellular response, either the organisms are destroyed or the infection remains localized. However, in the susceptible host, tissue destruction continues with recurrent septicemia. Granulomas are formed, and in acute brucellosis they may be found in the liver, spleen, lymph nodes and bone marrow. In chronic brucellosis they may also be found in subcutaneous tissue, testes, epididymis, ovary, kidney and brain. Recovery from infection is associated with development of cellular immunity, with activated macrophages as the cells responsible for the eventual elimination of the organisms. Because brucellae are intracellular parasites, chronic and latent infections also occur.

The incubation period is variable, ranging from about 2 weeks to several months. The onset of symptoms is usually insidious but may be sudden, with malaise, weakness, weight loss, headache, backache, chills, sweats and arthralgia occurring in most cases. The fever is intermittent and variable in degree. Chronic brucellosis may last for 1 to 20 years with relapses of different intensities. Fever, weakness, anxiety, mental depression and abscesses in tissue are characteristic. Relapses frequently occur, but they are generally less severe than the initial episode.

Complications resulting from brucellosis are varied. Infective endocarditis, meningitis, osteomyelitis, acute suppurative arthritis, bursitis and renal brucellosis, characterized by a diffuse interstitial nephritis or by abscess and renal calcification, may occur. Meningoencephalitis and associated neurologic disorders may also be produced.

Because of its various effects on the host, brucellosis mimics influenza, malaria, typhoid fever, typhus, tularemia, miliary tuberculosis and some noninfectious diseases. Thus laboratory confirmation and recognition of the animal source are important in the diagnosis of brucellosis.

Mechanisms of Pathogenicity

The ability of the *Brucella* to multiply within macrophages is considered to be an important virulence attribute and is associated with the cell surface since rough strains do not cause disease. Intracellular parasitism is thought to account for the ability of the *Brucella* to establish long-term infections and to survive in the presence of antibody.

Growth in fetal bovine tissue is quantitatively related to the amount of erythritol—a polyhydric, four-carbon alcohol—in these tissues. This carbohydrate enhances growth of the organisms in tissue and accounts for the predilection for these tissues. Erythritol is not found in human placenta, and infection of these tissues in man is rare.

Endotoxin is probably responsible for the fever characteristic of the disease. Hypersensitivity to endotoxin and to a brucella protein is produced and may play a role in the production of both fever and Jarisch-Herxheimer reaction, which may occur after administration of antibiotics. In chronic disease granulomas consisting of epithelioid cells, giant cells and lymphocytes are produced. The granulomas may undergo central necrosis and caseation. This tissue response suggests a role for delayed hypersensitivity in pathogenesis of the disease.

Immunity

Patients who have or have had brucellosis develop a delayed-type hypersensitivity that can be demonstrated by a skin test with an antigen termed brucellergen. This cellular hypersensitivity is thought to offer the host some means of protection against further infection.

Agglutinins, precipitins, opsonizing and bactericidal antibodies are also produced as a result of infection. Bactericidal antibody is effective in destroying extracellular organisms but is not effective against intracellular organisms. Measurement of agglutinating antibodies is useful in diagnosis of the disease. Immunity to brucellosis is poor, and second infections can occur. Recovery from brucellosis depends on the presence of activated macrophages.

A purified soluble protein antigen and a live attenuated vaccine (Rev. I) of *B. melitensis* have been tested and are effective in immunizing animals.

Prevention and Control

The incidence of brucellosis has markedly decreased in recent years due to the pasteurization of milk, the isolation and slaughter of infected animals, and the introduction of a live attenuated vaccine for cattle (*B. abortus* strain 19). Brucellosis resulting from ingestion of cheese imported from Mexico and Spain and made from unpasteurized goat milk has been reported, but this method of acquisition is rare.

Treatment

Antimicrobial therapy should be initiated as soon as brucellosis is suspected. The organisms are intracellular (mononuclear cells), and antibiotics that penetrate cells must be used. Tetracycline is the drug of choice with both streptomycin and tetracycline used in severe cases. Therapy must be prolonged in order to prevent relapses. Treatment may initially result in high fever, delirium or shock (Jarisch-Herxheimer reaction).

Laboratory Procedures

Specimens

Repeated blood cultures should be taken in the early febrile stage of the disease. Bone marrow, spleen and liver biopsies may also be used for isolation of the *Brucella*. Cerebrospinal fluid should be examined in patients with central nervous system symptoms.

Isolation and Identification

Specimens can be examined directly by gram stain and by fluorescent antibody staining (see Fig. 18–1). Cultures on blood agar should be incubated aerobically in 10% CO_2, and they may take as long as 30 days to be positive. Contaminated cultures should be inoculated on a selective medium, such as Weed's medium, or be injected into guinea pigs. Six weeks after inoculation of the animals, serum is collected for measuring *Brucella* agglutinins and tissues are cultured and examined for characteristic lesions. Identification is done by determining characteristics as shown in Table 18–1. Biotypes of each species exist, and reactions may vary from those shown in the table.

B. melitensis can be differentiated from *B. suis* and *B. abortus* using monospecific antiserum. *B. suis* and *B. abortus* share antigens, and these latter two species cannot be immunologically differentiated. *B. canis* does not agglutinate in the monospecific antiserum.

Serologic tests
Because of the difficulty in isolating these organisms, agglutinin titers are commonly used for diagnosis. A fourfold increase in agglutination titer to one of the species is considered significant. Presumptive diagnosis is based on an agglutination titer of 1:160 or greater. A prozone phenomenon may be observed with serum which contains IgG antibodies. The IgG antibodies bind to the antigen and prevent agglutination by IgM. Antiglobulin can be used to detect the IgG-antigen complex.

FRANCISELLA

General Characteristics
Francisella tularensis is a small (0.2×0.3–0.7 μm), pleomorphic, gram-negative, non-motile, obligate aerobe that appears as short rods or coccobacilli (Fig. 18–2). Capsules are not produced. Faint bipolar staining can be observed. The organism is slow growing and is fastidious, requiring cystine or cysteine for growth. This requirement aids in identification. Its optimal growth temperature is 35–37 C.

Species
Francisella tularensis is the only species in the genus *Francisella* that causes disease in both animals and man. *F. novicida* causes disease in animals but not in man.

Ecology
The source of the organisms is primarily the cottontail rabbit, but they are also found in birds (quail, pheasants), squirrels, woodchucks, skunks, foxes, muskrats, opossums, ticks, deerflies and fleas. The organisms are transmitted transovarially in ticks; thus the tick serves as a continual reservoir of infection. *F. tularensis* can parasitize about 100 different species of mammals and arthropods.

Antigens and Toxins
The cell wall contains several antigens. However, there is only one antigenic type of *F. tularensis*. A polysaccharide antigen produces an immediate-type hypersensitivity (wheal and flare). A protein antigen

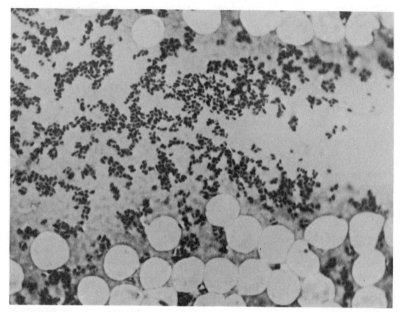

Fig. 18–2.—Giemsa stain of *F. tularensis* in blood of vole. Note short coccobacillary organisms. (Courtesy of Dr. William Jellison, Hamilton, Montana.)

shared with the *Brucella* accounts for immunologic cross reactions. A protein antigen is responsible for the development of delayed hypersensitivity. The cell wall contains endotoxin. No other toxins have been demonstrated.

Genetics
Smooth strains dissociate into rough strains with an associated loss of virulence.

Infections
Humans become infected by direct contact with infected animals, by insect bites (ticks or deerflies), by drinking contaminated water or ingesting improperly cooked meat from infected animals, or by inhaling contaminated aerosols.

There are two main types of tularemia in man: the glandular or ulceroglandular type and the typhoidal type (Fig. 18–3). The ulceroglandular type occurs in 70% to 80% of the patients with tularemia and is characterized by abrupt fever, rigors, headache, myalgia, prostration, splenomegaly and a papule at the site of entrance. Early in

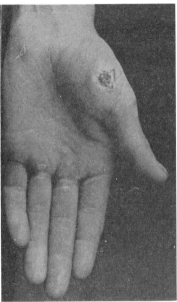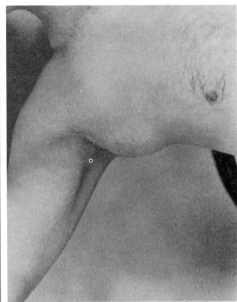

Fig. 18-3.—Ulceroglandular form of tularemia. Note ulcer on hand *(left)* and swollen axillary lymph node *(right)*. (Courtesy of Dr. William Jellison, Hamilton, Montana.)

the disease, a maculopapular rash may be present on the extremities and trunk. In 7 to 8 days the papule develops into an ulcer. By this time the regional lymph nodes are infected and are painful and swollen. The lymph nodes suppurate and may discharge purulent material. Usually there is no lymphangitis, and the point of entry may not be apparent. A bacteremia may occur and result in pneumonia. The symptoms of pneumonia may be minimal with only rhonchi and a mild bronchopneumonia. In other cases there may be a nonproductive cough with tracheobronchitis and pleural effusion. If an entire lobe is involved there is a nonproductive cough, severe respiratory distress, and pulmonary consolidation. The pneumonic type of disease occurs among clinical laboratory workers and research personnel who, in attempting to work with the organism, produce and inhale an aerosol of the organism. The pneumonic form has a high mortality; transmission to other persons rarely occurs.

In fatal cases of tularemia, local lesions are found in the liver, spleen and lymph nodes throughout the body. The overall duration of tularemia is approximately 1 month with adenopathy often remaining longer. Meningitis, osteomyelitis and endocarditis may also be produced.

The oculoglandular form of tularemia is due to the splashing of contaminated material, such as blood, into the eye. Initially, there is pain, photophobia, congestion, lacrimation and purulent discharge. The conjunctivas swell and granulomatous lesions may appear on the conjunctivas or cornea, which may ulcerate. The disease is similar to the ulceroglandular type, with enlargement of the regional lymph nodes (preauricular and cervical). In some cases an ulcer does not form and the disease is referred to simply as glandular tularemia.

Tularemia is difficult to diagnose and requires recognition of contact with animals or vectors. A delayed hypersensitivity reaction develops during the first week of the disease and is useful in diagnosing tularemia and in determining prevalence of the disease in a population group. Laboratory diagnosis is essential to differentiate tularemia from other infectious diseases with similar symptomatology. Ulceroglandular tularemia may resemble cat-scratch fever, sporotrichosis and infectious mononucleosis. The pneumonic form of tularemia must be differentiated from atypical pneumonia due to Q fever, psittacosis, mycoplasma, histoplasmosis, coccidioidomycosis or tuberculosis. The typhoidal form must be differentiated from typhoid fever, brucellosis, tuberculosis and other systemic infections.

Mechanisms of Pathogenicity

Francisella tularensis produces an endotoxin; no exotoxin has been found. The organisms multiply intracellularly, accounting for their ability to persist for months and even years in infected individuals. About 50 bacilli are needed to establish infection by the respiratory or intradermal route in man, but 10^7 organisms are required for infection by the oral route. The host response to infection is production of granulomatous lesions that appear as tubercles in the liver, spleen, kidney and lung. A delayed hypersensitivity reaction can be elicited in infected individuals and supports the histologic evidence suggesting that hypersensitivity may contribute to pathogenesis. An interesting observation is that strains of high virulence ferment glycerol and have citrulline ureidase activity, whereas strains of low virulence do not. The significance of this relationship is not yet apparent.

Immunity

Agglutinins appear during the second or third week of the disease and persist, but they seem to play little role in recovery from disease. Cellular immunity seems to be the most important factor associated with acquired immunity. People with tularemia develop delayed-type skin reactions that persist for years. An attenuated vaccine has been developed, but tularemia has been reported in immunized individuals. Relapses and reinfection also occur, which suggests that infection may produce only low levels of immunity.

Prevention and Treatment

Infected rabbits are the main source of infection. Tularemia can be prevented by adequately cooking infected animals and by wearing rubber gloves and glasses when skinning and dressing animals. Clothing should be secured around the ankles and wrists to prevent attachment of ticks, and workers should check periodically for attachment of ticks, particularly in the groin, axillae and scalp. Ticks should be carefully removed. Covering the tick with cloth soaked in ether, acetone or benzene should result in release in about 10 minutes. Touching the tick with a hot needle or cigarette may also cause release. Tweezers — not fingers — should be used to remove ticks. Removal should be with a straight rather than twisting motion. For treatment, streptomycin is the antibiotic of choice. Approximately 5% of the cases of tularemia are fatal if untreated. A live attenuated vaccine is available for individuals at risk from the disease.

Laboratory Procedures

Specimens for culture include material from the initial lesion and aspirates of enlarged regional lymph nodes. Sputum, gastric aspirates, pharyngeal washings, pleural fluids and bronchial secretions should be obtained from patients with pneumonic tularemia. Diagnosis depends on demonstration of organisms in the specimen by the gram stain and by fluorescent antibody test (see Fig. 18-2). Cultures must be inoculated on cysteine-glucose-blood agar plates because *F. tularensis* requires cysteine for growth. The organisms are difficult to culture and may take 2 to 3 weeks before growth is obtained. Intraperitoneal inoculation of guinea pigs with clinical specimens can be helpful in isolation. If *F. tularensis* is present, the animal will die in 5 to 10 days. Granulomatous lesions will be found in the spleen and liver and the organisms can be isolated from the spleen and blood. The identity of isolates from the patient and guinea pig can be confirmed by agglutination with specific antiserum. An increase in agglutinating antibody titer to *F. tularensis* using serum from the patient or the infected guinea pig is also considered confirmative. Antibodies usually are detectable in the second week of the disease. Because of cross-reactivity with the *Brucella*, parallel agglutination tests should also be done with *Brucella*.

Most laboratories are not equipped to culture and identify *F. tularensis*, and work with this organism should not be attempted by inexperienced personnel with inadequate facilities.

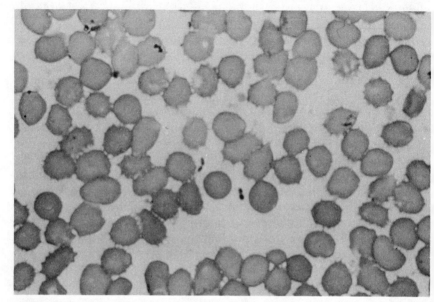

Fig. 18–4.—*Yersinia pestis* in peripheral blood. Note bipolar staining; Wayson's stain. (Courtesy of Allan M. Barnes, Ph.D., Chief, Plague Branch, Center for Disease Control, Fort Collins, Colorado 80522.)

YERSINIA

General Characteristics

Yersinia pestis is a pleomorphic, gram-negative coccobacillus (0.5–0.8×1.5–2.0 μm) that shows bipolar staining with Giemsa or Wayson's (carbol fuchsin-methylene blue) stain (Fig. 18–4). A capsule is produced in vivo and in young cultures. It is non-motile, and like other *Yersinia*, it is a member of the family Enterobacteriaceae. Like the enteric bacteria, it is a facultative anaerobe and grows on simple media. Optimal temperature for growth is 28 C, but growth at this temperature results in a loss of virulence. Growth at 37 C allows the organism to maintain its virulence.

Species

Several species of *Yersinia* cause disease in man and animals: *Y. pestis, Y. pseudotuberculosis* and *Y. enterocolitica. Y. pseudotuberculosis* and *Y. enterocolitica* are discussed in Chapter 14.

Ecology

Yersinia pestis normally causes a disease of wild rodents called sylvatic plague. The permanent reservoirs of infection are animals, such as field mice, that are resistant to plague. The bacilli cause chronic infections in these animals, with the flea serving as a vector for transmission between animals and for transmission to man. These animals include prairie dogs, ground squirrels, wood rats, mice, gerbils and wild rabbits. On occasion, the disease spreads from man to man by aerosols (pneumonic plague) or by the human flea.

In the United States, sylvatic plague occurs in Texas, New Mexico, Utah, California and Arizona. Most cases of plague occur in Southeast Asia.

Antigens, Toxins and Virulence Factors

Yersinia pestis is antigenically complex and contains a multitude of antigens. Some of these antigens are specific for *Y. pestis*. Others are shared with *Y. pseudotuberculosis* and other organisms. However, there is only one antigenic type of *Y. pestis*.

A protein capsule, designated fraction 1 (F1), allows the organisms to resist phagocytosis. The F1 antigen is produced in vivo and in vitro at 37 C, but not at 28 C or in fleas. Two other surface antigens, V and W, are also antiphagocytic. The V antigen is a cell-bound protein of about 90,000 daltons and is immunogenic. The W antigen is a lipoprotein with a molecular weight of 145,000 which is released into the medium during growth. The most virulent plague bacilli have all three antigens (V, W and F1).

Coagulase and fibrinolysin are also produced. Their role in human disease is unknown.

In addition to endotoxin, *Yersinia pestis* also elaborates a protein toxin (murine toxin) which is released on cell death. It is lethal for mice in microgram quantities, but other animals are resistant. It acts on mitochondrial membranes, hydrolyzing NAD to nicotinamide and thereby inhibiting respiration. Its role in human infections is still questioned. Recent reports suggest that the murine toxin alters the metabolic and calorigenic activity controlled by the sympathetic nervous system and that hypothermia is the determinant of lethality.

Genetics

Both smooth and rough forms of *Y. pestis* are virulent. Transfer in vitro results in loss of virulence. Bacteriophages that lyse *Y. pestis* and *Y. pseudotuberculosis* have been described. A bacteriocin (pesticin I) that inhibits growth of *Y. pseudotuberculosis* and *Y. enterocolitica* is produced. Pesticin production correlates with coagulase and fibrinolysin production. Strains that do not produce pesticin I and consequently coagulase and fibrinolysin are infectious but of lowered virulence.

Virulent strains also are able to absorb hemin and aromatic dyes with resultant colored colonies. Avirulent strains, which do not produce colored colonies, regain virulence if an excess of iron, sufficient to saturate serum transferrin, is present.

Transmission and Epidemiology

The epidemiology of plague is complex and the precise events that lead to epidemics are not clearly understood. A flea-rodent cycle is required to perpetuate the disease. The flea ingests the organisms by feeding on an infected host. The organisms multiply in the stomach of the flea, and the multiplication blocks the proventriculus. The cycle in arthropods requires about 2 weeks. During a subsequent meal, the organisms are regurgitated into the host (wild or domestic rodent or man). Transmission may also occur through contaminated mouth parts by feeding on an infected host.

If the rodent host is susceptible, an epidemic (epizootic) occurs in the rodent population with death. Resistant hosts develop a bacteremia but survive and thus become an excellent reservoir for the infection of fleas. Transfer of plague from the wild rodent (sylvatic plague) to the black rat via fleas results in urban plague. The black rat lives in association with man, and when large die-offs because of plague occur, the rat flea feeds on humans and human plague results.

In the United States, man acquires infection from rodents other than rats with squirrels, prairie dogs, field mice and chipmunks serving as the reservoirs. Human contact with these rodents, in particular prairie dogs and their burrows, may result in plague. Dogs and cats can serve as intermediaries in transmission by bringing infected rodents and their fleas to man.

Plague can be transmitted from human to human via two mechanisms: through the human flea and by inhalation. Only in certain parts of the world do humans carry fleas, and it is not considered a major means of spread of the disease. The second and most important means of transmission is via the respiratory route. In approximately 2% of bubonic plague cases, the organisms invade the lungs and are found in the sputum. The result is spread of the plague bacillus via inhalation (pneumonic plague). Plague in this case has a shortened course and is highly fatal (greater than 90% in untreated cases).

Infections

The disease develops about 2 to 6 days after a flea bite. Initially, a vesicular lesion is formed at the site of the bite. Organisms spread through the lymphatics producing a lymphadenitis and then localize and proliferate in the regional lymph nodes. A severe swelling of the

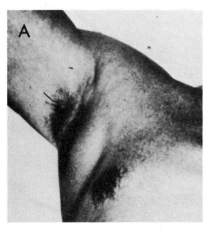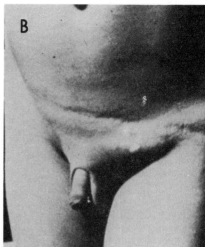

Fig. 18-5.—Axillary **(A)** and inguinal **(B)** buboes in patients with bubonic plague. (Courtesy of Allan M. Barnes, Ph.D., Chief, Plague Branch, Center for Disease Control, Fort Collins, Colorado 80522.)

lymph nodes occurs (referred to as a bubo). Depending on the site of the bite, buboes may appear near the inguinal or in the axillary lymph nodes (Fig. 18-5). The buboes are tender and generally painful. In fatal cases of bubonic plague, the organisms escape from the buboes and septicemia results. The organisms then proliferate in the spleen and liver, as well as in other lymph nodes. Clinical features include fever, generalized malaise, headache, shaking chills, severe prostration and disseminated intravascular coagulation. Vomiting, coma, convulsions and subcutaneous hemorrhaging can develop.

In some cases, the bacilli, as a result of septicemia, are deposited in other organs, including the lung, resulting in a severe pneumonia. Inhalation of plague bacilli from an aerosol generated by pneumonic patients also results in the pneumonic form of the disease. The pneumonic form may also follow pharyngeal plague. The incubation period for pneumonic plague is 2 to 3 days. The organisms spread throughout the lung, producing a hemorrhagic pneumonic process. Signs and symptoms include rigor, malaise, headache, nausea and a mucoid, bloody sputum containing numerous bacilli which are transmitted via aerosols generated by coughing. The pneumonic form has the highest mortality.

Septicemic plague is similar to the bubonic type in that it is initiated by a flea bite. In this form of the disease, the organisms fail to localize in the regional lymph nodes, and the result is a highly fatal disease with a shorter course than the bubonic type. Hemorrhages in the skin and mucous membranes result from intravascular thrombi.

Meningitis may occur in patients without evidence of an adenitis, or it may occur by hematogenous spread from an infected bubo.

Occasionally, the disease may be mild, and in some cases *Yersinia pestis* may be isolated from the oropharynx of healthy individuals. These people were in recent contact with plague victims and are considered transient carriers of the plague bacillus.

The symptoms of plague can be confused with those of tularemia, meningococcemia, gram-negative sepsis as caused by enterics, and rickettsial infection. The history of exposure to rodents, rabbits and fleas requires inclusion of *Y. pestis* in a differential diagnosis.

Mechanisms of Pathogenicity

Four factors are considered important in the pathogenesis of *Yersinia pestis*: antiphagocytic antigens, the ability to survive and multiply within monocytes, a murine toxin and classic endotoxin.

The ability of *Yersinia pestis* to survive in monocytes is important in establishing an infection. In the flea and the rat, the organisms do not synthesize the F1, V and W antigens. On injection of the organisms into a host via a rat flea, the organisms are phagocytized by both monocytes and neutrophils. The neutrophils kill the organisms, but in the monocytes they multiply and synthesize the F1, V and W antigens. These organisms subsequently resist killing by the neutrophils. Thus the ability to survive and multiply in monocytes is a major attribute of virulence.

The importance of the murine toxin in human disease is unknown. However, edema, hemoconcentration, the production of serosanguineous fluids and the necrosis of lymph nodes in human disease are similar to what is seen in animals injected with murine toxin.

A major factor related to the pathogenesis of plague is the classic endotoxin. Purpura, disseminated intravascular coagulation, fever, tachycardia and hypotension—all attributes of endotoxin—are the major clinical features associated with human cases of plague. Endotoxin can be demonstrated in blood and in cerebrospinal fluid (in patients with meningitis) by the *Limulus* tests.

Unlike other gram-negative bacteremias, the plaque bacillus can easily be demonstrated by direct staining and by colony counts of blood specimens. A unique aspect of the septicemic form of plaque is the large numbers of bacilli (up to 10^7/ml) in peripheral blood. Large numbers indicate a poor prognosis. This and other data indicate that the plague endotoxin may be less potent than other endotoxins. Although the LD_{50} for plague endotoxin is higher than that of other endotoxins, it is equally pyrogenic.

Immunity

Acquired immunity may depend on the development of antibodies to the F1, V and W antigens. Humoral antibodies promote opsonization by the neutrophils, enabling them to engulf and kill the bacilli. Antibody to the murine toxin does not confer protection. A live attenuated and a formalinized vaccine afford partial protection against plague and are used in areas where plague is endemic. Booster doses are required every 3–6 months to maintain immunity.

Prevention and Control

Sylvatic plague is endemic in certain wild rodent populations in the United States and other parts of the world. Immunization, with concurrent antibiotic prophylaxis, has been shown to help in stopping epidemics. Early treatment and quarantine of suspected cases are of paramount importance. Proper sanitation to control the rat population is necessary for long-term prevention of epidemics. Insecticides must be used to control the vector and its transfer between animals and man and animals.

Treatment

Early diagnosis and treatment with antibiotics are essential and must be initiated within 12 to 15 hours of the appearance of fever. The case fatality rate for untreated bubonic plague is 60% to 90%, but in the pneumonic form it approaches 100%. Streptomycin is the drug of choice, although trimethoprim has also been used successfully. Supportive therapy directed at failing circulatory and pulmonary function should be initiated. A Jarisch-Herxheimer reaction may occur with antibiotic treatment. Attending personnel must be extremely careful during patient contact and when handling exudates from infected persons so as to minimize chances of infection.

Laboratory Procedures

Specimens
Sputum, blood, pus aspirated from the site of infection, and throat swabs should be collected. For cases of meningitis, cerebrospinal fluid may be used. Bone marrow, lymph nodes and lung tissue from autopsies should also be collected.

Giemsa's or Wayson's stain of all specimens, including blood, should be done (see Fig. 18–4). Bipolar-staining, gram-negative rods are suggestive of *Yersinia pestis*. Specimens should be cultured on blood agar, MacConkey or deoxycholate agar, nutrient agar and meat infusion broth. Good growth should be obtained within 2 days. Quantitative blood cultures may be of significance in determining prognosis. Confirmation of *Y. pestis* is based on agglutination with specific *Y. pestis* antiserum, staining by fluorescent antiserum and susceptibility to specific bacteriophages. Patients with plague also demonstrate a rise in antibody titer to the F1 and murine toxin. *All specimens should be handled with extreme care, and inexperienced laboratory personnel should not attempt to isolate the organism.*

Endotoxin can also be assayed in cerebrospinal fluid and blood.

PASTEURELLA

Several species of *Pasteurella* are found in animals, but only one species, *P. multocida*, is associated with disease in man. Other species are *P. pneumotropica, P. haemolytica* and *P. ureae*.

Pasteurella multocida

Pasteurella multocida is a gram-negative, non-motile coccobacillus (0.15–0.25×0.3–1.25 μm) that shows marked bipolar staining. It is non-spore-forming, nonmotile and has an optimal growth temperature of 37 C. It grows readily on plain agar or blood agar, but it does not grow in the presence of bile. Hemolysins are not produced. Lactose is not fermented. The *Pasteurella* can be differentiated from the *Yersinia* by determining production of B-D-galactosidase. The *Yersinia* produce B-D-galactosidase. Five serologic types (A–E), based on capsular or O polysaccharides, are recognized. No toxins other than endotoxins have been described.

Pasteurella multocida is a parasite of animals that is acquired by man. It is found in the respiratory tract of animals such as dogs, cats, sheep, rats, cattle, swine and horses. In animals under stress it causes a hemorrhagic septicemia.

The organisms may be introduced into man by an animal bite. If infection results, there is local pain, swelling, discoloration and regional lymphadenitis. Pyarthrosis, synovitis and osteomyelitis may result. In addition to infection precipitated by animal bites, *P. multocida* may colonize the lungs of persons with compromised respiratory tracts. Sinusitis, otitis media, mastoiditis, pneumonia, empyema and bronchiectasis may result.

Pasteurella infections may also cause a septicemia with osteomyelitis, meningitis, endocarditis or pneumonia resulting. Infections of the alimentary tract may also be produced.

Penicillin is the drug of choice for treatment of infections caused by *P. multocida.*

PROBLEM SOLVING AND REVIEW

NO. 1. GIVEN: – The patient was a 45-year-old man who had worked in a meat packing plant for about 10 years. Prior to that he had worked on a farm. He had been ill for 5 weeks with chills and a temperature of 39.6 C. He complained of a headache, frequent sweating and anorexia. Upon examination he had a cervical lymphadenopathy and hepatosplenomegaly. Laboratory values reported were hemoglobin 12.0 gm/100 ml, leukocytes 6,000/cu mm with 45% neutrophils. Granulomas were present in the liver. Blood was obtained for culture and serologic testing. The laboratory reported growth in the blood culture, a *Brucella* agglutinin titer of 1:3,200 and a *Francisella tularensis* agglutination titer of 1:40.

PROBLEMS: – 1. What is the diagnosis and probable etiologic agent? 2. What is the probable source of the organism? 3. What is the basis for the diagnosis? 4. How do you explain the agglutination titer for *F. tularensis*? 5. If you gram stained the blood culture, what would you expect to find? (Ans. p. 353.)

NO. 2. GIVEN: – A 48-year-old man sought medical attention for an illness of 1 week's duration characterized by fever, chills, nausea and decreased appetite. Over the following 2 weeks he had a weight loss of 15 pounds, and he developed severe pain in the dorsum of the left foot. The patient spontaneously became afebrile and asymptomatic and was discharged without a specific diagnosis. For the next 3 months, he had repeated brief episodes of fever and diaphoresis. Examination at 4 months revealed spastic hemiparesis, mild splenomegaly, and cervical and supraclavicular lymphadenopathy. Information from the patient revealed that his pet beagle dog had given birth to two pups 2 months before the patient's onset of illness. One pup was stillborn, and the other died shortly after birth.

PROBLEMS: – 1. What is the suspected diagnosis? 2. How would you obtain information for a presumptive and confirmative diagnosis. 3. What would be the positive results? (Ans. p. 353.)

NO. 3. GIVEN: – A 51-year-old Californian was hospitalized with a 1-week history of fever, chills, malaise and diarrhea. Stool specimens were negative for enteric pathogens. The diarrhea gradually resolved but the fever continued. A large, tender axillary lymph node was noted, as was a scabbed erythematous lesion on the left hand. Three days before onset of symptoms the patient had been hunting. He shot, field dressed, and ate wild rabbit.

PROBLEMS: — 1. What is the probable diagnosis? 2. What is the source of the organism and portal of entry? 3. How would you prove the diagnosis? 4. What results would confirm your diagnosis? (Ans. p. 353.)

NO. 4. GIVEN: — A 13-year-old girl was admitted with fever and severe pain in the left axilla of 48 hours' duration. Her temperature was 39 C, pulse 88, and blood pressure 102/70. A tender 2×3-inch ill-defined mass was present in the left axilla. Two small macular areas were noted on the left upper arm. Three days before the onset of the patient's illness she and her family had camped near a prairie dog area in New Mexico.

PROBLEMS: — 1. What is the suspected diagnosis? 2. How would you obtain information for a presumptive and confirmed diagnosis? 3. What results would you expect if positive? (Ans. p. 353.)

SUPPLEMENTARY READING

BRUCELLA
Buchanan, T. M., Faber, L. C., and Feldman, R. A.: Brucellosis in the United States, 1960–72. An abattoir-associated disease. Part I: Clinical features and therapy, Medicine (Baltimore) 53:403–439, 1974.
Elberg, S. S.: Immunity to Brucella infection, Medicine (Baltimore) 52: 339–356, 1973.
Monroe, P. W., Silberg, S. L., Morgan, P. M., and Adess, M.: Seroepidemiological investigation of Brucella canis antibodies in different human population groups, J. Clin. Microbiol. 2:382–386, 1975.
Munford, R. S., Weaver, R. E., Patton, C., Feeley, J. C., and Feldman, R. A.: Human disease caused by Brucella canis. A clinical and epidemiological study of two cases, J.A.M.A. 231:1267–1269, 1975.
Spink, W. W.: The Nature of Brucellosis (Minneapolis: University of Minnesota Press, 1956).

FRANCISELLA
Buchanan, T. M., Brooks, G. F., and Brachman, P. S.: The tularemia skin tests, Ann. Intern. Med. 74:336, 1971.
Chafin, J. L., and Larson, C. L.: Infection-immunity in tularemia. Specificity of cellular immunity, Infect. Immun. 5:311–318, 1972.
Young, L. S., and Sherman, I. L.: Tularemia in the United States: Recent trends and a major outbreak, J. Infect. Dis. 119:109, 1969.

YERSINIA

Butler, T. A.: A clinical study of bubonic plague. Observations of the 1970 Vietnam epidemic with emphasis on coagulation studies, skin histology and electrocardiograms, Am. J. Med. 53:268–276, 1972.

Butler, T. A., Levin, J., Linh, N. N., Chau, D. M., Adickman, M., and Arnold, K.: Yersinia pestis infection in Vietnam. II. Quantitative blood cultures and detection of endotoxin in the cerebrospinal fluid of patients with meningitis, J. Infect. Dis. 133:493–499, 1976.

Wennerstrom, D. E., Brown, S. D., and Montie, T. C.: Altered lethality of murine toxin from Yersinia pestis under various metabolic conditions, Proc. Soc. Exp. Biol. Med. 154:78–81, 1977.

ANALYSIS

No. 1.—1. Brucellosis probably due to B. suis. 2. Contact with infected hogs during work. 3. High brucella agglutination titer. 4. Antibodies are produced which cross-react. 5. Gram-negative coccobacilli.

No. 2.—1. Brucellosis due to B. canis. 2. Obtain serum for serologic testing; cultures of blood and bone marrow. 3. Titer of 1:160 to Brucella canis indicates brucellosis (presumptive). Cultures reveal gram-negative rod that has biochemical and serologic characteristics of B. canis.

No. 3.—1. Tularemia. 2. The source of the organism is probably an infected rabbit. The organism entered the patient through a break in the skin (left hand). 3. Prepare gram and fluorescent antibody stains of enlarged lymph nodes and lesion. Cultures of lymph node, lesion and blood. Request agglutinin titers. 4. Stains should show small gram-negative rods with bipolar staining. Fluorescent antibody stains of tissue would be positive. Requirement of cysteine for growth of suspected F. tularensis. Positive reaction of isolate with specific antiserum to F. tularensis, as demonstrated by agglutination and fluorescent antiserum. Rise in agglutination titer of patient.

No. 4.—1. Bubonic plague. 2. Prepare smears of lesions and aspirates from lymph node. Culture lesion, aspirate from lymph node, and blood. Withdraw blood for serologic testing. 3. Gram-negative, bipolar rods in tissue (presumptive). Culture yields nonmotile, facultative, gram-negative rods with biochemical characteristics of Yersinia pestis. Isolate agglutinates with specific antiserum, and it is positive with Y. pestis fluorescent antibody serum. Isolate sensitive to Y. pestis phage. Patient shows rise in titer to Y. pestis as demonstrated by agglutination test.

19 / Haemophilus and Bordetella

OVERVIEW

Members of the genus *Haemophilus* are distinct from members of the genus *Bordetella* in nutritional and physiologic aspects and also with respect to the types of diseases they produce.

At one time *Haemophilus influenzae* was considered to be the etiologic agent of what is now known as swine influenza. However, it was established that *H. influenzae* was a secondary invader that caused disease only after the influenza virus caused significant damage to the upper respiratory tract. Then, as now, *H. influenzae* plays an important role in pulmonary disease after primary infection or insult to the respiratory tract and in diseases of the CNS in children.

Whooping cough, caused by *Bordetella pertussis*, although still important, no longer occurs with the same frequency as it did in the past. This is in part due to the development of an effective vaccine, the almost uniform vaccination of preschool children, and the use of antibiotics to prevent and treat the disease and reduce communicability.

HAEMOPHILUS

General Characteristics

The organisms are gram-negative coccobacillary to rod-shaped cells (0.2–0.3×0.5–2.0 μm) that may have thread-like and filamentous forms (Fig. 19–1). They are nonmotile. They grow optimally at 37 C and are facultatively anaerobic. Growth requires use of media containing hemin (X factor), NAD (V factor), or both.

Species

The genus *Haemophilus* contains several species that cause disease in man: (1) *H. influenzae* causes infections of the upper and lower respiratory tract, otitis media, acute epiglottitis, meningitis, osteomyelitis and cellulitis; (2) *H. aegyptius* cause conjunctivitis; (3) *H. ducreyi* causes chancroid (soft chancre), a venereal disease and (4) *H. parainfluenzae* can cause endocarditis and meningitis. *H. suis* is found in

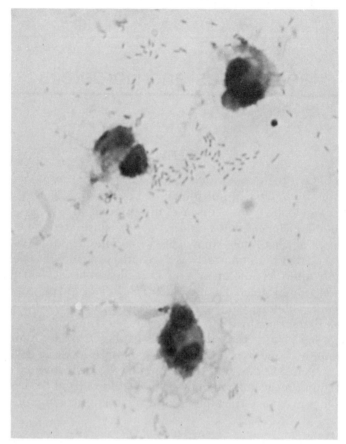

Fig. 19–1.—*Haemophilus influenzae* in cerebrospinal fluid. Note coccobacillary shape.

swine. *H. hemolyticus* is found in nasopharyngeal cultures and can be confused with beta-hemolytic streptococci because of production of a hemolysin. Neither *H. suis* nor *H. hemolyticus* causes disease in humans.

The various species of *Haemophilus* are identified by their requirements for X and V factors, CO_2 and by production of hemolysin (Table 19–1).

Fresh sheep blood is the source of X factor (hemin). To obtain V factor (NAD), the laboratory may take advantage of the excess production of NAD by *Staphylococcus aureus*. To do this a blood agar plate is first streaked with the clinical specimen, and then a strain of *Staphylococc-*

TABLE 19-1.—DIFFERENTIAL CHARACTERISTICS
OF *HAEMOPHILUS SPP.*

ORGANISM	REQUIREMENTS FOR GROWTH			HEMOLYSIS
	X	V	CO$_2$	
H. influenzae	+	+	−	−
H. aegyptius	+	+	−	−
H. hemolyticus	+	+	−	+
H. suis	+	+	−	−
H. ducreyi	+	−	+	+/−
H. aphrophilus	+	−	+	−
H. parahaemolyticus	+	−	−	+
H. parainfluenzae	−	+	−	−
H. paraphrophilus	−	+	+	−
H. paraphrohaemolyticus	−	+	+	+

cus aureus is streaked across the plate (Fig. 19-2). Since NAD is needed only when the cells are undergoing oxidative phosphorylation, the requirement for V factor can be obviated by growth anaerobically. The better growth of the *Haemophilus* near *S. aureus*, with reduced growth away from the *S. aureus* inoculum, indicates a requirement for V factor. This phenomenon is termed satellitism. An alternate method is to place a paper disk impregnated with NAD on a plate that has been inoculated with the *Haemophilus* sp. Growth will occur around the disk. Alternatively, the organisms can be isolated on "chocolate" agar (heated blood agar). Heating inactivates enzymes in the red blood cells, which destroys NAD thus assuring sufficient V factor for growth of the *Haemophilus* organisms.

Ecology

Haemophilus influenzae and *H. parainfluenzae* are both found as members of the normal flora of the upper respiratory tract. *H. influenzae* is found in 5% to 20% of the population, whereas *H. parainfluenzae* has been cultured from up to 25%. *H. aegyptius* and *H. ducreyi* are not found as normal flora. Except for *H. suis*, all species of *Heamophilus* are found only in man.

Cell Wall

The cell wall is that of a typical gram-negative cell wall.

Haemophilus Influenzae

Antigens

H. influenzae can be divided into six serologic groups (a-f) based on antigenicity of the capsular polysaccharide. The carbohydrates of

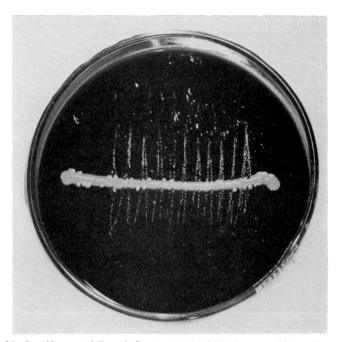

Fig. 19–2.—*Haemophilus influenzae* on blood agar. Note that growth occurs only near the line of *S. aureus* growth and around the colony of *S. aureus* near the periphery of the plate. This is the satellite phenomenon.

types a, b and c are polysugarphosphates and are immunologically related to some of the pneumococcal capsular polysaccharides. The capsule from type b, the major pathogen for humans, is a polyribosyl-ribitol phosphate. Nontypable strains lack a capsule. Somatic antigens are present, some of which are shared among all typable and untypable strains. Other somatic antigens show some specificity for types and strains.

Genetics

S → R dissociation results in a change in colony morphology and size and reflects loss of capsular polysaccharide and decreased virulence.

Transformation, transduction and R factor transfer have been described. The recent occurrence of ampicillin resistance in *H. influenzae* is due to acquisition of R factors. Transfer of R factors between *H. influenzae* type b and *H. parainfluenzae* has been shown.

Toxins

Haemophilus influenzae contains endotoxin and a lymphocyte blastogenic factor. In addition, a nondialyzable, heat-stable ciliostatic factor is produced early in the growth cycle. This factor causes a loss of cilia; it results in damage and sloughing of epithelial cells and may be important in pathogenicity.

A labile surface antigen, termed M, that is toxic for animals has also been described.

H. influenzae type b produces a thermostable protein (bacteriocin) that is toxic for serotypes of *H. influenzae* other than type b as well as for nontypable *H. influenzae*, other *Haemophilus* spp. and enteric bacteria. This bacteriocin may be important in helping the organism establish itself in the host.

Infections

H. influenzae infections are acquired by aspiration of organisms colonizing the respiratory tract (endogenous) or by contact with other carriers (exogenous).

Diseases caused by *H. influenzae* are associated with five major systems: pulmonary system (pneumonia, empyema, pharyngitis, sinusitis, epiglottitis, bronchiolitis, chronic bronchitis); central nervous system (meningitis); skeletal system (septic arthritis, osteomyelitis, periorbital and facial cellulitis); cardiovascular system (infective endocarditis, pericarditis) and urinary tract. The pulmonary and CNS forms of disease are discussed below.

In all cases the disease starts as a nasopharyngitis that spreads by direct extension to produce sinusitis or otitis media or via bacteremia to infect the CNS and other organs. Aspiration of secretions by the nonimmune child or by children and adults with compromised pulmonary tracts leads to pulmonary disease. Disease occurs most frequently in young children and older adults.

PULMONARY DISEASE. — The initial nasopharyngitis commonly occurs after viral infection and may lead to pneumonia and empyema.

The symptoms of pneumonia are typical of a bacterial infection except for the absence of pleuritic pain. Exacerbations of chronic bronchitis in chronic obstructive pulmonary disease may be incited by or may be due to infection with *H. influenzae*.

Bacteremia following infection of the respiratory tract can lead to endocarditis and meningitis.

EPIGLOTTITIS AND OBSTRUCTIVE LARYNGITIS. — This severe disease has an acute onset with fever, sore throat, barking cough and absence of hoarseness. The patient may progress within a few hours from a normal state to a state of toxicity, prostration, severe dyspnea and cyanosis. The throat is inflamed and the epiglottis appears beefy red, swollen and stiff. Epiglottitis can result in airway occlusion by the swollen epiglottis being pulled down by inspiration. A septicemia may be present and treatment must be promptly initiated. Epiglottitis may also occur in patients with meningitis. Acute epiglottitis occurs in children between 2 and 7 years of age.

MENINGITIS. — The disease occurs most frequently in children between 6 weeks and 2 years of age. It follows a bacteremia that results from infection of the respiratory tract. *H. influenzae* type b is the most important cause of meningitis in infants and children. The symptoms of meningitis are variable and depend on age, duration and severity of infection. In an infant, symptoms of meningitis may not be obvious. The child may only show fever, alternating restlessness and drowsiness. The child may vomit and cry when handled and the respiratory symptoms may be mild or absent. Older infants show the classic symptoms of fever, vomiting, stiff neck, headache, occasional delirium and positive Kernig's and Brudzinski's signs. Examination of the cerebrospinal fluid reveals many polymorphonuclear leukocytes and microorganisms (see Fig. 19 – 1).

Mechanisms of Pathogenicity

To cause disease, the organism must be able initially to compete with bacteria constituting the normal flora of the upper respiratory tract. *H. influenzae* serotype b produces a bacteriocin that may contribute to its ability to compete with other bacteria, including other types of *H. influenzae.*

The presence of a capsule enables the organism to resist phagocytosis and survive in the host environment. The capsule, like the pneumococcal capsule, is soluble and diffuses in body fluids. The ability of the soluble capsular material to react with antibody, thereby reducing the amount available for opsonization, favors survival of the organism and thus subsequent growth of the organism and disease.

A ciliostatic factor may be important in pulmonary infection and in exacerbation of disease in patients with chronic bronchitis. The loss of cilia and the damage to epithelial cells may be associated with the symptoms and the pathologic features of these diseases. Although the role of the blastogenic factor in disease and immunity is unknown, lymphokines which cause cytotoxicity might be involved. However, proof is lacking. An endotoxin is produced, but its role in diseases caused by *H. influenzae* is unknown.

Immunity

Two factors are important in determining the host-parasite relationship: (1) the presence of an encapsulated strain and (2) the presence or absence of antibody. Of the six serogroups of *H. influenzae* (a–f), serotype b is most important in human disease and about 80% of the en-

:apsulated strains found in the upper respiratory tract are type b. However, nonencapsulated strains are most frequently isolated from :he upper respiratory tract. The capsule is antiphagocytic and antibody :o the capsule equates with immunity. Children up to 6 weeks of age ιre generally immune to infection because of placental transfer of an-:ibody. Susceptibility to infection begins at about 6 weeks as maternal ιntibody is lost and continues for the first 2-5 years of life until im-nunity is naturally acquired. Immunity, as a result of subclinical in-:ections or by immunization with cross-reacting antigens from other ›rganisms, remains throughout adulthood but decreases in older per-;ons. Under normal circumstances, infections occur primarily in ⁄oung children who lack immunity.

Other host factors are also important in determining whether infec-:ion will occur. Infection in adults is associated with impairment of 1ormal host defense mechanisms, such as occurs in the lung following ⁄iral pneumonia or in those who have chronic debilitation of the ower respiratory tract, e.g., chronic bronchitis, bronchiectasis. Immu-1odeficiency diseases also predispose to infection.

The presence of bactericidal antibody and immunity to *H. influen-:ae* type b has, in the past, been believed to result from subclinical or :linical disease. Recent studies have shown a cross-reacting antigen n several genera of microorganisms, including *E. coli*. Oral feeding of ιdults with a strain of cross-reacting *E. coli* results in a good antibody ·esponse to the capsular antigen of type b *H. influenzae*. It is now pro-›osed that natural immunity in animals and man is associated with :arriage of organisms (*E. coli* and other) that contain the cross-reacting ›olyribitol phosphate antigen. This work suggests a new and exciting ιpproach to immunization against this and other diseases.

Immunization of humans with capsular polysaccharide has been ιttempted. The antigen is nontoxic and highly immunogenic in adults. Iowever, the most susceptible group, children, either do not respond ⁄ith antibody or give a low and unsustained response.

Prevention

Vaccines are not available at present for prevention of the disease. .mmunization against viral influenza minimizes secondary infections n the young and elderly and in persons with compromised respiratory racts.

Treatment

The antibiotics of choice for treatment are ampicillin and chloram-phenicol. Recently, there have been reports of ampicillin-resistant *Haemophilus influenzae*.

Other Haemophilus Spp

Haemophilus parainfluenzae

Haemophilus parainfluenzae is a member of the normal flora of the upper respiratory tract and is found in the oropharynx of about 30% of the people. It is recognized infrequently as a pathogen for man; however, it has been found as the etiologic agent in bacterial endocarditis and in meningitis in children.

Haemophilus aegyptius (Koch-Weeks Bacillus)

H. aegyptius is similar to *H. influenzae* both in colonial morphology and in its requirements for growth (X and V factors; see Table 19–1) In general, X- and V-requiring *Haemophilus* isolated from the eye are called *H. aegyptius*, whereas those isolated from other sources are called *H. influenzae*. *H. aegyptius* is the etiologic agent of epidemic conjunctivitis, also known as "pinkeye," an infection that occurs in school-age children. Treatment is with local ophthalmic antibiotic ointment or solution.

Haemophilus ducreyi

Haemophilus ducreyi differs microscopically from other species of *Haemophilus*. The organisms have a larger diameter, appear in short to long chains and may be found as groups of parallel organisms.

H. ducreyi causes chancroid, a venereal disease that accounts for less than 10% of all venereal disease. This organism gains access through abraded skin, invades the dermis and produces a soft and tender ulcer with a ragged, irregular margin (soft chancre), which localizes in the regional lymph node. The bubo that forms may rupture and cause satellite lesions. Injection of killed *H. ducreyi* intradermally

TABLE 19–2.—DIFFERENTIATION OF HARD
AND SOFT CHANCRE

HARD CHANCRE	SOFT CHANCRE
Indurated	Not indurated
Not painful	Painful
Single lesion	Multiple lesions
Edge of lesion is clearly demarcated	Edge of lesion is undermined
Smooth base	Pebbled base
Initial lesion usually on glans penis	Initial lesions usually on genital areas other than glans penis
Lesions may occur on mucus membranes	Lesions occur primarily on skin
Treponema observed by darkfield microscopy of lesion exudate	Gram-negative rods observed by stains of lesion exudate
Caused by *T. pallidum*	Caused by *H. ducreyi*

results in a delayed hypersensitivity (Frei test) reaction. This hypersensitivity persists for years. The lesions can be differentiated from those caused by *Treponema pallidum* (chap. 20) as shown in Table 19–2.

Treatment is by aminoglycosides or tetracycline.

Several other species of *Haemophilus*—*H. aphrophilus, H. paraphrophilus, H. paraphrohaemolyticus*—have been isolated from patients with endocarditis, pharyngitis, brain abscess, inflamed appendix and urinary tract infection. However, these species are infrequently encountered.

Haemophilus (Corynebacterium) vaginale
The classification of this organism is uncertain, and it is recognized as belonging to either the genus *Haemophilus* or the genus *Corynebacterium*.

The organism is a small, nonmotile bacillus (0.3–0.6 × 1–2 μm) showing club formation and metachromatic granules. The gram stain reaction is variable. In cultures it is usually gram positive, whereas in tissue it is usually gram negative. It does not require X and V factors for growth and thus is not believed to be in the genus *Haemophilus*. Catalase is not produced; starch is fermented.

INFECTION.—The organism is associated with vaginitis and nongonococcal urethritis (Fig. 19–3). The vaginitis produced by *H. vaginale* is characterized by a pasty discharge associated with the vaginal wall and a distinctive odor. The organism does not invade the tissue but apparently grows in vaginal secretions, altering their consistency and elevating vaginal pH. *H. vaginale* is found in the vagina of 10% to 15% of women without disease. In persons with disease, it is frequently found in combination with other organisms such as *Trichomonas vaginalis, N. gonorrhoeae, Candida albicans* and herpesvirus. Neonatal sepsis due to *H. vaginale* has also been reported. The organism colonizes the male urethra and is transmitted sexually.

Ampicillin can be used for treatment.

Laboratory Procedures

Haemophilus influenzae and H. parainfluenzae
The usefulness of the gram stain is again emphasized with this group of organisms (see Fig. 19–1). Specimens of cerebrospinal fluid, sputum, exudate from the epiglottitis and the middle ear should be gram stained and cultured immediately. The observation of pleomorphic gram-negative coccobacillary rods with an elongated form (thread form), particularly in children under the age of 3, should sug-

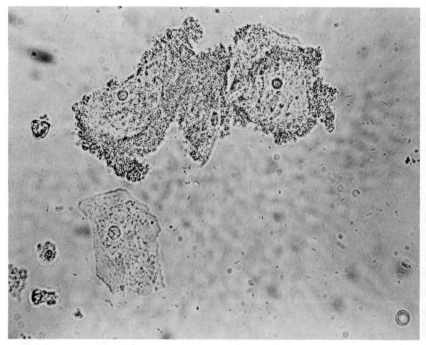

Fig. 19–3.—Clue cells, epithelial cells with masses of adherent bacteria, in *H. vaginale* vaginitis. Normal epithelial cells in lower left. (Courtesy of Dr. Herman L. Gardner, Burton, Texas.)

gest *H. influenzae*. The specimen is cultured on "chocolate" agar or blood agar streaked with *S. aureus* or with a disk containing V factor. Differentiation among the *Haemophilus* is done by determining the requirement for X and V factors and hemolysis (see Table 19–1). Serotyping of *H. influenzae* is done by the quellung test and by agglutination. Blood should also be cultured. Counterimmunoelectrophoresis has been successfully used to detect the polyribosyl-ribitol antigen in patients with meningitis, arthritis, epiglottitis and pericarditis.

Haemophilus ducreyi

The chancre should be cleaned with a wet sterile gauze. Fluid expressed from the edge of the lesion should be collected for gram stain and culture and is the specimen of choice. Alternatively, aspirate from the bubo may be stained, but this specimen is not as good as exudate from the chancre. Gram stain of the smear will show bacilli intracellularly and extracellularly. *H. ducreyi* are thicker than other species of *Haemophilus* and they are found singly, in short and long chains, and in groups in parallel rows. They may show bipolar staining. Cultures of the material on blood agar plates (20–30% rabbit blood) and in clotted rabbit or human blood (3 ml) should be made. Smears of the clotted blood should be made after 24 hours' incubation gram stained, and subcultures should also be made. *H. ducreyi* can exist along with other venereal disease agents, and mixed infections must be considered.

Haemophilus aegyptius
Conjunctival smears should be gram stained, cultured and identified as described for *H. influenzae*. *H. influenzae* may be differentiated from *H. aegyptius* by testing for indole production; most strains of the former produce indole.

Haemophilus (Corynebacterium) vaginale
Vaginal and cervical swabs should be obtained and a gram stain and wet mount (either saline or 10% KOH) prepared. The specimen is examined for clue cells, squamous epithelial cells with adhered masses of gram-negative pleomorphic coccobacilli (see Fig. 19–3). Papanicolaou smears of the cervix may also be examined for clue cells.

Cultures should also be done on potato-starch-dextrose agar, chocolate agar, and blood agar and incubated at 37 C in 5% to 10% CO_2. Isolated colonies are identified by determining reactions in fermentation and other mediums.

BORDETELLA

General Characteristics
The *Bordetella* are gram-negative, short coccobacilli (0.2×0.5–1.0 μm) found singly or in pairs. The organisms do not produce spores; they are strict aerobes and grow at 35 to 37 C. They are nonmotile except for *B. bronchiseptica*. The organisms are not fastidious, but *B. pertussis* requires potato-glycerol agar with 30% fresh rabbit blood to bind unsaturated fatty acids, sulfur and sulfides, and thereby to detoxify the medium. This special medium, Bordet-Gengou agar, is used for primary isolation and growth. The organisms are quite sensitive to drying, and cultures from clinical sources must be promptly plated.

Species
The genus *Bordetella* contains three species, all of which cause disease in man: *B. pertussis, B. parapertussis* and *B. bronchiseptica*. Differentiation is based on a requirement for enriched medium for growth, urease production and motility. *B. pertussis* requires Bordet-Gengou medium for growth; it is nonmotile and does not produce

TABLE 19-3.—CHARACTERISTICS OF *BORDETELLA* SPECIES

	B. PERTUSSIS	B. PARAPERTUSSIS	B. BRONCHISEPTICA
Does not require Bordet-Gengou agar for growth	+	−	−
Urease production	−	+	+ (4 hr)
Nitrate reduction	−	−	+
Motility	−	−	+

urease or reduce nitrates (Table 19–3). Further differentiation among species is done by fluorescent antibody techniques using specific antisera.

Ecology

B. pertussis and *B. parapertussis* are found only in man. *B. bronchiseptica* causes bronchopneumonia in animals and can cause a whooping cough-like disease in man. Transmission is via aerosols from infected persons to nonimmune persons.

Antigens

The *Bordetella* have a genus-specific, heat-stable O antigen and a common heat-labile agglutinogen. Specific heat-labile agglutinogens associated with K antigen are found in each species. Six agglutinogens (referred to as factors) specific for *B. pertussis* are used to determine serotypes. Each serotype contains more than one agglutinogen.

Genetics

After isolation and transfer on media, *B. pertussis* undergoes an S→R change referred to as phase variation. Shift in colony types from S→R or phase I to IV is associated with a decrease in virulence and immunogenicity. The decrease in virulence and immunogenicity is related to loss of protective antigen, histamine-sensitizing factor and some envelope polypeptides.

Surface Structure and Toxins

CAPSULE.—Antiserum to the capsule does not elicit a quellung reaction, and the function of the capsule is not known.

PILI.—Filaments observed on the cell surface are now thought to be pili. They agglutinate erythrocytes and probably serve as adherence factors.

HEAT-LABILE TOXIN.—This toxin, which is inactivated by heating at 56 C for 15 minutes, is found in the cytoplasm. It is found in all three species of *Bordetella* and is cytotoxic for tissue culture, ciliostatic and may promote adherence of organisms to epithelial cells. Death of mice follows intravenous and intraperitoneal injection, and dermonecrosis results after injection into the skin.

ENDOTOXIN. — The endotoxin has properties in common with endotoxin from other organisms.

LEUKOCYTOSIS AND LYMPHOCYTOSIS-PROMOTING FACTOR (LPF). — This protein of approximately 70,000 daltons has been isolated as a single band on gel electrophoresis. It induces a leukocytosis and a lymphocytosis and has histamine-sensitizing activity; it causes hypoglycemia and refractoriness to the hyperglycemic effect of epinephrine. Recently, it has been reported to be a T-cell mitogen. The histamine-sensitizing activity sensitizes mice so that they become hyperreactive to pharmacologic agents such as serotonin, bradykinin and histamine. The mechanism of action of LPF is not known, but it may block the intracellular accumulation of cyclic AMP.

Infections

Whooping cough (pertussis) occurs only in young children, with about half of the cases occurring in children under 4 years of age. About two thirds of the deaths occur in children under 1 year of age. The organism is highly communicable with an attack rate of 90% in unimmunized children. Epidemics occur every 2–4 years. Many patients may not have typical pertussis but can transmit the organism to others.

The incubation period is 10–16 days. Three distinct stages occur during the disease process; the catarrhal, the spasmodic or paroxysmal, and the convalescent stage, each of which lasts about 2 weeks.

Catarrhal Stage

This primary stage is characterized by slight fever (rarely exceeds 39 C), mild coughing and sneezing and lasts about 2 weeks. The symptoms are generally mild and resemble those of the common cold. Large numbers of organisms can be found in the sputum and in droplet nuclei generated by coughing and sneezing, so the disease is easily transmitted during this stage.

Spasmodic or Paroxysmal Stage

The spasmodic stage lasts about 2 weeks and is characterized by violent, repetitive coughing. With time the coughing episodes become more frequent and violent with 10 to 20 episodes per day. At the end of each coughing episode, the patient drools ropy, foamy mucus and may vomit. Coughing occurs with equal frequency during the night and day. The inspiration of air following repetitive coughing results in the characteristic whoop. The intense prolonged spasm may be serious enough to cause cyanosis, convulsions and coma. One of the striking features of the disease in this stage is a leukocytosis with a lymphocytosis.

Convalescent Stage
During this stage the disease resolves, but coughing may persist for months in the absence of B. pertussis. Mild upper respiratory tract infection may trigger paroxysmal coughing. However, because pertussis is an inflammation of the tracheobronchial tree, secondary infections with viruses or other bacteria can occur. Most of the secondary bacterial infections are due to the pneumococcus, beta-hemolytic streptococci and H. influenzae. Secondary infection probably accounts for most of the deaths associated with this disease.

Mechanisms of Pathogenicity

Incubation Period
It is clear from observation of the natural disease and from experimental studies that the organism has a predilection for ciliated epithelial cells of the bronchi. The attachment of the bacteria is to the cell surface and not to the cilia. Pili have been described, but their role as adherence factors has not been proved. Experimental infections in man have been produced with as few as 140 organisms.

Catarrhal Stage
Several microbial products can be associated with this stage of pertussis. Histologically, necrosis of the ciliated bronchial epithelium is observed during this stage and may be related to the heat-labile toxin, the endotoxin, or both.

Spasmodic or Paroxysmal Stage
Matting of the ciliated epithelia may be due to the presence of capsular material. The cell LPF causes lymphocytosis in animals and is presumed responsible for the unique lymphocytosis that occurs during this phase of whooping cough in humans. The mechanism for lymphocytosis has been reported to be due to redistribution of lymphoid cells in the blood with failure of the circulatory lymphocytes to reenter the lymphoid system. In addition, LPF has also been reported to be a T-cell mitogen. The patient is sensitive to histamine, and the LPF has associated histamine-sensitizing activity

Sensitization of the host to histamine, liberation of histamine from damaged tissue and matting of cilia may in part account for the violent cough.

Immunity

A vaccine consisting of killed phase I (encapsulated) *B. pertussis* is available and is an effective immunogen. The pertussis immunogen is administered to children along with alum-precipitated tetanus and diphtheria toxoid. The vaccine is termed DPT (diphtheria-pertussis-tetanus) vaccine. Immunization should be initiated at 6 to 12 weeks of age with three injections at monthly intervals. Boosters should be given at 1, 3, and 5 years. Further immunizations with *B. pertussis* are not done because of the infrequent occurrence of disease in older children and because of reaction to the vaccine (fever, convulsions and encephalopathy).

The vaccine is composed of phase I organisms containing specified agglutinogens. Data from some countries indicate a change in predominant serotypes. The reasons are unknown, but the change may be due to natural antigenic shifts or to lack of specific agglutinogens in the vaccines being used. Immunity is serotype-specific and successful immunization requires that prevalent serotypes be included in the vaccine.

Both IgG and IgA specific for *B. pertussis* have been demonstrated in human pulmonary secretions. IgA may prevent adherence of *B. pertussis* to epithelial cells and cilia; IgG plays a more important role in long-lived resistance. Recovery from the disease is associated with immunity, but it is short-lived.

Treatment

The antibiotic of choice for treatment of pertussis is erythromycin (10–14 days). Supportive therapy consists of maintenance of an airway, nutritional intake and acid-base balance. Hyperimmune human γ-globulin can be used to abort or modify the disease but is rarely used.

Unimmunized contacts should be treated with erythromycin. Immunized contacts under the age of 4 should receive a booster immunization as well as erythromycin.

Other Bordetella

B. parapertussis and *B. bronchiseptica* can cause a milder form of whooping cough. The organisms resemble *B. pertussis* and can be differentiated by serologic and biochemical testing.

Laboratory Procedures

The recommended specimen is a swab of the posterior pharyngeal wall. Specimens should be obtained during the catarrhal stage or as early as possible during the spasmodic or paroxysmal stage. A gram stain of the pharyngeal swab should be done. The presence of large numbers of small gram-negative coccobacilli in a young child without a history of appropriate immunization should suggest infection with *B. pertussis*. A feature unique to whooping cough is the leukocytosis characterized by lymphocytosis, which differentiates this disease from other bacterial infections. The lymphocytosis occurs in the majority of patients over 6 months of age but in only about one fourth of those under 6 months.

B. pertussis is quite susceptible to drying, and clinical specimens must be promptly inoculated or placed in a transport medium. For culture, penicillin G (0.5 units/ml) is incorporated into the Bordet-Gengou agar or a drop of penicillin G (1,000 units/ml) is placed on the surface of the Bordet-Gengou (B-G) agar plate. To inhibit growth of other microorganisms from the pharyngeal surface, one should pass the pharyngeal swab through the penicillin before streaking the plate.

An older method of culture is the cough plate. A plate of B-G agar is held 6 inches from the patient's mouth during a spasmodic cough. The pharyngeal swab method is the recommended method. B-G agar is not routinely available in most laboratories. The physician must alert the laboratory so that the appropriate medium is available before collection of the specimen.

The cultures are incubated at 37 C; colonies of *B. pertussis* appear in 2 to 4 days as small, smooth colonies with pearl-like luster surrounded by a narrow fuzzy zone of beta-hemolysis.

Final identification is by agglutination with specific antiserum. The fluorescent antibody test can be used to identify organism in smears and from isolated colonies.

PROBLEM SOLVING AND REVIEW

No. 1. GIVEN: — An 8-month-old child was brought to the emergency room by his mother. The child was in acute respiratory distress. He had a fever and barking cough (croup). Examination revealed that the throat was inflamed and the epiglottis was fiery red, swollen and stiff. Blood examination showed a marked leukocytosis with increased numbers of polymorphonuclear leukocytes. Blood cultures were obtained, and after incubation a gram stain showed very small coccobacillary rods. After admittance, the child became toxic, had dyspnea, became cyanotic and died.

PROBLEMS: — 1. What is the probable etiologic agent? 2. What is the source of the organism? 3. What is the disease? 4. What is the approach to therapy? (Ans. p. 372.)

NO. 2. GIVEN: — A 2-year-old child was admitted to the hospital with complaints of headache, nuchal rigidity and positive Kernig's sign. The child had a mild pharyngitis and otitis media. A spinal tap showed increased pressure. The cerebrospinal fluid was turbid, and a gram stain showed gram-negative rods with an occasional thread form.

PROBLEMS: — 1. What is the suspected etiologic agent? 2. What is the most probable serotype? 3. How is this determined? 4. What is the primary site of infection? 5. Why did this child become infected? 6. What is the probable cause of the otitis? (Ans. p. 372.)

NO. 3. GIVEN: — A 4-year-old child, acutely ill, was brought to the physician's office. The mother stated that the child had had a "cold" with some cough for about a week. While being examined the child began to cough spasmodically. A white blood cell count was reported as 16,000 white blood cells per cubic millimeter with 90% lymphocytes. There was no history of any immunization. A pharyngeal swab was taken and a gram stain showed gram-negative coccobacilli. Other children in the family also had "colds."

PROBLEMS: — 1. What is the probable etiologic agent? 2. What is the portal of entry? 3. To what microbial activity can you relate the spasmodic cough? 4. What is the mechanism of transmission? 5. Why does the patient have a lymphocytic response? 6. How could this have been prevented? 7. Does this child present a risk to others? Why? (Ans. p. 373.)

SUPPLEMENTARY READING

Aftandelians, R. V., and Connor, J. D.: *Bordetella pertussis* serotypes in a whooping cough outbreak, Am. J. Epidemiol. 99:343–346, 1974.
Dahlgren, J., Tally, F. P., Brothers, G., and Ruskin, J.: *Haemophilus parainfluenzae* endocarditis, J. Clin. Pathol. 62:607–611, 1974.
Denny, F. W.: Effect of a toxin produced by *Haemophilus influenzae* on ciliated respiratory epithelium, J. Infect. Dis. 129:93–100, 1974.
Dunkleberg, W. E., Jr., Skaggs, R., and Kellogg, D. S., Jr.: Method for isolation and identification of *Corynebacterium vaginale* (*Haemophilus vaginalis*), Appl. Microbiol. 19:47–52, 1970.
Handzel, Z. T., Argaman, M., Parke, J. C., Jr., Schneerson, R., and Robbins,

J. B.: Heteroimmunization to the capsular polysaccharide of *Haemophilus influenzae* type b induced by enteric cross-reacting bacteria, Infect. Immun. 11:1045–1052, 1975.

Holt, R. N., Taylor, C. D., Schneider, H. J., and Hallock, J. A.: Three cases of *Haemophilus parainfluenzae* meningitis, Clin. Pediatr. 13:666–668, 1974.

Kong, A. S., and Morse, S. I.: The *in vitro* effects of *Bordetella pertussis* lymphocytosis promoting factor on murine lymphocytes. II. Nature of the responding cells, J. Exp. Med. 145:163–174, 1977.

Monif, G. R. G., and Baer, H.: *Haemophilus (Corynebacterium) vaginalis*, Am. J. Obstet. Gynecol. 120:1041–1045, 1974.

Morse, S. I., and Morse, J. H.: Isolation and properties of the leukocytosis and lymphocytosis-promoting factor of *Bordetella pertussis*, J. Exp. Med. 143:1483–1501, 1976.

Olson, L. C.: Pertussis, Medicine (Baltimore) 54:427–469, 1975.

Schneerson, R., Argaman, M., and Handzel, Z. T.: *Haemophilus influenzae* type b: Disease and immunity in humans, Ann. Intern. Med.: 78:259, 1973.

Schneerson, R., and Robbins, J. B.: Induction of serum *Haemophilus influenzae* type b capsular antibodies in adult volunteers fed cross-reacting *Escherichia coli* 075:K100:B5, N. Engl. J. Med. 292:1092–1096, 1975.

Sell, S. H. W.: The clinical importance of *Haemophilus influenzae* infections in children, Pediatr. Clin. North Am. 17:415–426, 1970.

Sell, S. H. W., and Karzon, D. T.: *Haemophilus influenzae* (Nashville: Vanderbilt University Press, 1973).

Smith, R. F., Rodgers, H. A., Hines, P. A., and Ray, R. M.: Comparisons between direct microscopic and cultural methods for recognition of *Corynebacterium vaginale* in women with vaginitis, J. Clin. Microbiol. 5:268–272, 1977.

Thorne, G. M., and Farras, W. E., Jr.: Transfer of ampicillin resistance between strains of *Haemophilus influenzae* type b, J. Infect. Dis. 132:276–281, 1975.

Venezia, R. A., and Robertson, R. G.: Bactericidal substance produced by *Haemophilus influenzae* b, Can. J. Microbiol. 21:1587–1594, 1975.

Vosey, W. E., McKenzie, W. J., and Lambe, D. W., Jr.: *Corynebacterium vaginale (Haemophilus vaginalis)* in women with leukorrhea, Am. J. Obstet. Gynecol. 126:574–578, 1976.

Wallace, R. J., Musher, D. M., and Martin, B. R.: *Haemophilus influenzae* pneumonia in adults, Am. J. Med. 64:87, 1978.

Wardlaw, A. C., Parton, R., and Hooker, M. J.: Loss of protective antigen, histamine-sensitizing factor and envelope polypeptides in cultural variants of *Bordetella pertussis*, J. Med. Microbiol. 9:89–100, 1975.

ANALYSIS

No. 1.—1. *H. influenzae*. 2. Throat of patient. 3. Acute obstructive epiglottitis. 4. Airway maintenance; ampicillin.

No. 2.—1. *H. influenzae*. 2. Type b. 3. Capsular swelling test. 4. Pharynx or ear (otitis media). 5. Lack of immunity. 6. *H. influenzae*.

No. 3. — 1. *Bordetella pertussis*. 2. Upper respiratory tract. 3. Leuko-cytosis and lymphocytosis promoting factor, matting of cilia by cap-sule. 4. Airborne droplets. 5. Due to LPF. 6. Immunization with per-tussis vaccine. 7. Yes. Communicability rate is high.

20 / Spirochetes, Treponemes, Borrelia and Leptospira

SPIROCHETES

Overview

The spirochetes consist of a large group of organisms with similar morphological features. Unlike other bacteria, the axial filaments or flagella are surrounded by an outer envelope or sheath. Some of the spirochetes such as *Treponema pallidum* cannot grow in culture, and under natural conditions they infect only man. The leptospira and borrelia, however, can be cultured in vitro and cause diseases of animals transmissible to man. Much work needs to be done in defining not only the structure of these organisms but also their antigens and mechanisms of pathogenicity.

One of the diseases of major impact in the world is syphilis, and much effort has been put into control of this disease. The infrequently seen diseases caused by *Borrelia* and *Leptospira* are probably more common than is recognized, and the physician and microbiologist must recognize the importance of these organisms in human disease. Recently, an outbreak of tick-borne relapsing fever at Grand Canyon National Park was reported and involved 62 persons, including employees and guests.

General Characteristics

Spirochetes are slender, flexuous, helically coiled bacteria with one or more turns in the helix (Figs. 20–1, 20–2). The cells consist of a protoplasmic cylinder intertwined with one or more axial fibrils that originate from subterminal disks located at either end of the cylinder. The organisms are covered by an outer envelope or sheath. They are motile, non-spore-forming and may be aerobic, facultatively anaerobic or anaerobic. Free-living, commensal and parasitic forms exist.

Genera

Three genera of spirochetes are important in diseases of man: *Treponema, Leptospira,* and *Borrelia.* The spirochetes are gram-negative

375

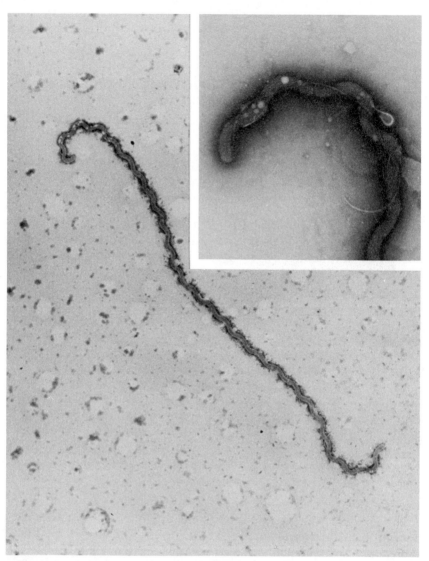

Fig. 20–1.—Negatively stained electron micrograph of *Leptospira interrogans* showing coiled protoplasmic cylinder, axial filaments and hooks. The protoplasmic sheath has been removed. Inset in upper right is an enlargement of hook. Note axial filaments and points of insertion. (Courtesy of D. Bromley and N. Charon, Dept. of Microbiology, West Virginia University Medical Center.)

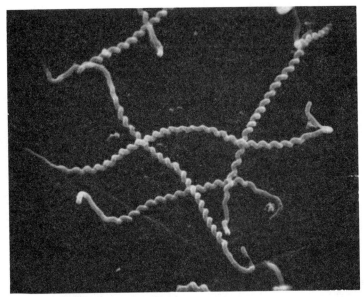

Fig. 20-2. — Scanning electromicrograph of *Leptospira interrogans*. (Courtesy of O. Carelton, P. Allender and N. Charon, West Virginia University.)

bacteria but cannot be visualized by usual staining techniques because of their size.

Some of the characteristics of pathogenic spirochetes belonging to these three genera are shown in Table 20-1.

Ecology

The leptospira are found as saprophytes in soil and water (*Leptospira interrogans* —biflex complex) or as parasites causing disease in man and animals (*Leptospira interrogans* —parasitic complex). They are not part of the normal flora of man or animals.

The *Borrelia* spp. are pathogens of animals and man which are transmitted via lice or ticks. Nonpathogenic borrelia are found as part of the normal flora of the mouth and intestinal tract.

The treponemes are also found as part of the normal flora of the oral cavity and intestinal and genital tracts of man and animals. Some species, which are not part of the normal flora, are pathogenic for man. The pathogenic species cannot be grown in vitro.

Structure

The structure of the spirochetes is unique. These bacteria contain the usual cytoplasmic membrane and a cell wall that encloses the cy-

TABLE 20-1.—DIFFERENTIAL CHARACTERISTICS
OF SPIROCHETES

	LEPTOSPIRA	BORRELIA	TREPONEMA
Length:	15–18 μm	4–30 μm	6–15 μm
Width:	0.1–0.2 μm	0.4–0.5 μm	0.1–0.2 μm
Appearance:	Many closely wound spirals with hooked ends	Few, wavy loose and irregular spirals	5–20 rigid and regular spirals
No. of axial filaments:	2 (one from each end)	15–20	1–8
In vitro growth:	Yes	Yes	No
How observed:	Silver stain, darkfield	Wright's stain	Silver stain, darkfield
Oxygen requirements:	Aerobic	Anaerobic or microaerophilic	Anaerobic
Type of metabolism:	Respiratory	Fermentative	Fermentative
Reservoir:	Animals	Animals, insects	Man, animals°

°Treponemes from animals do not cause disease in man.

toplasm and constitutes what is termed the protoplasmic cylinder. The axial filaments, which are also referred to as flagella, vary in numbers and are similar in structure and function to other bacterial flagella. In treponema the shaft of the flagella is sheathed but the sheath is absent on *Borrelia*. The protoplasmic cylinder and axial filaments are enclosed in an envelope, termed the outer sheath, composed of protein, lipids and carbohydrates.

The cell wall composition differs among the spirochetes. All three genera contain muramic acid. The diamino acid in the peptidoglycan of *Leptospira* is diaminopimelic acid, whereas ornithine is present in the *Borrelia* and *Treponema*.

Endotoxin has been demonstrated in *Leptospira*, *Treponema* and *Borrelia*.

TREPONEMES

Species

Three species of treponemes are associated with human disease: *T. pallidum* causes syphilis, *T. pertenue* causes yaws and *T. carateum* causes pinta. The pathogenic treponemes cannot be cultured in vitro but can be grown in the skin, eyes and testes of a rabbit. Nichol's strain of *T. pallidum* is a laboratory strain propagated in rabbits. Reiter's treponeme, a nonpathogenic, culturable treponeme, is used in serologic testing. Speciation of the nonculturable pathogens is based on the type of disease produced in humans. The ability to produce cutaneous lesions in rabbits, hamsters and guinea pigs may also be used but is not practical in the usual laboratory. The culturable *Treponema* spp. are differentiated by physiologic tests.

Antigens

The antigenic compositions of the treponemes have not been well studied. Infection results in the production of antibodies that react with tissue lipid and with specific treponemal antigens. Cross-reactive antigens are shared among the pathogenic and nonpathogenic species.

Syphilis

Humans are the only hosts for *T. pallidum*. The organism enters the host through minute breaks in the epithelium, and direct contact is necessary for infection.

Primary Syphilis

The incubation period for primary syphilis is 9–90 days (average 3 weeks). The initial lesion, a chancre, is found at the point of inoculation (Fig. 20–3). The lesion is usually single, but multiple lesions have been reported. It occurs on the external genitalia or mucous

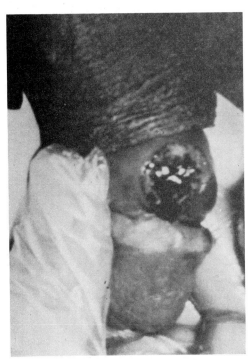

Fig. 20–3. — Syphilitic chancre. (Reproduced with permission of the VD Control Division, Bureau of State Services, Center for Disease Control, Public Health Service, Department of Health, Education and Welfare.)

membranes and begins as a papule that undergoes necrosis resulting in a firm, nontender, cutaneous ulcer. A yellow serous discharge rich in treponemes is present. The base of the lesion is smooth and the borders are smooth, not undermined and hemorrhagic. Local lymphadenitis and lymphangitis may occur. The chancre lasts 1–14 days and eventually heals. About 5% of chancres occur extragenitally. The lesion in women is often on the cervix or vaginal wall.

Secondary Syphilis

Secondary syphilis usually occurs 6–8 weeks after exposure and lasts 3 weeks to 3 months. At onset the symptoms resemble those of influenza, i.e., there may be fever, malaise and gastrointestinal manifestation. The lymph nodes are swollen, painless and have a rubbery hard feeling. A mucocutaneous rash which is usually bilaterally symmetrical and has a predilection for the soles and palms occurs (Fig. 20–4). These lesions, which are follicular-papular, are of the same size and have a coppery hue. White mucous patches may occur on the mucous membrane. The lesions in secondary syphilis are infectious. Several episodes of secondary disease may occur before the patient progresses to the latent form of the disease.

Latent Syphilis

In this stage positive serologic tests are obtained in the absence of clinical signs and symptoms, and with or without a history of infection.

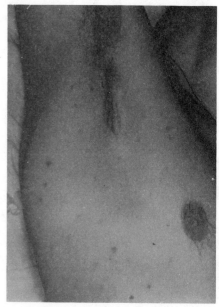

Fig. 20–4.—Typical rash of secondary syphilis. (Courtesy of Dr. William Welton, Department of Medicine, West Virginia University Medical Center.)

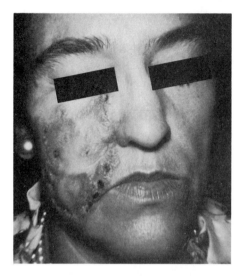

Fig. 20–5. – Gumma on face of patient with syphilis. (Courtesy of Dr. William Welton, Department of Medicine, West Virginia University Medical Center.)

One of the difficulties in detection and diagnosis during this stage is that 40–60% of persons with syphilis have no recognizable primary or secondary stage and seek help only when irreparable disease occurs.

Late Syphilis (Tertiary)

Late syphilis, the most destructive phase, occurs 2–10 years after the initial infection and affects about one third of the untreated patients. A granulomatous lesion, called a gumma, is found in the skin, soft tissue, mucous membranes, bone or viscera (Fig. 20–5). The gumma is composed of epithelial cells and giant cells surrounded by macrophages, lymphocytes and plasma cells. Few spirochetes are found in the lesion. Gumma growth can be stopped with penicillin, and the lesion readily heals. In addition, more destructive, diffuse lesions may involve primarily the walls of blood vessels, CNS, and musculoskeletal system. The diffuse lesions may not be obvious until irreparable damage has been done. Such lesions are characterized as perivascular infiltrates of lymphocytes, plasma cells and macrophages. The invasion of blood vessels results in cerebral hemorrhage, aortic valvular disease and aortic aneurysm. CNS syphilis involves the meninges (meningitis), parenchymal tissue of the brain (paresis), spinal cord (tabes dorsalis) and sometimes destroys the optic nerve with resultant blindness.

Prenatal Congenital Syphilis

Transmission of *T. pallidum* from the infected mother to the fetus via a spirochetemia can result in death in utero or shortly after birth.

In some infants, lesions similar to those of secondary syphilis may occur within a few weeks after birth. At 2 to 30 years of age, the lesions associated with late syphilis in the adult may be present.

Growth of the spirochete in utero results in Hutchinson's triad: malformed incisors, interstitial keratitis and eighth nerve deafness. Treatment of the mother within the first trimester of pregnancy prevents perinatal syphilis.

Mechanisms of Pathogenicity

Recently, attachment of *T. pallidum* to cultured animal cells has been demonstrated. The treponemes attach to the cell surface via the

Fig. 20–6.—Scanning electron micrograph of rabbit testicular tissue infected with *T. pallidum*. Note attachment of organism by tapered ends to surface of host cell. (From Hayes, N. S., Muse, K. E., Collier, A. M., and Baseman, J. B.: Infect. Immunol. 17:174–186, 1977. By permission of authors and publisher.)

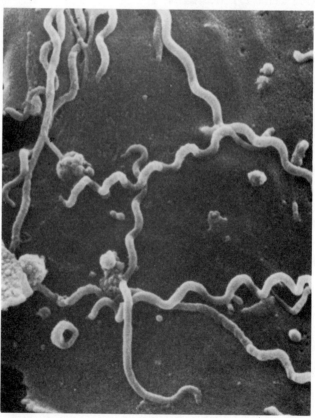

tapered end of the parasite (Fig. 20–6). The chemical nature of the bacterial structure and the host cell structure involved are unknown. Killed treponemes attach and detergent treatment reduces the ability of the organisms to attach without affecting motility. Antisera from convalescent rabbits prevent attachment without causing lysis, immune immobilization or agglutination. Avirulent treponemes do not adhere to cell cultures. The significance of attachment in infections with *T. pallidum* is not known but may explain the association of the organism with specific tissue sites.

After entry and establishment in the host, the organisms proliferate, spread through the lymphatics and produce a spirochetemia. The variable incubation period for development of the primary lesion is probably related both to the size of the infecting inoculum and to the organism's long generation time of approximately 30 hours. The infectious dose for man is low and is estimated at 57 organisms. The lesions are probably due to an inflammatory response to the spirochete and may be augmented by both immediate and delayed hypersensitivity. Serum IgE is higher in patients with primary syphilis than in nonsyphilitic patients. In early syphilis, reactivity of lymphocytes from patients with syphilis to *T. pallidum* antigen in leukocyte migration and lymphocyte transformation tests is decreased and correlates with the progression of primary and secondary syphilis. Treatment results in an increased responsiveness of lymphocytes from patients with syphilis. In later stages of syphilis, cell-mediated immunity is evident and may be important in development of the tissue destruction characteristic of this stage.

Both the primary and secondary lesions are similar and contain numerous spirochetes, mononuclear leukocytes, lymphocytes and plasma cells. There is also a swelling of capillary endothelium. Necrosis is minimal or absent and the lesions heal without scarring. The primary and secondary lesions are highly infectious.

The gumma, which is a granulomatous reaction, is thought to be an immunologic host response. No toxins have been described.

Immunity

Humoral antibody, both IgM and IgG are produced during infection. IgM antibody disappears with treatment but IgG antibody remains for life. Persons with untreated syphilis show some relative resistance to reinfection as evidenced by absence of a chancre upon reinfection. However, syphilitics who receive treatment during the secondary or tertiary form of syphilis are susceptible to reinfection. Experimentally, passive transfer of serum to animals causes a delay in development of lesions, which suggests that humoral immunity might be important. In addition, plasma cells are abundant in the lesions found in man, which suggests local production of antibody. However, antibody is present during disease and appears to have no effect on the disease process. Lymphocyte reactivity of both humans and animals is suppressed during early syphilis suggesting defective T-cell function during disease. It is clear that a good understanding of immunity in this important disease is lacking.

Prevention

The methods used for prevention of syphilis are the same as those used for prevention of gonorrhea. Prompt reporting, identification and treatment of the infected persons and contacts are important.

Treatment

Penicillin is the drug of choice. In primary and secondary syphilis, a single injection of 2,400,000 units of benzathine penicillin G or aqueous procaine penicillin G, 600,000 units daily for 8 days (total 4.8 megaunits) is used. For congenital syphilis the treatment is benzyl-penicillin or aqueous procaine penicillin, 50,000 units/kg body weight daily for 10 days. Other antibiotics (tetracycline, erythromycin) can be used in the penicillin-sensitive patient. Serologic testing should be used to monitor the effect of treatment.

Treatment of gonorrhea with penicillin adequately treats incubating syphilis, but treatment of syphilis is not adequate for gonorrhea.

Laboratory Procedures

MICROSCOPIC OBSERVATIONS. — Exudate from the chancre or skin eruption should be examined by darkfield microscopy. A positive darkfield examination is a positive diagnosis of primary, secondary or early congenital syphilis or of an infectious relapse. Darkfield examinations may be negative when patients are receiving treatment, when the lesion is fading or healing, and in very early or late syphilis. Three preparations, one each on consecutive days, should be examined.

Serologic Tests for Syphilis

Serologic tests for syphilis (STS) are of two kinds, nonspecific (nontreponemal) and specific (treponemal). The nonspecific serologic tests are those which use a cardiolipin-lecithin antigen that is nontreponemal in origin and detect an antibody termed reagin. The specific tests use antigens from *T. pallidum* or whole organisms and detect antitreponemal antibody.

Examples of nonspecific tests are the Venereal Disease Research Laboratory (VDRL) test and the Rapid Plasma Reagin Card (RPR) test, which are flocculation tests. These tests are extremely sensitive, although biologic false positive tests can occur. They are used for screening asymptomatic patients and large populations and also for gauging the effectiveness of therapy in treated patients. A declining titer indicates a therapeutic response, whereas an increased titer indicates continued infection.

Treponemal tests for syphilis are highly sensitive and highly specific. They are used to confirm positive reagin tests and to diagnose congenital syphilis and false negative reactions (late syphilis). Several examples of these specific tests are the *Treponema pallidum* immobilization (TPI), the microhemagglutination (MHA-TP) and the fluorescent treponemal antibody-adsorption (FTA-ABS) test. The FTA-ABS test is of value in confirming the nonspecific test and in diagnosing congenital and late syphilis. In this test the antigen is *T. pallidum* (Nichol's strain) obtained from infected rabbit testes and fixed to a glass slide by acetone or methanol. The patient's serum is diluted 1:5 in a reagent termed FTA sorbent, an extract of Reiter's treponeme that is used to remove nonspecific treponemal antibodies (other than those against *T. pallidum*). The sorbed serum is then added to the slide containing fixed *T. pallidum*, and any antibodies in the serum will react with *T. pallidum*. This reaction is observed by reacting the fixed *T. pallidum* − anti-*T. pallidum* preparation with a fluorescein-conjugated antihuman globulin antiserum. Fluorescence indicates a positive reaction. The test can be quantitated by using dilutions of the patient's serum. No test currently available can differentiate infections due to *T. pallidum, T. pertenue* and *T. carateum*. The FTA-ABS test detects antibodies of all immunoglobulin classes. A modified test using fluorescein-labeled anti-IgM has been developed.

False positive reactions, particularly with the nonspecific treponemal serologic tests, occur in about 1% of the population, most frequently in drug addicts, persons with collagen disease or hepatitis and others.

Generally, serologic tests become positive about 7 to 14 days after appearance of the chancre. The longer the chancre is present, the more likely the serologic test will be positive. The FTA-ABS is positive in all stages of syphilis. The IgM-FTA-ABS is useful in detecting congenital syphilis; IgM antibody in infant blood indicates active antibody production by the fetus and thus infection.

Nontreponemal tests may not be reactive in early primary syphilis, latent syphilis and late syphilis. Because false positive reactions occur, verification should be obtained by a test with specific treponemal antigen (FTA-ABS).

With adequate treatment, the nontreponemal serologic tests should be negative as follows: 6–12 months after primary syphilis, 12–18 months after secondary syphilis. The antibody titer may either fall or remain stable after syphilis of 2 years or more duration. A positive test on cerebrospinal fluid is diagnostic of CNS syphilis.

The specific tests for syphilis (FTA-ABS) are used to confirm positive nontreponemal tests, to confirm late syphilis in patients with nonreactive nontreponemal tests, and to diagnose syphilis in asymptomatics or in others who are nonreactive to nontreponemal tests or who have a child with congenital syphilis. The specific treponemal tests remain positive for a long time.

Nonsyphilitic Treponematoses

Yaws is a nonvenereal disease found in the tropics. It is caused by *T. pertenue*, an organism indistinguishable from *T. pallidum*. The disease is primarily seen in individuals under the age of 20. Flies may act as the vector; the infection may also be transmitted by direct contact.

The primary lesion, or yaw, occurs 3–4 weeks after exposure. It is a painless red papule surrounded by a zone of erythema. The papule ulcerates, becomes encrusted and heals. Secondary lesions, similar to the primary lesions, occur 6 weeks to 3 months later, and successive crops appear over a period of months or years. Tender hyperkeratotic lesions (crab yaws) appear on the soles of the feet. The late lesions are gummas of the skin and bones. Yaws can be treated effectively with penicillin.

Pinta, another nonvenereal disease found in the tropics, is transmitted by direct contact and possibly by flies. It is caused by *T. carateum*, which is morphologically and serologically similar to the pathogenic treponemes. The primary lesions produced by *T. carateum* are small, erythematous papules that are scaly and indurated and occur within days to months after inoculation. The primary lesions enlarge, may coalesce and are usually red to violet in color. The secondary lesions are similar to the primary but may be slate blue, gray or black. The late lesions may occur up to 10 years after primary lesions and are depigmented and hyperkeratotic.

Penicillin is the drug of choice for treatment.

Bejel is a nonvenereal disease found in Africa and the eastern Mediterranean countries. It is a childhood disease caused by *T. pallidum* and is called endemic syphilis. Bejel probably is acquired from an infected mother by a nursing infant. The lesions and disease are identical to venereal syphilis. A primary lesion is seldom observed. The secondary lesions are found primarily on the lips, tongue, palate and larynx. The late lesions (gummas) are found primarily in the skin and bones.

BORRELIA

Species
The *Borrelia* cause relapsing fever and are transmitted to man via arthropod vectors. *Borrelia recurrentis* is transmitted by lice *(Pediculus humanus)*; the other *Borrelia* are transmitted by ticks. *Borrelia* cannot be differentiated on the basis of biochemical and serologic criteria, and speciation is dependent on determination of the species of tick *(Ornithodorus)* that serves as the vector. Table 20–2 contains a partial list of *Borrelia* spp. and their arthropod vectors. The louse-borne *Borrelia recurrentis* causes epidemic relapsing fever. Tick-borne *Borrelia* causes epidemic and sporadic outbreaks of relapsing fever. In the United States, three species of ticks are known to be vectors. *O. turicata* and *O. parkeri* are found in semiarid areas, and *O. hermsi* is found in forested areas. The rodent reservoir can be ground squirrels, prairie dogs, chipmunks, goats, sheep and other rodents.

Antigens
One of the striking features of the *Borrelia* spp. is their ability to undergo antigenic variation within the host. The variation is due to the selection of organisms by antibody produced to organisms containing a specific antigen. Antigens which are shared between organisms of different antigenic phases and also different species have been described.

Relapsing Fever
The incubation period for relapsing fever is between 2 and 15 days. The first phase of the disease is characterized by sudden onset of fever

TABLE 20–2.—SPECIES OF *BORRELIA* AND THEIR ARTHROPOD VECTORS

SPECIES	VECTOR
B. recurrentis	Pediculus humanus (louse)
B. hermsii	Ornithodorus hermsi
B. duttonii	O. moubata
B. turicatae	O. turicata
B. parkeri	O. parkeri

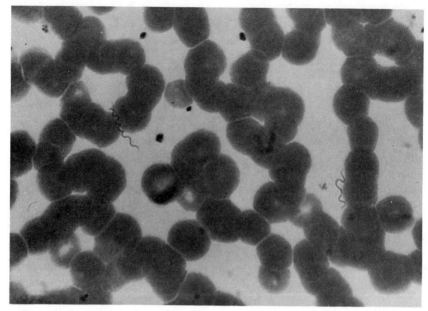

Fig. 20–7.—*Borrelia hermsii* spirochete in peripheral blood smear of patient with tick-borne relapsing fever. Wright's stain. (From Boyer, K. M., et al.: Am. J. Epidemiol. 105:469–479, 1977. By permission of the authors and journal.)

(usually near 40.4 C), shaking chills, severe headache, delirium or mental lethargy, muscle, joint, and bone pain, and extreme muscular weakness. Eye pain, photophobia, liver and spleen tenderness are also common. Other manifestations, such as a transient macular rash on the torso and cough, also occur. During the afebrile period the spirochetes are readily detected in the blood (Fig. 20–7). The fever persists from 3 to 6 days and is followed by an afebrile period of 5 to 10 days. *Borrelia* cannot be detected in the blood during the afebrile period. The hallmark of relapsing fever is recurrent episodes similar to the first febrile phase. Subsequent attacks are usually shorter and milder, and fewer spirochetes are found in the blood in these later episodes than in the first phase. Each relapse is caused by a distinct antigenic type, and between 1 and 9 episodes can occur. Relapsing fever brought on by the louse-borne *Borrelia recurrentis* generally has fewer relapses than that caused by the tick-borne *Borrelia*. Complications may include iritis and iridocyclitis, which may result in eye damage, in addition to bronchitis, pneumonia, nephritis, endocarditis and neurologic complications. Recovery from each relapse is cor-

related with the appearance of specific antibody which with complement is responsible for clearing the spirochetes from the blood.

Epidemic relapsing fever (louse-borne) occurs most frequently during the winter months when lice reside in heavy clothing and is usually seen in populations where there is overcrowding, malnutrition
and poor personal hygiene. Case fatality rates may be as high as 40%
in untreated cases and approximately 4% in treated cases. Myocarditis
is the most common cause of death.

Endemic relapsing fever (tick-borne) occurs most frequently during
the summer months. Mortality is 2–5%, but among children less than
1 year old it is greater than 20%.

Mechanisms of Pathogenicity

The factors related to pathogenicity of the *Borrelia* are not known.
The disease is due to proliferation of the organisms in the blood and
the host response via antibody production. Antibody to the *Borrelia*
causes lysis of organisms, release of endotoxin and fever. Antigenic
variants that survive the first immune response proliferate, and the
host again responds with production of antibody, with subsequent lysis of organisms, release of endotoxin and characteristic symptoms.

EPIDEMIC RELAPSING FEVER (LOUSE-BORNE). – Epidemic relapsing fever is characterized by man-to-man transmission of *B. recurrentis* via the body louse. *B. recurrentis* is ingested by *Pediculus humanus* during a blood meal on an infected human. Approximately 1 mg of
blood is taken up by the louse, and at least 10^6 *Borrelia* must be ingested before the louse can transmit the spirochetes to man. After entering
the midgut, the spirochetes penetrate the gut wall and enter the hemolymph where they multiply. The louse remains infected for life
(27–50 days), and there is no transovarial transmission. The bite is not
sufficient to transmit the disease to man, and man acquires the infection via contamination of skin with infected hemolymph of crushed
lice. Infected lice are unable to pass the *Borrelia* to subsequent generations.

ENDEMIC RELAPSING FEVER (TICK-BORNE). – Ticks are responsible for transmitting the infection to man. The ticks that carry *Borrelia*
do not always cause painful bites and the host may be unaware of their
presence. The feeding time for these ticks on man is approximately 30
minutes to 1 hour. The bite of the tick is sufficient to transmit the spirochetes into the human circulatory system. During the meal, tick saliva and coxal fluid containing the spirochete are excreted. Unlike the
louse, the tick vector can pass the *Borrelia* to subsequent generations
by transovarial transmission with no effect on the tick.

Prevention
    Prevention is accomplished by rodent and insect control and measures (proper clothing, use of insecticides) to eliminate arthropod bites.

Treatment
    Tetracycline is the antibiotic of choice. General supportive therapy, e.g., fluid and electrolytes, should be given. The Jarisch-Herxheimer reaction may result if treatment is given during a febrile period.

Laboratory Diagnosis
    Direct examination of Wright- or Giemsa-stained blood films is the general method for detecting cases of relapsing fever, along with mouse and guinea pig inoculations. Finding stainable spirochetes in the blood of infected individuals is considered sufficient for laboratory identification of *Borrelia*. Stained blood films from the infected animals should be examined 1–10 days after inoculation. Culture of blood in special media can also be attempted. Antibodies to *Proteus* OX-K often appear during the disease and can be measured.

LEPTOSPIRA

Species
    Leptospirosis is a zoonosis caused by *Leptospira interrogans*–parasitic complex. Dogs, cattle, rats, mice, skunks, swine, and many other animals are infected by *Leptospira*, which then infects humans who come in contact with urine from these animals. Specific species of animals tend to be infected by a particular serotype of *L. interrogans*. For example, dogs (serovar *canicola*), cattle (serovar *pomona*), rats (serovar *icterohaemorrhagiae*) and mice (serovar *ballum*) are likely to be infected by specific serovars. However, most serovars are able to infect a number of animal species (Table 20–3).

Antigens
    Leptospira interrogans is antigenically complex and can be divided into serogroups and serovars, a partial list of which are shown in Table 20–3. The term *serovar* is used to describe antigenically different organisms and is analogous to serotype. Some antigens are specific for a serovar and others are shared among several *Leptospira* (serogroup antigen).
    The outer sheath of the *Leptospira* is highly antigenic, and removal reduces agglutinability with specific antiserums. Serovar-specific li-

TABLE 20-3.—HOST AND SEROVAR DISTRIBUTION OF
LEPTOSPIRES ISOLATED IN THE UNITED STATES

SEROGROUP	SEROVAR	HOSTS°
Icterohaemorrhagiae	*Icterohaemorrhagiae*	Man, dog, cattle, *rats*, mouse, raccoon, muskrat, fox, opossum, skunk, marmot, nutria
Canicola	*Canicola*	Man, *dog*, cattle, pig, skunk, raccoon, armadillo
Ballum	*Ballum*	*Mice*
	Arborea	Mouse, opossum, rat
	Undetermined	Rats, mice, shrew, fox, bobcat, skunk, rabbit, snake
Autumnalis	*Fort-bragg*	Man
	Autumnalis	Opossum, raccoon
	Orleans	Nutria
	Louisiana	Armadillo
Pomona	*Pomona*	Man, *cattle*, *pig*, dog, horse, goat, skunk, bobcat, raccoon, opossum, woodchuck, fox, deer, armadillo, mouse
Australis	*Australis*	Raccoon, opossum, fox, skunk
	Undetermined	Beaver, nutria
Grippotyphosa	*Grippotyphosa*	Cattle, raccoon, skunk, foxes, vole, opossum, mice, squirrel

°Known major hosts are italicized.

popolysaccharides located in the sheath elicit leptospirocidal and protective antibody. The flagella or axial filaments are serologically heterogenous.

Leptospirosis

Leptospira are shed in the urine of infected animals and are usually transmitted to other hosts via this medium. Man acquires the infection by coming in direct contact with infected animals, their urine, or soil and water contaminated with urine. The organisms enter the host circulatory system via a surface abrasion or through the mucous membranes of the eyes, nose and mouth. A lesion is not produced at the point of entry. The incubation period is from 4 to 19 days. Depending on the serovar and the host, leptospirosis has many possible manifestations. Generally, leptospirosis consists of two stages. The first stage lasts from 4 to 7 days and is characterized by septicemia (leptospiremia). Symptoms are abrupt in onset and include severe headache, a rapidly rising temperature, muscle soreness and tenderness, either diarrhea or constipation, and conjunctival infection. Other manifestations include joint pains, photophobia, rash, pneumonitis, proteinuria and bradycardia. The second phase begins after a brief afebrile period and coincides with increasing antibody levels, disappearance of leptospires from the blood, and development of leptospiruria due to multiplication of the leptospires in the renal tubes. The main manifestations of this phase may include fever, meningitis, uveitis, and hepatomegaly with hepatic tenderness and mild icterus. Leptospires can be isolated from the cerebrospinal fluid in cases of meningitis and from the eyes in cases of uveitis during this phase. Phase two may persist for up to 30 days, but this phase is inapparent in 35% of all cases. Recovery is generally complete. In approximately 5% to 10% of cases of leptospirosis, a severe disease called Weil's disease occurs and is characterized by a second phase of fever, jaundice, anemia, renal failure and leukocytosis. Death occurs in 10% to 15% of cases of Weil's disease and is attributed to acute renal failure. Serotype *icterohaemorrhagiae* is most often associated with this disease.

Leptospira of the serogroup *autumnalis* are associated with pretibial fever. The characteristic sign is a symmetrical rash limited to the pretibial area. Symptoms include fever, headache, leukopenia and splenomegaly. The rash may resemble that of erythema nodosum and may sometimes be urticarial.

The incidence of leptospirosis is highest during the summer and fall months. Those in risk occupations include sewer workers, abbatoir workers, farmers and veterinarians. In recent years the disease has been reported in children, housewives and students more frequently than in persons involved in risk occupations. Dogs are most frequently the source. Recent epidemics have involved persons swimming in ponds and streams contaminated by urine from infected animals. Because leptospirosis has so many possible manifestations, many cases are actually misdiagnosed. Leptospirosis should be considered in any case of unknown fever with or without hepatitis, meningitis or encephalitis.

Mechanisms of Pathogenicity

The factors involved in the pathogenesis of leptospirosis are unknown. The leptospires are thought to be able to invade host tissues due to the low antibody titer initially present in a susceptible host. It is also thought that they are able to survive and cause infection in the renal tubules in immune hosts as a result of isolation of the kidney from the complement system. However, it is not clear how the organisms which are initially in the blood gain access to the renal tubules. Some studies suggest that the leptospires travel to the tubules by way of the interstitial spaces and through the tubular epithelial cells or between adjacent cells. Other work suggests that they may migrate from the interstitial space to the tubular lumen via lysosomal vacuoles. Recent histopathologic studies suggest that the production of interstitial edema, probably resulting from endothelial damage or an inflammatory response due to a toxin may enable the organisms to pass through the tissues. It was found in these studies that the basement membrane around the cells of the proximal tubules was thicker but less election-dense. This suggested that the effectiveness of the basement membrane as a barrier to infection was reduced, thus permitting the organisms to enter the space between tubular epithelial cells and then the lumen.

A cytotoxic protein has been isolated from culture fluids. This protein is found in larger amounts in virulent strains than in avirulent strains. A hemolysin is also produced which is presumably responsible for intravascular hemolysin and anemia.

Immunity
IgM antibody is found within a week after onset and at termination of the first phase of the disease and is associated with absence of fever and leptospires in the blood. Immunity is serovar-specific and second attacks rarely occur. In endemic areas, vaccination of animals with killed leptospires of the prevailing serovar protects and minimizes the opportunity for human exposure.

Prevention and Treatment
Penicillin is the treatment of choice and must be given early in the course of the disease. Its effectiveness is questionable, but it decreases the severity of stage II leptospirosis. Supportive measures such as dialysis have been shown to be effective in the treatment of severe cases of Weil's disease.

Vaccines are available for immunization of animals. Immunity is serotype-specific.

Laboratory Diagnosis
Direct examination of blood, urine and cerebrospinal fluid is of questionable value, as fibrils present in these fluids can resemble *Leptospira* and confuse the identification of these organisms. Cultures

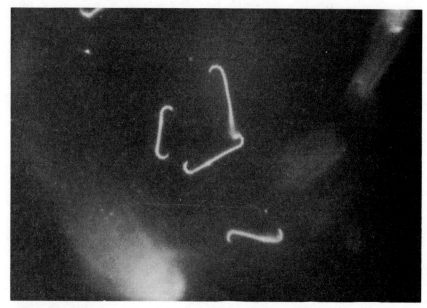

Fig. 20–8. — *Leptospira interrogans.* Darkfield microscopy. (Courtesy of D. Bromley and N. Charon, Dept. of Microbiology, West Virginia University Medical Center.)

of blood and cerebrospinal fluid (if indicated) should be obtained during the first week of the disease. After the first week, urine should be cultured. Physicians should notify the clinical laboratories to be sure that appropriate culture media are available. Cultures should not be expected to show growth for at least 7 days and should be observed for as long as 42 days. Darkfield microscopy of the cultures will show typical leptospiral forms (Fig. 20–8). A number of serologic methods are available for diagnosis, including agglutination, complement fixation, sensitized red cell agglutination and lysis. The microscopic agglutination test is serovar-specific and is the standard reference test for demonstrating leptospiral antibody. The complement fixation and sensitized red agglutination and lysis tests are genus-specific. A fourfold rise in titer is indicative of *Leptospira* infection.

Animal inoculation may be used to isolate the organisms or to provide serologic evidence for the presence of *Leptospira.*

PROBLEM SOLVING AND REVIEW

No. 1. Given: — A married professional man reported to his physician with the complaint of "flu." He had a lymphadenitis and a rash.

His white blood cell and red blood cell counts were normal, and he had a slight fever.

It was found that the patient's wife was in the first trimester of pregnancy. He had attended a convention about 6 weeks prior to the onset of symptoms and admitted intercourse with what he described as a refined young woman. He recalled no penile lesion, and none was noted upon examination.

PROBLEMS: — 1. What is the probable diagnosis? 2. How would you prove the diagnosis? 3. What is the treatment? 4. What would happen if he did not receive treatment? 5. Will treating the mother prevent congenital syphilis? 6. What else would you do? (Ans. p. 396.)

No. 2. GIVEN: — A 12-year-old girl became ill with chills, headache and fever (temperature 40 C) that lasted 3 days. After the fever subsided, the girl felt completely well, but 2 weeks later she had a febrile episode of 2 days' duration. A third febrile episode occurred 2 weeks after the second one. A history of the girl revealed that she and her parents had stayed in a cabin on the North Rim of the Grand Canyon 3 days prior to the first illness.

PROBLEMS: — 1. What is the suspected diagnosis? 2. What is normally done to prove the diagnosis? 3. How did the patient most likely become infected? 4. What is the treatment of choice: (Ans. p. 396.)

No. 3. GIVEN: — A 48-year-old man was admitted to the hospital with symptoms of nausea, vomiting, diarrhea and fever. Three days later he appeared lethargic, his scleras were icteric, and rales were noticed in the left lung. The liver edge was tender. On the 8th day of symptoms his temperature dropped from 39.5 to 37.3 C, while serum bilirubin rose from 8.6 mg/100 ml on admission to 19.0 mg/100 ml. Blood-streaked sputum was also noticed at this time. He remained afebrile for 3 days. On the 13th day the temperature spiked to 38.9 C, and serum bilirubin was 5 mg/100 ml. The patient continued to improve, the second febrile period lasting only 3 days. Convalescent serum, drawn on the 16th day, had antibodies directed to serotype *icterohaemorrhagiae* (titer 1:6,400). The patient lived in a slum tenement infested with rats.

PROBLEMS: — 1. Is there evidence of leptospirosis? 2. If so, what is the evidence? 3. What is the genus and species? 4. What is the probable source of the disease? 5. What is the disease? 6. Should cultures have been taken? If so, what cultures and when? (Ans. p. 396.)

●SUPPLEMENTARY READING

Boyer, K. M., Munford, R. S., Maupen, G. O., Pattison, C. P., Vox, M. D., Barnes, A. M., Jones, W. L., and Maynard, J. E.: Tick-borne relapsing fever: An interstate outbreak originating at Grand Canyon National Park, Am. J. Epidemiol. 105:469–479, 1977.

Canale-Parola, E.: Physiology and evolution of spirochetes, Bacteriol. Rev. 41:181–204, 1977.

Feigen, R. D., and Anderson, D. C.: Human leptospirosis, CRC Crit. Rev. Clin. Lab. Sci. 5:413–467, 1975.

Hayes, N. S., Muse, K. E., Collier, A. M., and Baseman, J. B.: Parasitism by virulent *Treponema pallidum* of host cell surfaces, Infect. Immun. 17: 171–186, 1977.

Heimoff, L. L.: The diagnosis of syphilis, Bull. N.Y. Acad. Sci. 52:863–870, 1976.

Hunter, E. F.: The fluorescent treponemal antibody–absorption (FTA-ABS) test for syphilis, CRC Crit. Rev. Clin. Lab. Sci. 5:315, 1975.

Johnson, R. C.: *The Biology of Parasitic Spirochetes* (New York: Academic Press, 1976).

Kelley, R. T.: Borrelia, in Lennette, E. H., Spaulding, E. H., and Truant, J. P. (eds): *Manual of Clinical Microbiology* (Washington: American Society for Microbiology, 1974).

Marshall, R. B.: The route of entry of leptospires into the kidney tubule, J. Med. Microbiol. 9:149–152, 1976.

Musher, D. M., Schell, R. F., Jones, R. H., and Jones, A. M.: Lymphocyte transfer in syphilis: An *in vitro* correlate of immune suppression *in vivo*, Infect. Immunol. 11:1261–1264, 1975.

Newman, R. B.: Laboratory diagnosis of syphilis, CRC Crit. Rev. Clin. Lab. Sci. 5:1, 1974.

Weiser, R. S., Erickson, D., Perine, P. L., and Pearsall, N. N.: Immunity to syphilis: Passive transfer in rabbits using serial doses of immune serum, Infect. Immun. 13:1402–1407, 1976.

ANALYSIS

No. 1.—1. Syphilis. 2. Darkfield on exudate from rash; VRDL serology. 3. Penicillin. 4. He would have a 30% chance of developing late syphilis with cardiovascular or neurologic disease. 5. Yes. 6. Report case to state health department. Try to obtain names of all sexual contacts. Initiate treatment.

No. 2.—1. Relapsing fever. 2. Stain of blood during febrile periods. The presence of loosely coiled spirochetes indicates relapsing fever. 3. Probably by a tick, as ticks are known to reside for long periods of time in cabins in this area. 4. Tetracycline.

No. 3.—1. Yes. 2. Serologic response. 3. *Leptospira interrogans*. 4. Rats and consequently rat urine. 5. Weil's disease. 6. Yes. Blood should have been obtained on admission. Urine should have been cultured during the relapse.

21 / Rickettsia, Coxiella and Rochalimaea

OVERVIEW

The *Rickettsia* are a unique group of bacteria in that they are, with one exception, obligate intracellular parasites. Unlike the viruses they are metabolically active, yet they cannot reproduce independently of the host cell. Little is known about the mechanisms by which they cause disease. A toxin, hemolysin, and several antigens have been described, but their role in disease and immunity is unknown.

The most important rickettsial infection in the United States (Rocky Mountain spotted fever) is misnamed. Although first recognized in that region, currently a majority of these cases occur in the East and Midwest. The number of reported cases of Rocky Mountain spotted fever increased from 268 in 1966 to 844 cases in 1975.

GENERAL CHARACTERISTICS

The rickettsiae are gram-negative, nonmotile, coccobacillary organisms ($0.3 \times 1.0 - 2.0$ μm) that, unlike most bacteria, have a prolonged generation time of about 7 hours (Fig. 21-1). With one exception, *R. quintana*, growth cannot be obtained on artificial media, and inoculation into guinea pigs, tissue culture or the chick embryo yolk sac is required for replication, isolation and identification. *R. quintana* can be grown on blood agar. The rest of the rickettsiae are obligate intracellular parasites.

The rickettsiae have a cell wall typical of gram-negative bacteria, but it cannot be easily visualized by gram staining, so the Gimenez (modified Macchiavello) stain is used instead. With this stain, the rickettsiae are found in the cytoplasm of the host cell and stain red against a green background. The cell walls contain muramic and diaminopimelic acids as well as protein and polysaccharide.

The rickettsiae are similar to bacteria not only on a morphological basis but also on a metabolic basis. However, unlike bacteria, they can

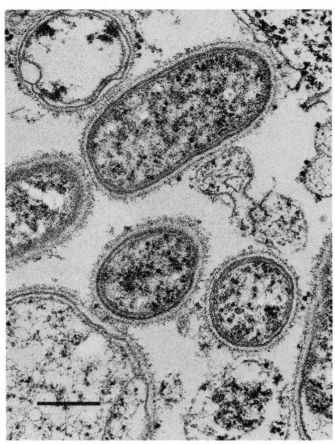

Fig. 21-1.—Electron micrograph of encapsulated *Rickettsia prowazekii* from extract of infected chicken embryo fibroblasts in tissue culture. Bar represents 0.25 μm. (Courtesy of Drs. D. J. Silverman and C. L. Wisseman, Jr., Department of Microbiology, University of Maryland School of Medicine.)

use ATP directly as an energy source and are permeable to nucleotides. Table 21-1 compares the rickettsiae with other microorganisms.

GENERA

The rickettsiae comprise a large group of organisms that infect endothelial cells. There are three genera: *Rickettsia, Rochalimaea* and

TABLE 21-1.—CHARACTERISTICS OF *RICKETTSIA* AND OTHER MICROORGANISMS

	RICKETTSIA	OTHER BACTERIA	CHLAMYDIA	VIRUSES
Nature of cell wall:	Gram negative	Gram positive or negative	Gram negative	Not applicable
Nucleic acids:	RNA, DNA	RNA, DNA	RNA, DNA	RNA or DNA
Multiplication:	Binary fission	Binary fission	Binary fission	–
Inclusions in vivo:	Cytoplasmic	None	Cytoplasmic	Nuclear and cytoplasmic
Growth:	Obligate° intracellular parasite	In vitro and in vivo	Obligate intracellular parasite	Obligate intracellular parasite
Generation time:	7 hr	10 min	2-3 hr	–
Metabolically active:	+	+	+	–
Inhibited or killed by antibiotics	+	+	+	–

°Except *Rochalimaea quintana.*

Coxiella. With the exception of *Rochalimaea quintana,* they can be propagated only in vivo. Unlike the *Rickettsia* and *Rochalimaea,* the *Coxiella* are resistant to heat and drying. *Coxiella burnetii* can be transmitted by aerosols and by ingestion, but all of the other rickettsiae require an arthropod vector for transmission to man.

SPECIES

More than seven species of rickettsia are associated with disease of man. Some of these are listed in Table 21-2.

TABLE 21-2.—*RICKETTSIA* ASSOCIATED WITH DISEASES OF MAN

DISEASE	GENUS AND SPECIES
Epidemic typhus	*R. prowazekii*
Brill-Zinsser disease	*R. prowazekii*
Endemic (murine) typhus	*R. typhi*
Rocky Mountain spotted fever	*R. rickettsii*
Rickettsialpox	*R. akari*
Scrub typhus	*R. tsutsugamushi*
Q fever	*Coxiella burnetii*
Trench fever	*Rochalimaea quintana*

TABLE 21-3.—VECTORS AND RESERVOIRS
FOR *RICKETTSIA*

DISEASE	VECTOR	RESERVOIR
Epidemic typhus	Human louse	Man
Brill-Zinsser disease°	Human louse	Man
Endemic typhus	Flea, rat louse	Rat, squirrel
Spotted fever	Dog tick, wood tick	Rodent, tick†
Tick typhus	Tick	Rodent
Rickettsialpox	Mite	Mite,† mouse
Scrub typhus	Mite	Mite,† rat, shrew
Q fever	Tick	Rodent, cattle, sheep
Trench fever	Louse	Man

°Reactivation of epidemic typhus.
†Transovarial transmission.

ECOLOGY

Transmission of all rickettsiae, except the organism causing Q fever, requires direct contact with an arthropod vector that has fed on an infected rodent, human or other animal reservoir. Transovarial transmission of rickettsiae responsible for scrub typhus, spotted fever and rickettsialpox has been shown in mites and ticks. Q fever is transmitted to man, not directly by a tick, but by contact with infected animal products or tissues. However, Q fever is transmitted to animals by ticks. The reservoirs and vectors are listed in Table 21-3.

ANTIGENS

Rickettsiae can be isolated from infected yolk sacs and used for preparation of ether-soluble group antigens and ether-insoluble type-specific antigens. The insoluble type-specific antigens are protein and are located in the cell wall and differentiate species and strains. The antigens are used for measuring antibody in infected persons. Antisera can be prepared in animals for use in immunofluorescence studies of rickettsiae and for agglutination, complement fixation and neutralization antibody tests.

The *Coxiella* differ from other rickettsiae in that they undergo phase variation, which is analogous to the S→R variation seen with other bacteria. The organisms are in phase I upon isolation from man but convert to phase II upon growth in chick embryos. This results in antigenic change as well as other changes. Phase I organisms contain two antigens and do not react with antisera against phase II. Vaccines prepared from phase I are much better immunogens than phase II vaccines.

INFECTIONS

Epidemic typhus and Brill-Zinsser disease

The etiologic agent, *Rickettsia prowazekii*, is transmitted from man to man by the human louse. The rickettsiae, obtained by feeding on an infected person, multiply in the gut of the louse and after 5 to 10 days' growth, they appear in the feces of the louse. When the louse feeds on man, it defecates, and the irritation of the bite causes the host to scratch, permitting entry of the rickettsiae.

Typhus is abrupt in onset with fever, severe headache and rash. The fever may peak on the first day or it may take several days to peak. The headache is intense and persists day and night. The patient may have a slight cough with patchy pulmonary consolidation.

Four to seven days after the onset of symptoms, a rash that consists of discrete pink macules first appears on the shoulders and upper trunk and then spreads over the body in 1 to 2 days. It rarely appears on the face, palms or soles. The macular rash darkens and then becomes maculopapular; it occasionally progresses to petechial hemorrhagic or confluent forms with gangrene of the feet. In fatal cases, profound stupor, a drop in blood pressure, peripheral vascular collapse and severe renal failure may be observed.

Brill-Zinsser disease is a relapse of epidemic typhus that occurs years after the primary attack. The rickettsiae remain in the reticuloendothelial system, and, under conditions that result in depression of host resistance, the disease recurs. The clinical features are those of epidemic typhus except they are milder. However, the headache is as intense as in epidemic typhus. The disease is shorter in duration, lasting 7–11 days, and the fever is irregular. The rash may be absent and complications are rare except in older persons. Brill-Zinsser disease must be considered in any person with fever and headache, with or without a rash, who was born in Russia or Eastern Europe during or before World War II.

Patients with Brill-Zinsser disease produce antibodies earlier than patients with epidemic typhus with a rise in antibody demonstrable about 4 to 5 days after onset of disease. Unlike primary infections with *R. prowazekii*, which causes an initial IgM response, antibody in Brill-Zinsser disease is of the IgG class and represents an anamnestic response.

Endemic Typhus (Murine Typhus)

Endemic or murine typhus is similar to epidemic typhus in manifestations of disease except it is milder. The onset is gradual and the fever

is lower (39 C) and remittent. The maculopapular rash is not as extensive. The etiologic agent, R. *typhi*, is maintained in rats and is transmitted to man by the rat flea. The flea defecates as it feeds on man or
rats, and because of the skin irritation, the infective feces are rubbed
into the bite.

Scrub Typhus

Scrub typhus is characterized by an initial lesion at the site of a mite
bite that ulcerates and is covered with a scab (eschar). Regional lymphadenopathy, fever, and severe headache are characteristic of the infection. A macular rash appears between the 5th and 8th days of illness; it then becomes maculopapular and extends to the extremities.
The disease must be differentiated from dengue, leptospirosis, malaria and typhoid fever.

The etiologic agent, R. *tsutsugamushi*, is found in mites (chiggers).
Rodents are infected with the rickettsiae and act as a continuing reservoir. The organisms are also maintained in the mite population by
transovarial transmission. Man is accidentally infected when he enters a mite-infested area.

Rocky Mountain Spotted Fever

Rocky Mountain spotted fever (RMSF) is characterized by intense
headache, often frontal, fever and a rash. The rash is the earliest diagnostic sign, appearing first and characteristically on the wrists and
ankles and then spreading up the extremities (Figs. 21–2, 21–3). The

Fig. 21–2.—Typical rash of Rocky Mountain spotted fever. (Courtesy of
Dr. Edmund Flink, Department of Medicine, West Virginia University Medical
Center.)

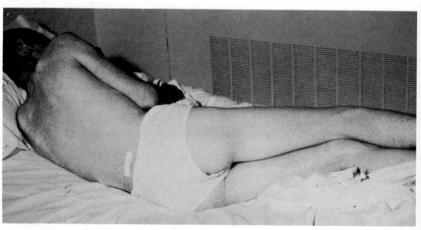

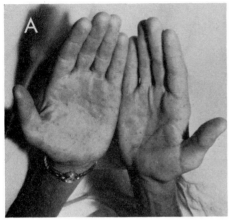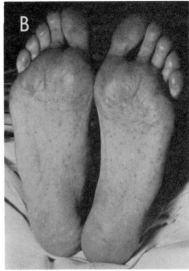

Fig. 21–3.—Rash on palms of hands **(A)** and soles of feet **(B)** of patient with Rocky Mountain spotted fever. (Courtesy of Dr. Edmund Flink, Department of Medicine, West Virginia University Medical Center.)

distribution of the rash helps differentiate RMSF from other exanthomatous diseases. The patient is restless, apprehensive and irritable and may become mentally confused with subsequent delirium and coma. Muscle tenderness is common and a stiff neck may be present. RMSF must be differentiated from measles, measles encephalitis, meningococcemia and endemic typhus.

The etiologic agent, *R. rickettsii,* is transmitted to man by the dog and wood tick. The dog tick is the main vector for Rocky Mountain spotted fever in the eastern United States; in the West, the vector is primarily the wood tick, *Dermacentor andersoni.* The tick becomes infected by feeding on wild and domestic animals. The organisms multiply in the ovaries and salivary glands of the arthropod, and the tick transmits the disease to man while taking a blood meal. The tick must remain attached to man for 4 to 6 hours before the rickettsiae can be transmitted. Crushing of infected ticks during removal results in contamination of the tick bite and infection of the host. The infection is transmitted transovarially in the tick population.

Tick Typhus

A number of diseases similar to Rocky Mountain spotted fever are caused by rickettsiae that are antigenically similar to *R. rickettsii.* The

diseases are milder and differ from RMSF by the presence of an eschar at the site of the tick bite. These infections are not found in the
United States and are known by various names, some referring to the
geographic regions in which they are found (Siberian tick typhus,
Queensland tick typhus, Fièvre boutonneuse, South African tick bite
fever, etc.).

Rickettsial pox

The primary lesion is an erythematous papule at the site of the mite
bite which vesiculates and then develops into an eschar. Within a
week after development of the eschar, the patient complains of chills
(2–3 per day), sweats, headache, backache, malaise and has a fever.
One to two days after the onset of fever, discrete maculopapular lesions appear which progress to central vesiculation. The rash may be
found on any part of the body. The vesicles dry and scabs are formed;
these slough off and leave a brownish discoloration. The disease may
be confused with varicella (chickenpox). This infection does not result
in death.

The etiologic agent, *R. akari*, is transmitted from the mouse mite
when the mites are forced to feed on man because of a decrease in the
mouse population. The rickettsiae are found in the oral secretions of
mites that have fed on infected mice or that have been infected transovarially.

Q Fever

Q fever is a self-limiting disease characterized by malaise, fever,
frontal headache, chills and pneumonia. Hepatitis and endocarditis
may also result. The onset is abrupt and, unlike all other rickettsial
diseases, there is no rash. Inapparent infection is common. The disease must be differentiated from brucellosis, typhoid fever, infectious
hepatitis, leptospirosis and other rickettsial diseases. In those cases
with pneumonia, Q fever must be differentiated from mycoplasmal,
chlamydial, viral and fungal pneumonias.

Coxiella burnetii, the etiologic agent, is maintained in wild animals
and is transferred to cattle and sheep by infected ticks. Man acquires
the disease by inhaling aerosols containing *C. burnetii* or by ingesting
milk from infected animals. Unlike other rickettsiae, *C. burnetii* is
resistant to drying and aerosols can be generated in handling of wool
and from dried secretions and excreta from infected animals.

Trench Fever

This disease is characterized by an abrupt onset with chills and fever, headache and pain associated with the tibia. The symptoms sub-

side and recur in cycles of 3 to 5 days. A rash is present during febrile periods. The disease recurs over a 3 to 5-week period. The etiologic agent, *Rochalimaea quintana*, is transmitted by lice feeding on man. The louse acquires the rickettsia by feeding on an infected human and maintains the organism for life. Trench fever is usually found in soldiers in time of war. *Rochalimaea quintana* is the only rickettsia pathogenic for man that can be cultured on blood agar. Because of in vitro growth and proliferation in the lumen of the louse gut, a separate genus *Rochalimaea* has been created.

A summary of the epidemiologic and disease characteristics of the rickettsial diseases is shown in Table 21 – 4.

MECHANISMS OF PATHOGENESIS

Most of the clinical manifestations of rickettsial disease can be associated with their predilection for endothelial cells of small blood vessels with resultant growth in and destruction of these cells. The hyperplasia and local thrombus formation lead to obstruction of flow. The influx of inflammatory cells around small blood vessels (angiitis) in skin, brain and myocardium accounts for the rash, stupor and terminal shock.

Little is known about the mechanism by which these organisms damage the host cell and cause disease. Injection of large numbers of rickettsiae into animals results in damage to endothelial cells, leakage of plasma, a decrease in blood volume and shock, which suggests that a toxin may cause cell destruction. The toxin is a lipopolysaccharide with biologic activities similar to those of endotoxin. In vitro hemolysis of sheep and rabbit cells but not human cells can be produced by infectious preparations of typhus rickettsiae. Many hemolysins affect cells other than by causing lysis; thus the hemolysin may be important in the disease process via a mechanism other than erythrocyte hemolysis.

Rickettsiae readily enter macrophages and replicate in the cytoplasm. It is suggested that this property protects the organisms against host factors that might result in their destruction. Some differences exist among the rickettsiae in their pattern of replication. *R. prowazekii* multiplies in the cytoplasm and is released by cell lysis. However, *R. rickettsii* grows in the cytoplasm and nucleus and is constantly being removed from the cytoplasm without causing detectable damage to the host cell. The early and rapid spread of *R. rickettsii* may account for the shorter incubation period of Rocky Mountain spotted fever and the more extensive tissue damage as compared with epidemic typhus.

TABLE 21-4.—EPIDEMIOLOGY AND SOME CHARACTERISTICS
OF RICKETTSIAL INFECTIONS

DISEASE	GEOGRAPHIC OCCURRENCE	ESCHAR	RASH	
			DISTRIBUTION	TYPE
Typhus group				
Primary epidemic typhus	Worldwide	None	Trunk to extremities	Macular, maculopapular
Brill-Zinsser disease	Worldwide	None	Trunk to extremities	Macular, maculopapular
Murine typhus	Scattered pockets worldwide	None	Trunk to extremities	Macular, maculopapular
Spotted fever group				
Rocky Mountain spotted fever	Western hemisphere	None	Extremities to trunk, palms and soles	Macular, maculopapular, petechial
Tick typhus	Mediterranean, Africa, Asia	Frequent	Trunk, extremities, face, palms, soles	Macular, maculopapular, petechial
Rickettsialpox	U.S., Russia, Korea	Usually present	Trunk, face, extremities	Papular, vesicular
Scrub typhus	Japan, S.W. Asia, W. and S.W. Pacific	Frequent	Trunk to extremities	Macular, maculopapular, evanescent
Q fever	Worldwide	None	None	None
Trench fever	Europe, Mexico, Central & S. America	None	Trunk to extremities	Macular

TABLE 21-5. — SEROLOGIC TESTS AND INFECTIVITY
OF *RICKETTSIA*

	RICKETTSIAL COMPLEMENT FIXATION			WEIL-FELIX AGGLUTINATION			GUINEA PIG REACTION
	GROUP ANTIGEN			PROTEUS			
	TYPHUS	RMSF	Q FEVER	OX-19	OX-2	OX-K	
Epidemic typhus	+	0	0	+++	+	0	Fever only
Endemic typhus	+	0	0	0 or +++		0	Scrotal swelling
Murine typhus	+	0	0	+++	+	0	Swelling, necrosis
RMSF	0	+	0	+++	+++	0	Swelling
Tick typhus	0	+	0	+++	+++	0	Swelling
Rickettsialpox	0	+	0	0	0	0	Swelling
Scrub typhus	0	0	0	0	0	+++	—
Q fever	0	0	+	0	0	0	Fever only

IMMUNITY

Several antibodies are formed in response to infection or immunization with the rickettsiae. As usually occurs after infection, IgM antibodies are produced first. However, Brill-Zinsser disease is a recurrence of epidemic typhus and results in an IgG response. This difference in immunoglobulin class is useful in distinguishing between epidemic typhus and Brill-Zinsser disease. After infection with certain rickettsiae, antibodies to strains of *Proteus*, designated OX-K, OX-2 and OX-19, are produced. This agglutination of *Proteus* is termed the Weil-Felix reaction. The differential response to these heterophile antigens helps in differentiating among the various rickettsial diseases (Table 21-5). In addition, specific antibody to the rickettsia is produced. It is detectable during the 2d week of the disease with maximum titers during the 15th to 20th day.

A number of serologic tests have been devised using antigens prepared from the rickettsia. The complement fixation test is most commonly used. Epidemic and murine typhus rickettsia share a common antigen as do members of the spotted fever group (see Table 21-5). Rickettsia that cause Q fever and trench fever have specific antigens. The complement fixation test cannot be used for diagnosis of scrub typhus; instead, the indirect fluorescence test is used.

Antibody is important in control of the disease. In the absence of antibody, the rickettsia readily penetrate the phagocytic cell membrane, enter the cytoplasm, replicate and destroy the cell. If antibody is present, opsonization and subsequent phagocytosis occur and the phagocytosed rickettsia are destroyed within the phagolysosome. Antibody, however, does not affect multiplication of rickettsia in non-phagocytic cells.

In human typhus convalescent serum macrophage cytophilic antibody, which enhances phagocytosis and causes intravacuolar killing, has been demonstrated. Delayed hypersensitivity is produced in some rickettsial infections and blast transformation has also been reported, suggesting a role for cellular immunity.

PREVENTION AND CONTROL

In 1975 there were 44 cases of endemic (murine) typhus and 844 cases of Rocky Mountain spotted fever reported to the Center for Disease Control. No deaths from endemic typhus were reported, but there were 49 deaths from Rocky Mountain spotted fever. Control of rickettsial diseases is directed at the reservoir and the vector. Rodent control minimizes the role of the reservoir and the probability of contact with the vector. Individuals in tick-infested areas should wear loose-fitting clothing and should periodically check for attachment of ticks to their skin. Pasteurization of milk prevents the spread of Q fever, but abattoir workers and farmers may be exposed to the organism from infected animals. A killed vaccine is available for Rocky Mountain spotted fever. It is not considered very effective and its use is limited to groups at high risk. Newer and better vaccines are being evaluated.

TREATMENT

Tetracyclines and chloramphenicol are the drugs of choice. Treatment should be prolonged to avoid recurrence. Mortality in untreated Rocky Mountain spotted fever is about 20%, but in persons more than 40 years old it approaches 50%. Rickettsialpox is benign and chemotherapy is not necessary.

LABORATORY DIAGNOSIS

Rickettsiae are identified by injecting guinea pigs intraperitoneally with whole or clotted blood obtained from the patient during the febrile stages of the disease or with tissue obtained at autopsy. Figure 21-4 summarizes the laboratory approach to diagnosis of rickettsial diseases. If the blood clot is used, the serum is saved for immunologic studies. The temperature of the guinea pig is measured daily, and the testes are observed for scrotal swelling and necrosis. Serum from the infected guinea pig should also be collected for immunologic studies.

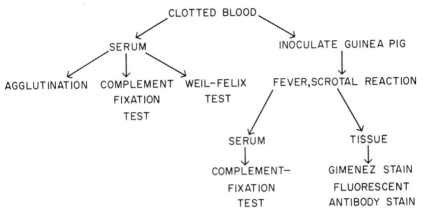

Fig. 21–4. — Laboratory diagnosis of rickettsial disease.

A complement fixation test using antigens prepared by yolk sac culture should be done with serial blood specimens to detect a rise in antibody titer. Tissue from the guinea pig can be stained by the Gimenez modification of the Macchiavello stain or with fluorescein-labeled antibody. Tissue from the patient, reservoir or arthropod vector can also be examined for rickettsiae by use of fluorescent antibody.

Serum specimens from the patient should also be studied immunologically. Complement-fixing antibodies can be measured. In addition, infection with rickettsiae can result in production of agglutinating antibody to strains of *Proteus* (Weil-Felix test). Three stains, *Proteus* OX-19, OX-2 and OX-K, are used, but it should be remembered that agglutinins for *Proteus* can also be produced by homologous infections. Antibody to *C. burnetii* can be detected by an agglutination test using phase I antigen.

Table 21–5 lists the results expected in serologic studies of the rickettsia and gives the reaction expected after inoculation of guinea pigs with rickettsia.

Rochalimaea quintana (the organism causing trench fever) can be isolated by growth on blood agar.

Most laboratories do not have the expertise to diagnose rickettsial diseases. State health laboratories and the Center for Disease Control can be of assistance.

PROBLEM SOLVING AND REVIEW

No. 1. GIVEN: A 5-year-old child was admitted to the hospital with complaints of severe headache for several days. A rash was present on the palms, soles, wrists and arms. The child was acutely ill and stuporous. The parents and child lived in a town of about 60,000 people. The mother stated that the family had returned a week earlier from a vacation at a state park in Virginia where they had camped and hiked. The family had a dog, which accompanied them on their vacation.

PROBLEMS: — 1. What must be considered in the differential diagnosis? 2. What laboratory work-up would you request to reach a diagnosis? Indicate tests and specimens. The laboratory report indicates that organisms were not found on gram stain and cells were not present in the CSF. Blood cultures were negative. The Weil-Felix test was positive for *Proteus* OX-19 and OX-2. The CF test was also positive. 3. What is the probable diagnosis? 4. What is the genus and species of the etiologic agent? 5. What is the probable source(s) of the organism? 6. How could the disease have been prevented? 7. Is a vaccine available for prevention? (Ans. p. 411.)

NO. 2. GIVEN: — A 32-year-old man was admitted to the service of a large city hospital with headache, fever (39 C) and a maculopapular rash. The patient reported that the rash had first appeared on his chest and abdomen and then on his arms and legs. No rash was apparent on his face, palms or soles. About 12 days before he became ill, he was bitten by a rat while sleeping. The patient had never been outside the United States.

PROBLEMS: — 1. What diseases must be considered in the differential diagnosis? 2. Why did you not consider epidemic typhus or Brill-Zinsser disease? 3. What specimens would you send to the laboratory and what test would you request? No organisms were observed on gram stain of cerebrospinal fluid. Cultures for *S. typhi* were negative. Agglutinins for *Salmonella typhi* O and H antigen were 1:20 and 1:10, respectively. The complement fixation test for the typhus group antigen was positive and agglutinins for *Proteus* OX-19 and OX-2 were present. Scrotal swelling was reported in the inoculated guinea pig. 4. What is the diagnosis and what is the etiologic agent? 5. How was the organism acquired? 6. What is the reservoir? 7. How could the disease be prevented? (Ans. p. 411.)

SUPPLEMENTARY READING

Beaman, L., and Wisseman, C. L.: Mechanisms of immunity in typhus infections. VI. Differential opsonizing and neutralizing action of human typhus rickettsia-specific cytophilic antibody in cultures of human macrophages, Infect. Immun. 14:1071–1076, 1976.

Brezina, R., Murray, E. S., Tarizzo, M. L., and Bögel, K.: Rickettsia and rickettsial diseases, Bull. W. H. O. 49:433–442, 1973.

Hattwick, M. A. W., Brien, R. J. O., and Hansen, B. F.: Rocky Mountain spotted fever: Epidemiology of an increasing problem, Ann. Intern. Med. 84: 732–739, 1976.

Kishimoto, R. A., Veltri, B. J., Shirey, F. G., Canonico, P. G., and Walker, J. S.: Fate of Coxiella burnetii in macrophages from immune guinea pigs, Infect. Immun. 15:601–607, 1977.

Krauss, H., Schiefer, H. G., and Schmatz, H. D.: Ultrastructural investigations on surface structures involved in Coxiella burnetii phase variation, Infect. Immun. 15:890–896, 1977.

Vinson, V. W.: Rickettsiae, in Rose, N. R., and Friedman, H. (eds.): Manual of Clinical Immunology (Washington, D.C.: American Society for Microbiology, 1976).

Weiss, E.: Growth and physiology of rickettsiae, Bacteriol. Rev. 37:259–283, 1973.

Wisseman, C. L., Edlinger, E. A., Waddell, A. D., and Jones, M. R.: Infection cycle of Rickettsia rickettsii in chicken embryo and L-929 cells in culture, Infect. Immun. 14:1052–1064, 1976.

Woodward, T. E., Pedersen, C. E., Jr., Oster, C. N., Bagley, L. R., Romberger, J., and Snyder, M. J.: Prompt confirmation of Rocky Mountain spotted fever: Identification of rickettsiae in skin tissues, J. Infect. Dis. 134:297–301, 1976.

ANALYSIS

No. 1:–1. Measles, measles encephalitis, meningococcemia and Rocky Mountain spotted fever. 2. (a) CSF for gram stain and cell count. (b) Hemagglutination titer for measles antibody. (c) Blood for rickettsial complement fixation, Weil-Felix test, and for isolation of rickettsia. 3. Rocky Mountain spotted fever. 4. Rickettsia rickettsii. 5. Ticks acquired from hiking through tick-infested territory or from ticks attached to the dog. 6. Wearing proper clothing to prevent ticks attaching to skin. Inspecting skin and carefully removing ticks. Removing ticks from the dog. 7. Yes, but it is used only for those whose occupations put them at risk of infection.

No. 2:–1. Meningococcemia, measles, typhoid fever, murine typhus. 2. Patient had not been out of the United States. 3. Cerebrospinal fluid for gram stain and culture (bacterial meningitis). Blood and stool for culture of S. typhi. Blood for isolation of rickettsiae and for serologic tests (complement fixation and Weil-Felix). 4. Endemic (murine typhus); R. typhi. 5. Rat fleas. 6. Rats. 7. Rat and flea control methods.

22 / Chlamydia and Mycoplasma

CHLAMYDIA

Overview

This genus of obligately intracellular organisms once considered to be viruses are now classed as bacteria on the basis of exhibiting binary fission, presence of a bacterial cell wall structure, ribosomes and susceptibility to antibiotics. On a worldwide basis, the chlamydiae are important human pathogens; they cause ornithosis, trachoma, inclusion conjunctivitis, lymphogranuloma venereum and a nongonococcal urethritis. They also cause a variety of infections in birds and mammals.

General Characteristics

The *Chlamydia* are intracellular, inclusion-forming, gram-negative, coccoid organisms that contain both DNA and RNA but are unable to sustain growth outside of tissue cells. They require ATP for growth, which they obtain from the host by their intracellular existence. Cytochromes have not been demonstrated and metabolic reactions are essentially anaerobic. The organisms go through a developmental cycle that begins with a small elementary body (infectious form) coming in contact with the cell membrane. The membrane invaginates with the chlamydiae being taken into the cell in a phagocytic vesicle. The elementary body (250–350 nm), which is contained within a cytoplasmic vesicle, enlarges to form the initial, noninfectious body. The initial body divides by binary fission and aggregates into a large inclusion body (600–1000 nm). The inclusion body then breaks up by some mechanism into numerous elementary bodies, and these are released to invade other cells. Inclusion bodies are demonstrable in all chlamydial diseases (Fig. 22–1). Chlamydiae can be cultivated in the yolk sac of chick embryos, in tissue culture and in mice and guinea pigs. The chlamydiae are susceptible to sulfonamides and a number of antibiotics, including tetracyclines, penicillin, chloram-

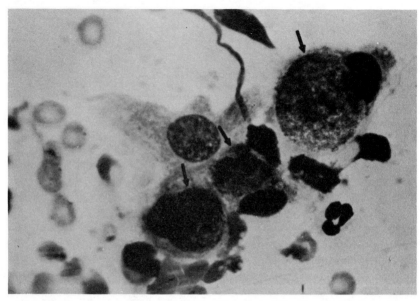

Fig. 22–1.—Smear from human conjunctiva stained with Giemsa. Three intracellular inclusions *(arrows)* compress the cell nucleus. Each inclusion is in the late stage of development prior to release of the elementary bodies. (From Grayston, J. T., and Wang, S.: J. Infect. Dis. 132:87, 1975. By permission of authors and journal.)

phenicol and erythromycin, but not streptomycin. The two species, *C. trachomatis* and *C. psittaci,* have a common complement-fixing, acidic polysaccharide antigen.

Species

Within the cytoplasmic vesicle *Chlamydia trachomatis* forms compact inclusions (microcolonies) that compress the cell nucleus. These inclusions contain glycogen and can be stained with iodine. Growth in the yolk sac of chick embryos can be inhibited by sulfadiazine and helps in differentiating *C. trachomatis* from *C. psittaci.* Propagation in the lungs of mice or guinea pigs is possible, and eye infections can be produced in primates. *C. trachomatis* can be isolated from infectious material using tissue culture, particularly with irradiated McCoy cells. Fifteen serotypes have been differentiated using immunofluorescent techniques, and antibodies to these types can be detected in the serum or tears of patients. *C. trachomatis* is primarily a human pathogen, causing trachoma, inclusion conjunctivitis, lymphogranuloma venereum and urethritis. Transmission is by direct contact; there is little information on carrier rates.

TABLE 22-1.—DIFFERENTIAL CHARACTERISTICS
OF CHLAMYDIAL SPECIES

CHARACTERISTIC	C. TRACHOMATIS	C. PSITTACI
Cytoplasmic inclusions	+	+
Have rigid wall	+	−
Contain glycogen	+	−
Stain with iodine	+	−
Yolk sac growth inhibited by sulfadiazine and cycloserine	+	−

Chlamydia psittaci forms inclusions (microcolonies), but the vesicle ruptures early, releasing chlamydiae in various stages of development into the cell cytoplasm. The inclusions are not stained by iodine, and growth in the chick embryo is not inhibited by sulfadiazine. Propagation is possible in mice, guinea pigs and a variety of tissue culture cells. *C. psittaci* can be differentiated serologically from *C. trachomatis* using sorbed antisera, and there is no significant DNA homology between the two species. *C. psittaci* also has a broad host range among birds and mammals, causing pneumonitis, polyarthritis, enteritis or encephalitis. From birds man contracts ornithosis, which can then be transmitted from person to person via droplets.

Table 22-1 contains a summary of some of the differences between the two chlamydial species.

Chlamydioses

Trachoma

This disease of the eye was described in Egypt 15 centuries before Christ, and it remains a worldwide problem—particularly in the Middle East, Africa and India where it is endemic. Transmission in endemic areas is from eye to eye. Trachoma is a chronic follicular conjunctivitis with pannus formation (growth of new vessels into the cornea) and the development of conjunctival scars (Fig. 22-2). Recovery does not provide immunity and vaccines are unsuccessful. There is evidence that repeated exposure results in sensitization and a more severe infection.

In nonendemic areas trachoma occurs as a sporadic eye disease dependent on genital tract-to-eye transmission. The types of eye diseases resulting from this form of transmission include (1) neonatal inclusion conjunctivitis, an acute papillary conjunctivitis that usually heals spontaneously without scars or pannus, (2) adult inclusion conjunctivitis with follicles and sometimes corneal opacities and (3) a classic trachoma disease as described above. Some authors consider

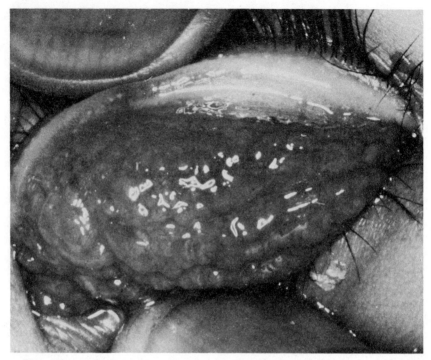

Fig. 22–2.—Follicular conjunctivitis due to *C. trachomatis*. Note the "cobblestone" appearance of clinical trachoma. (Courtesy of J. T. Grayston, School of Public Health and Community Medicine, University of Washington.)

inclusion conjunctivitis and trachoma to be stages of the same disease. Serotypes A, B, Ba and C of *C. trachomatis* predominate in trachoma of endemic areas, whereas serotypes D, E, F and G are more frequently isolated from sporadic cases in nonendemic areas. Eyelid scrapings stained with Giemsa often show the large purple inclusions. The chlamydiae can be isolated by inoculating chick embryos or tissue culture and then identified serologically; also serotype-specific antibodies can be demonstrated in serum or tears by means of the immunofluorescent technique. Treatment is with topical and/or systemic tetracyclines or sulfonamides.

Nongonococcal Urethritis

Nongonococcal urethritis (NGU) is an inflammatory disease associated with a persistent urethral discharge of uncertain etiology, although *Mycoplasma*, herpesvirus and *Chlamydia* have been implicated. There is increasing evidence that *C. trachomatis* is of major importance in NGU, and in one survey of over 200 patients, chlamydiae were isolated from 57% of the cases. Cervicitis in women may be caused by any one of a number of organisms, but in a study of over 600 nongonococcal cases, chlamydiae were isolated from 37% of the infections.

Lymphogranuloma Venereum

Lymphogranuloma venereum (LGV) begins as a small (2–3 mm), painless vesicular lesion on or about the genitals followed by a regional lymphadenitis. The nodes become tender, inflamed, elongated masses that may resolve but more often develop into abscesses that form draining fistulas; intrapelvic and perianal nodes may be involved in women, resulting in proctocolitis. Rectal strictures may develop in both men and women. The incubation period is 1–4 weeks, and early symptoms—fever, headache and myalgia—may be reported. LGV is a worldwide venereal disease that has increased in incidence in the United States since the Vietnam War. Treatment with sulfonamides, tetracyclines or erythromycin is usually successful. LGV is caused by strains of *C. trachomatis*, serotypes L_1, L_2 or L_3, characterized by ease of cultivation, infectivity for mouse brains and absence of growth inhibition by neuramidinase (these organisms can also cause inclusion conjunctivitis and urethritis). LGV is usually diagnosed on clinical grounds. Isolation of the chlamydiae can be attempted by inoculating yolk sacs of chick embryos or tissue cultures with exudate from buboes or blood; smears can be stained or examined by immunofluorescence for inclusions. A rise in antibody titer can be detected with the complement fixation or immunofluorescent test with the latter being more specific. A protein antigen common to *C. trachomatis* has been purified and appears to be highly specific by counter immunoelectrophoresis for detection of antibody in patients with lymphogranuloma venereum. A hypersensitivity develops in 2 to 6 weeks and can be determined by the Frei test. This test consists of an intradermal injection of 0.1 ml of antigen prepared from chlamydiae grown in the chick yolk sac; a positive test is a 5-mm area of induration, indicating either a past or present infection. A control injection of egg protein is given to be certain that the reaction is not due to a hypersensitivity to chicken products. The Frei test is not often used, and the antigen is not available commercially.

Ornithosis

Ornithosis is a pneumonitis contracted from birds infected with *C. psittaci*. At one time, psittacine birds (parrots, parakeets, cockatoos) were considered the prime source and the disease was referred to as psittacosis or parrot fever. As other domestic and wild birds became implicated, the name ornithosis was applied. Humans contract the infection either from aerosols from infected birds or from patients. *C. psittaci* enters through the respiratory tract, producing a pneumonitis with a severe cough, and spreads via the blood to involve other organs, particularly the liver and spleen. The incubation period varies from 1 to 3 weeks. Initially the patient may have fever, myalgia and a frontal headache. The disease may be mild, severe and last about 3 weeks, or fatal (5–20%). Clinical diagnosis is difficult because the pneumonia is similar to that seen in infections caused by respiratory viruses, *Mycoplasma pneumoniae*, and other bacteria. Inclusion bodies can be demonstrated in the monocytes or macrophages of the sputum, but a definitive diagnosis usually requires isolation of the chlamydiae or demonstration of a fourfold rise in antibody titer with the complement fixation test. For isolation, sputum or blood is inoculated into the yolk sac of embryonated eggs, mice or tissue culture; the isolated *C. psittaci* is then identified serologically. Tetracyclines are the antibiotic of choice for treatment.

Mechanisms of Pathogenicity

The chlamydiae are intracellular organisms. The mechanisms by which they cause disease are not understood. The intracellular growth suggests that part of the host response may be the result of competition between the host and parasite for nutrients. The chlamydiae are cytotoxic for macrophages, and experimental infection has shown that macrophages can be "transformed" into giant epithelioid cells. Stimulation of fibroblast growth has also been reported. The severe disease in patients with trachoma and lymphogranuloma venereum may result from an exaggerated host response. There may also be a difference in virulence, which could account for the more severe pathologic features associated with some types.

Laboratory Procedures

The laboratory aids to diagnosis of chlamydial infections include examination of direct smears, cultivation and identification of the organisms and determination of antibody titers in the serum or tears of patients.

Materials

These should be collected before the use of antimicrobial agents, and as they are frequently contaminated with bacteria, they are usually added to a collecting medium that contains streptomycin. Care should be taken in handling all such material, particularly from suspected cases of ornithosis, as it can be infectious. Depending on the type of infection, materials could include eyelid (conjunctival) scrapings, urogenital swabs, sputum, lymph node exudate, biopsy tissue, blood or serum.

Smears

Preparations can be made from most of the above materials as well as from yolk sac or tissue culture cells infected with the specimens from the patients. The smears are stained by Giemsa (purple inclusions), Macchiavello (red inclusions) or Castaneda (blue inclusions) techniques: the inclusions are intracellular (see Fig. 22–1). Smears can also be examined by the immunofluorescent techniques using conjugated antisera for specific identification of the inclusions. Immunofluorescence is more sensitive than Giemsa staining for examining epithelial scrapings from the eye and genital tract.

Cultivation

Most of the clinical materials can be inoculated directly into the yolk sac or embryonated eggs, incubated and harvested in 5 to 7 days (serial passages may be necessary to demonstrate the chlamydiae). Irradiated or 5-iodo-2-deoxyuridine-treated McCoy or HeLa cell cultures are inoculated and incubated at 35 C for 2 to 3 days; serial transfers are usually necessary to demonstrate the organisms. For both procedures, identification is by the demonstration of inclusions in stained smears and specific serologic identification by immunofluorescence or the complement fixation test. Mice can be inoculated intracerebrally or intraperitoneally for isolation.

Antibody Determination

Serum is collected during the acute and convalescent stages (tears from patients with suspected trachoma or inclusion conjunctivitis can be used), and complement fixation tests are done using known antigens. A microimmunofluorescent test is also used as follows. Small dots of known antigen are placed on a slide. These are covered with the serum or tears, then washed and stained with conjugated antihuman globulin (indirect method, chap. 4); the antigen reacting with the antibody will fluoresce. In both procedures a fourfold rise in titer is considered diagnostic; a single titer of 1:64 or higher supports a diagnosis of an active LGV infection.

MYCOPLASMA

Overview

In 1898 the causal agent of contagious bovine pleuropneumonia was isolated and the organism was referred to as a pleuropneumonia-like-organism, or PPLO (chap. 3; L-forms). These pleomorphic bacteria were eventually called *Mycoplasma* (fungus form) with the distinguishing features of: (1) being the smallest free-living microorganisms (300 – 1,000 μm), (2) having a nonrigid cell wall (resistant to penicillin), (3) being bound by a single triple-layered membrane containing cholesterol and (4) requiring a sterol component in media used for growth. The genus contains approximately 40 species that infect humans, animals and birds; in humans one species, *M. pneumoniae*, can cause pneumonia, tracheobronchitis, otitis media and bullous myringitis, but the role of other species such as *M. hominis* and the T-strains *(Ureaplasma urealyticum)* is still uncertain.

Species

Mycoplasma pneumoniae grows rather slowly, forming small beta-hemolytic colonies (Fig. 22–3); it ferments glucose and reduces tetrazolium salts. It is antigenically distinct and can be identified by the fluorescent antibody technique (chap. 4). It adsorbs to the surface of red cells and ciliated epithelium through neuraminic acid receptor sites.

Mycoplasma hominis is morphologically similar but does not ferment glucose or reduce tetrazolium. It adsorbs to HeLa cells and chick embryo cells but not to ciliated epithelial cells; neuraminic acid

Fig. 22–3.—Colonies of *Mycoplasma pneumoniae* growing on brain heart infusion agar. Note the raised center, which is described as a "fried egg" appearance. (Courtesy of R. W. Veltri, Department of Otolaryngology and Microbiology, West Virginia University.)

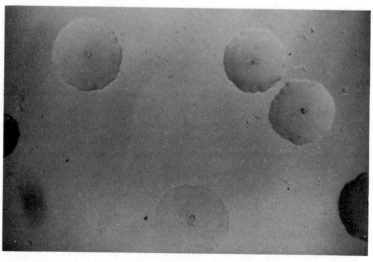

is not the receptor site. T-strains *(Ureaplasma urealyticum)* produce very small colonies on solid media and split urea.

These species are associated with disease in humans and have been isolated from the oropharynx *(M. pneumoniae)* and the genitourinary tract (particularly *M. hominis* and T-strains). Other species associated with humans include *M. orale* and *M. salivarium* in the oropharynx and *M. fermentans* in the genitourinary tract.

Infections

Pneumonia (primary atypical pneumonia; PAP)

Pneumonia caused by *M. pneumoniae* occurs worldwide, but outbreaks are recorded most often in schools, military installations and universities. It most frequently affects persons 5–25 years old, in contrast to pneumococcal pneumonia, which occurs at the extremes of life, and respiratory syncytial and parainfluenza virus infections, which are most prevalent in pre-school-age children. The incubation period varies from 3 to 4 weeks with an onset of sore throat, cough, malaise, fever and nonpleuritic chest pains. Chest roentgenograms show patchy bronchopneumonic infiltrates persisting for several days. Earache due to mycoplasmal infection of the tympanic membrane (myringitis) is a common complication. An exanthem that lasts 7–14 days and involvement of the central nervous system have been reported; pathogenesis of these neurologic sequellae is unclear. Pathologically, there is a thickening of bronchiolar walls due to infiltration of lymphocytes, macrophages and plasma cells, and the alveoli are infiltrated with mononuclear cells. In addition to pneumonia, the mycoplasmae can cause pharyngitis, tracheobronchitis and otitis media. There have also been reports implicating *M. pneumoniae* as the etiologic agent of arthritis. Clinically, none of the above infections can be differentiated from those due to other bacteria or viruses; thus a specific diagnosis of a *Mycoplasma* infection depends on the results of laboratory procedures. *Coxiella, Chlamydia,* respiratory viruses and, under certain conditions, other bacteria can cause clinically similar respiratory infections.

Genitourinary Infections

M. hominis and *Ureaplasma urealyticum* colonize the genitourinary tracts, particularly of women. These mycoplasma have thus been associated with nongonococcal urethritis in men and vaginitis, cervicitis, salpingitis, septic abortion, infertility and stillbirths in women. Subcutaneous abscesses and conjunctivitis have been reported in neonates. However, the exact etiologic role is presently tenuous because of conflicting epidemiologic and clinical studies.

Mechanisms of Pathogenicity

The mechanism by which *M. pneumoniae* causes disease is not clear. The organisms do not invade tissue but adsorb preferentially to ciliated epithelium. The spherule-shaped microorganisms have a tip-like structure by which they attach to a neuramidinase-sensitive site on the respiratory epithelium. The organisms then lose their spherule shape and become filamentous. Within 24 hours after adsorption, there is a decrease in RNA and protein synthesis in the epithelial cells, followed by a loss of ciliary activity and loss of the apical portion of the ciliated epithelium. The means by which ciliary activity is lost and cytotoxicity is produced is unknown. Clearly, attachment is a key step as avirulent cells, which do not attach, do not cause cellular changes. The metabolic alterations and cytopathology may be due to perturbation in host membrane, competition between the mycoplasma and host cell for nutrients, transfer of "toxic" products to the host cell or the effect of mycoplasma enzymes on host cell membrane. In tissue cultures arginine is depleted by *M. pneumoniae*, suggesting a nutritional effect.

Membranes of virulent *M. pneumoniae* have been reported to be cytotoxic. *M. pneumoniae* produces beta-hemolysis due to production of peroxide. It is suggested that the peroxide may play a role in the pathogenesis of disease by altering the surface of epithelial cells, but proof is lacking.

Ureaplasma urealyticum (T-strains) produces urease, and some work suggests that ammonia produced by the action of urease is responsible for cytotoxicity, i.e., ciliostasis, loss of cilia and loss of epithelium.

Prevention and Treatment

Killed and attenuated vaccines have been used to prevent mycoplasmal infections. Antibody is produced and protection against bronchitis and pneumonia has been reported. Vaccination also reduced the hospital stay in immunized volunteers who contracted pneumonia.

Tetracyclines and erythromycin are the antibiotics of choice for mycoplasmal infections. The mycoplasmae may persist after treatment but the disease is eliminated. Because the mycoplasmae lack cell walls, penicillin and congeners are not effective.

Laboratory Procedures

The materials usually collected include throat swabs, sputum, throat washings, joint fluids, urine or urethral swabs. As the mycoplasmae are very susceptible to drying, the swabs should be placed in Stuart's transport medium containing penicillin.

The medium used for cultivation is a heart infusion broth or agar, containing serum, yeast extract, thallium acetate and penicillin. The specimens are inoculated into broth and diphasic medium (agar slant covered with broth) and incubated at 37 C; subcultures are made onto agar plates from both media at 4, 7, 14, 21, and 28 days. In 4 to 7 days the colonies will be 0.05–0.6 mm in diameter and will have a dense central area surrounded by a less dense periphery, giving the colony a "fried egg" appearance. M. pneumoniae colonies often lack the peripheral zone. T-strains form small (15–20 μm) colonies and grow best in a 95% N–5% CO_2 atmosphere.

Identification is made by the growth inhibition test using species-specific antisera. The unknown culture is streaked onto the surface of an agar plate, and disks impregnated with specific antisera are placed on the agar surface. After 4 to 7 days of incubation there will be a zone of no growth 5 mm or larger around the disk containing the antiserum specific for the unknown isolate. The direct fluorescent antibody procedure can also be used for identification. M. pneumoniae will differentially absorb to guinea pig erythrocytes. This is demonstrated by flooding a plate with an erythrocyte suspension; after 15 minutes, the colonies are washed with dilute Dienes stain and examined microscopically to determine if the erythrocytes are adsorbed to the Mycoplasma colonies. M. pneumoniae will also reduce tetrazolium.

Serologic tests

The procedure of choice is the complement fixation test using a killed suspension of Mycoplasma. The patient's serum is collected during the acute and convalescent stages of the infection; a fourfold increase in titer is diagnostic. Other serologic procedures include the indirect hemagglutination, mycoplasmacidal and radioimmunoprecipitation test. Of historical interest are the streptococcal MG agglutination (chap. 5) and the cold hemagglutination tests. Positive reactions are due to antibodies stimulated by an antigen common to M. pneumoniae, Streptococcus MG and group O red cells. These two procedures were the principal serologic tests for primary atypical pneumonia until it was shown that similar agglutinins were demonstrable in other types of infections, and that the tests were positive in only half of the proven cases of M. pneumoniae infections.

PROBLEM SOLVING AND REVIEW

No. 1. GIVEN:—A 6-year-old girl was brought into the emergency room with tearing, redness and some exudate in the right eye. She had been complaining for some time and had been told she had a mild "pink eye," but eye drops containing an antibiotic brought no relief. Instead, the tearing and inflammation became progressively worse and blurring and difficulty with vision developed. The eye examination revealed both follicular and papillary hypertrophy, and with magnification a micropannus was detectable. Scrapings were obtained from the lid and stained with Giemsa; there were some possible intracellular inclusions but they were not definitely identifiable. Blood was taken to determine the antibody titer. The girl was from Taiwan and had moved to this country with her family about 2 years previously. The father had complained of an intermittent urethral discharge during the previous few months and the mother indicated she had had some vaginal discharge during the preceding 2 years; these had been attributed to the use of tap water from the city. All three family members were started on oral tetracyclines, and two younger children were scheduled for periodic eye examinations.

PROBLEMS:— 1. What is the probable cause of the eye disease? What is the name of the disease? What causes "pink eye"? 2. How was the infection probably contracted? Could tap water have been the source? 3. What additional laboratory procedures could be done? 4. How can the organism be cultured and identified? Is it a bacterium, virus or rickettsia? (Ans. p. 425.)

No. 2. GIVEN:—A 20-year-old male student was transferred to the hospital because of progressive pneumonia. Ten days before admission he had developed fever, malaise and a nonproductive cough. He was given oral penicillin but had been admitted because of persistent fever (40.6 C), chills and a right perihilar infiltrate. He had rales over the right upper thorax. The white blood cell count was 8,000/cu mm (62% polymorphonuclears, 8% bands and 30% lymphocytes). Sputum smear was nondiagnostic. He was treated with chloramphenicol for 2 days and then tetracycline for 1 day. His temperature remained elevated; he developed pleuritic pain and the sputum became blood tinged. At this point he was transferred to another hospital. Findings were similar to those previously reported.

PROBLEM:— 1. What specimens should be sent to the laboratory? Any special request? 2. The cultures were reported as negative; the ɔre-immune serum was 1:2 for *M. pneumoniae* (complement fixation) ɪnd 1:64 on the convalescent serum. What is your diagnosis? 3. What ₅s the drug of choice? 4. What bacterial factors might be related to the ɟisease and its symptoms? 5. What two strains of *Mycoplasma* are ⁻ound as normal flora? (Ans. p. 426.)

SUPPLEMENTARY READING

ɔaldwell, H. D., and Kuo, C.-C.: Serologic diagnosis of lymphogranuloma venereum by counter immunoelectrophoresis with a *Chlamydia trachomatis* protein antigen, J. Immunol. 118:442–445, 1977.

ɔrawford, Y. E.: *A Laboratory Guide to the Mycoplasmas of Human Origin*, Great Lakes, Ill.: NAMRU-4, 1972.

ɔenney, F. W., Clyde, W. A., and Glezen, W. P.: *Mycoplasma pneumoniae* disease: Clinical spectrum, pathophysiology, epidemiology and control, J. Infect. Dis. 123:74–92, 1971.

ɔrayston, J. T., and Wang, S.: New knowledge of chlamydiae and the diseases they cause, J. Infect. Dis. 132:87–105, 1975.

ɟu, P. C., Collier, A. M., and Baseman, J. B.: Interaction of virulent *Mycoplasma pneumoniae* with hamster tracheal organ cultures, Infect. Immun. 14:217–224, 1976.

ʋaniloff, J., and Morowitz, H. J.: Cell biology of the mycoplasma, Bacteriol. Rev. 36:263–290, 1972.

ʋcCormack, W. M., Brauan, P., Lee, Y., Klein, J. O., and Kass, E. H.: The genital mycoplasmas, N. Engl. J. Med. 288:78–89, 1973.

ʋoulder, J. W., Hatch, T. P., Byrne, G. I., and Kellogg, K. R.: Immediate toxicity of high multiplication of *Chlamydia psittaci* for mouse fibroblasts (L cells), Infect. Immun. 14:277–289, 1976.

ʀazin, S.: The mycoplasmas, Microbiol. Rev. 42:414, 1978.

ʃchachter, J.: Chlamydial infections, N. Engl. J. Med. 298:428, 1978.

ʃchachter, J., Hanna, L., Hill, E. C., Massad, S., Sheppard, C. W., Conte, J. E., Cohen, S. N., and Meyer, K. F.: Are chlamydial infections the most prevalent venereal disease? J.A.M.A. 231:1252–1255, 1975.

ʃtorz, J.: *Chlamydia and Chlamydial-Induced Diseases* (Springfield, Ill.: Charles C Thomas, Publisher, 1971).

ANALYSIS

NO. 1.–1. *Chalmydia trachomatis. Trachoma. Haemophilus aegyptius.* 2. Probably by hands or fomites contaminated by one or both parents. There is no evidence of transmission by water. 3. The tears could be tested for antibodies and eyelid smears examined by the direct fluorescent antibody technique; the serum antibody titer in this patient was 1:64 for type B. 4. Material from the eyelids or exudate is collected on swabs and inoculated into the yolk sac of embryonated eggs or irradiated McCoy tissue culture cells. After several passages, the organism is identified by the presence of cytoplasmic inclusions and by FA. It is a bacterium because it contains ribosomes and a cell wall and reproduces by binary fission.

No. 2. – 1. Throat culture, sputum, bronchial washings and blood. 2. *M. pneumoniae* pneumonia. 3. Tetracycline or erythromycin. 4. Production of a ciliostatic factor. 5. *Mycoplasma hominis, Mycoplasma salivarius, Mycoplasma orale.*

23 / Bacteria Rarely Encountered

OVERVIEW

There are a number of microorganisms rarely encountered in clinical practice and, unfortunately, seldom considered in differential diagnosis. However, this does not detract from their importance because they often pose diagnostic problems and can cause death.

Recently, an outbreak of respiratory illness occurred and after much effort directed toward isolating microorganisms, a bacterium was isolated. There is now evidence that this "rare" and new organism probably has been involved in other respiratory disease outbreaks.

ORGANISM CAUSING LEGIONNAIRES' DISEASE

The agent responsible for Legionnaires' disease is a pleomorphic, gram-negative rod ($0.3-0.4 \times 2-3$ μm). The rods may be up to 20 μm long and are often curved, and the cells are frequently vacuolated (Fig. 23-1). These organisms were initially recovered by inoculating a guinea pig intraperitoneally with suspensions of lung from patients who had died from pneumonia. The organism was then cultured from embryonated eggs and on a few occasions directly from human lung tissue on Mueller and Hinton agar supplemented with 1% hemoglobin and 1% IsoVitaleX. Growth was not obtained on trypticase soy or blood agar not in thioglycollate broth.

Antisera have been prepared using organisms from the yolk sac. The antiserum is specific for the organism and can be used to detect the organism in tissue by the indirect immunofluorescence test and for measuring serologic response in patients.

Legionnaires' disease is a pneumonia that was first noted in a group attending the 1976 convention of the American Legion in Philadelphia. The epidemic of 180 cases of respiratory disease affected 148 conventioneers and 31 nonconventioneers. The case fatality rate was 29% in those with preexisting illness, such as cardiopulmonary disease, diabetes and malignancy, and 5% for those without pre-

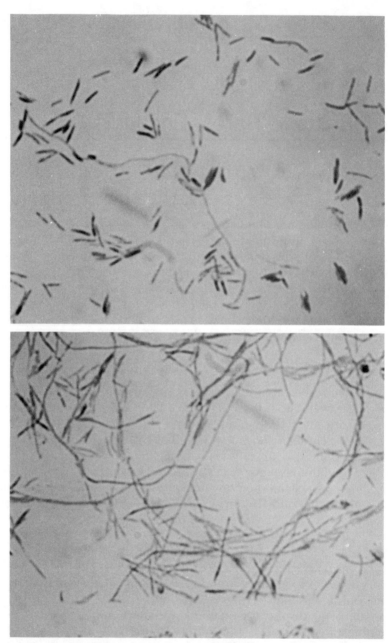

Fig. 23–1.—Stained smears of two isolates of the organism responsible for Legionnaire's disease. Note the pleomorphism and uneven staining. (Courtesy of Dr. Robert E. Weaver, Clinical Bacteriology Branch, Center for Disease Control, Atlanta.)

existing disease. The organism is not spread from person to person but is probably spread via air or water.

The disease begins 2–10 days after exposure with initial symptoms of malaise, muscle aches and a slight headache. Within a day after onset of the disease, the patient has a rapidly rising temperature and shaking chills. The temperature may increase to 39–41 C. A leukocytosis may be found. A nonproductive cough is reported, which with progression of the disease becomes productive. The sputum is not usually purulent. Chest roentgenograms show a patchy interstitial infiltrate or areas of consolidation that may increase in size. Pleural effusions were minimal in the Legionnaires' epidemic. Overall mortality is about 15% with death due to respiratory failure or shock. The mechanism of pathogenicity is not known.

There is serologic evidence that an antigenically similar bacterium was responsible for earlier outbreaks of disease in Pontiac, Michigan (Pontiac fever), the District of Columbia and Philadelphia. Epidemics of pneumonia, apparently caused by the same bacterium isolated from patients with Legionnaires' disease, have been reported in at least 11 states and from other countries. Pontiac fever differs clinically from Legionnaires' disease in that it is an acute febrile illness without pneumonia.

The organism is not resistant to antibiotics. In vitro determination of minimal inhibitory levels showed only resistance to vancomycin and borderline resistance to tetracycline and methicillin. The case fatality rates in patients treated with tetracycline or erythromycin were low. Clinical studies, in vitro testing and protection studies in infected eggs and guinea pigs suggest that erythromycin is the drug of choice.

There are no firm guidelines for isolating and identifying this unnamed organism. There have been only a few reports of direct isolation from pleural fluid or lung tissue. Tissue should be inoculated intraperitoneally into guinea pigs. One to two days after inoculation, the guinea pigs develop a febrile illness characterized by watery eyes and prostration. Guinea pig spleen tissue from moribund animals should then be inoculated into the yolk sac of 7-day-old embryonated eggs. Four to six days after inoculation, the yolk sacs from dead eggs can be smeared and stained by the Gimenez method and observed for bacilli.

Cultures of sputums, transtracheal aspirates, bronchial washings, tissue from the patient and infected animals should be done on Mueller-Hinton agar with 1% hemoglobin and 1% IsoVitaleX. After several passages on agar, growth can be obtained in 48 to 72 hours. Incubation should be at 35 C in 5% CO_2 for 10 days. The organism can be best visualized in tissue by the Dieterle-silver impregnation technique.

Antibody in paired serums can be determined using smears of the infected yolk sac and indirect immunofluorescence. The organism can also be identified by indirect immunofluorescence.

AEROMONAS AND PLESIOMONAS

The genus *Aeromonas* contains three species of gram-negative, non-spore-forming rods: *A. hydrophila, A. punctata* and *A. salmonicida. Plesiomonas shigelloides* was at one time considered a species of *Aeromonas*; but, because of biochemical differences and differences in number and distribution of flagella, it was placed in a different species. All except *A. salmonicida* have been associated with human disease.

The aeromonads and *Plesiomonas* are found in soil and water; they cause infections of fish, frogs, snakes and lizards. The source of infection for man is usually water, but infections associated with soil contamination and puncture wounds have been reported.

These organisms are associated with many different diseases: meningitis; endocarditis; infection of skin, soft tissue, muscle and bone; and a cholera-like diarrhea. Strains associated with cholera-like disease are enteropathogenic as measured by the ileal-loop reaction. In most cases, infections from this group of organisms are limited, but sepsis with a mortality rate slightly over 50% has been reported. Sepsis usually occurs in compromised patients, with the source usually being organisms from the gastrointestinal tract.

Treatment of these infections has generally been sulfamethoxazole-trimethoprim. Chloramphenicol and gentamicin have been used in meningitis. The organisms are sensitive in vitro to a number of antibiotics.

OTHER BACTERIA

Actinobacillus actinomycetemcomitans is a nonmotile, gram-negative rod that forms an adherent colony with a darkened, "star-like" area in the center. It has been isolated from patients with actinomycosis in which it is closely associated with the sulfur granules of *Actinomyces israelii*. In addition, it has been isolated from patients with endocarditis and abscesses, including those of the brain. Humans have usually been successfully treated by surgical drainage plus ampicillin.

Bartonella bacilliformis is a motile, pleomorphic, gram-negative rod that is difficult to culture. In Giemsa-stained smears from the blood of infected humans, the organism is present in or on the red blood cells. The organism is found in man and in the arthropod vector *Phlebotomus*. Bartonellosis (Carrión's disease) occurs at elevations of 2,500–8,000 feet above sea level in the Andes of Columbia, Ecuador and Peru. It is transmitted by the sand fly, *Phlebotomus* spp., and occurs in two clinical forms. Oroya fever is a febrile, hemolytic anemia in which the organisms are readily demonstrable on the red cells in stained smears. Verruca peruana, the cutaneous form, is characterized by the development of generalized reddish purple, vascular papules that may recur over periods of several months. The cutaneous form may follow Oroya fever. If the disease is not treated, mortality is about 40%, but verruca peruana responds well to antibiotics such as penicillin and tetracyclines. However, as concurrent *Salmonella* infections are common, chloramphenicol is the drug of choice.

Calymmatobacterium granulomatis (Donovania granulomatis) is a gram-negative, encapsulated, nonmotile rod that is morphologically similar and antigenically related to *Klebsiella pneumoniae*. Initial cultivation is possible in the yolk sac of the chick embryo, but the organ-

Fig. 23–2.—Perianal granuloma inguinale which appears as a red, elevated granulomatous lesion. Smears of this lesion were positive for Donovan bodies. (Courtesy of J. Goldberg, Community and Family Practice, Stritch School of Medicine, Loyola University.)

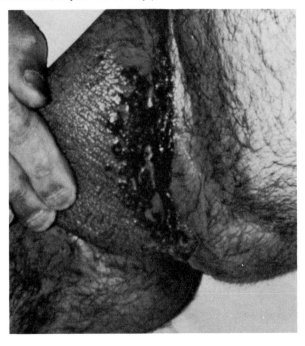

ism can then be transferred to blood agar or other special mediums. It causes the venereal disease granuloma inguinale, which begins as a painless genital nodule, and then ulcerates and spreads by direct extension to involve adjacent areas of the skin about the genitals and groin. Anal lesions can also occur (Fig. 23–2). Scrapings or punch biopsy specimens from these lesions stained with Wright's stain show the encapsulated rods within large mononuclear cells which are called Donovan bodies; this is the principal means of diagnosis (Fig. 23–3). Antigenic extracts from the organisms give a positive skin and complement fixation test, but the antigens are not readily available so the tests are not usually done. Tetracyclines and erythromycin are the antibiotics of choice. Penicillin is not effective.

Erysipelothrix rhusiopathiae is a gram-positive rod with a tendency to form long, nonbranching filaments. It does not produce a capsule or flagella and it is one of the few gram-positive bacteria to form H_2S in triple sugar iron medium. It causes the disease erysipeloid. Man contracts erysipeloid through contact with fish, shellfish, swine (the cause

Fig. 23–3.—Smear from granuloma inguinale stained with Wright's stain. Note the encapsulated *Calymmatobacterium granulomatis*. These "Donovan bodies" are located within the large mononuclear leukocyte. (Courtesy of J. Goldberg, Community and Family Practice, Stritch School of Medicine, Loyola University.)

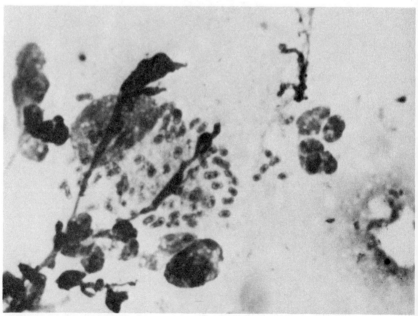

of swine erysipelas), poultry, bones, shells or hides, with the organisms entering the skin through cuts or abrasions. It is an occupational disease in buttonmakers, fishmongers, butchers and furriers. At the site of inoculation, usually the hands, a purplish red area of inflammation develops which spreads over adjacent areas and has a raised advancing edge. As the lesion spreads, the central portion heals. Unlike erysipelas, there is no lymphadenitis or lymphangitis. The infection is usually self-limiting or subsides in about 3 weeks. A bacteremia may occur, resulting in a septic arthritis or endocarditis. Penicillin is the antibiotic of choice.

Flavobacterium spp. are gram-negative, usually motile rods (often long and thin) that form pigmented colonies on solid media. They are widely distributed in soil, water and vegetable matter. Most species do not grow at 37 C and are thus not associated with humans. *F. meningosepticum* can cause meningitis and bacteremia, particularly of newborns or infants. This organism is nonmotile, produces a yellow colony and ferments a number of carbohydrates with acid, not gas; acid production may be delayed several days. On blood agar the organism produces a greenish discoloration around the colony.

Streptobacillus moniliformis is a gram-negative, nonmotile rod, forming nonbranching filaments that frequently have a series of bulbous swellings (*moniliformis* means necklace-shaped). In culture, this organism can spontaneously convert to L-forms (chap. 2) ("L" named for the Lister Institute). Isolation of *S. moniliformis* requires a medium enriched with blood or serum; in serum broth the organisms form characteristic "puffball" colonies. They have been isolated from rats, mice, weasels, cats and turkeys. *S. moniliformis* causes an arthritis in mice and turkeys; in humans it causes rat bite fever and is transmitted through rat bites, but bites of other animals have been implicated. This means of transmission is more likely to occur in children and in areas of crowding and poor sanitation. The bite usually heals but within a week the individual develops fever, chills, malaise with regional lymphadenitis and a generalized rash. About half the patients develop a nonsuppurative migrating polyarthritis. Endocarditis, pneumonia or brain abscesses can occur. Blood cultures are the laboratory procedure of choice. Agglutinin titers of 1:80 are an aid to diagnosis. Penicillin or tetracyclines are effective for treatment. The term *Haverhill fever* (after a milk-borne epidemic in Haverhill, Mass.) is applied to cases in which an animal bite cannot be established. Foods contaminated by mice or rats are the presumed source. Rat bite fever can also be caused by *Spirillum minus*, in which the history and symptoms are almost identical to streptobacillary fever, except that arthritis does not occur. This infection is also called Sodoku. This organism has not yet been cultivated.

Chromobacterium violaceum is a motile, gram-negative coccobacillary rod (0.6–0.9 × 1.5–3.0 μm) that may or may not produce a violet pigment. All strains isolated from humans with infection are pigmented, but experimental studies show that nonpigmented strains are as virulent for mice as the pigmented strains. The organism has been isolated from soil and water.

About 20 cases of human infection have been reported. The infection usually begins as a skin lesion or appears as a localized adenitis that rapidly progresses to overwhelming sepsis with necrotizing metastatic lesions. The organisms can be isolated from the initial lesion and from blood cultures.

SUPPLEMENTARY READING

Block, P. J., Fox, A. C., Yoran, C., and Kaltman, A. J.: *Actinobacillus actinomycetemcomitans* endocarditis: Report of a case and review of literature, Am. J. Med. Sci. 266:387–392, 1973.

Chandler, F. W., Hicklin, M. D., and Blackman, J. A.: Demonstrations of the agent of Legionnaires' disease in tissue, N. Engl. J. Med. 297:1218–1220, 1977.

Davis, W. A., Kane, J. G. and Garagusi, V. F.: Human aeromonas infections: A review of the literature and a case report of endocarditis, Medicine 57:267, 1978.

Fraser, D. W., et al.: Legionnaires' disease. Description of an epidemic of pneumonia, N. Engl. J. Med. 297:1189–1197, 1977.

Goldberg, J.: Studies on granuloma inguinale. IV. Growth requirements of *Donovania granulomatis* and its relationship to the natural habitat of the organism, Br. J. Vener. Dis. 35:266–268, 1959.

Grieco, M. H., and Sheldon, C.: *Erysipelothrix rhusiopathiae*, Ann. N.Y. Acad. Sci. 174:523–532, 1970.

King, E. O.: Studies of a group of previously unclassified bacteria associated with meningitis in infants, Am. J. Clin. Pathol. 31:241–247, 1959.

McDade, J. E., et al.: Legionnaires' disease. Isolation of a bacterium and demonstration of its role in other respiratory diseases, N. Engl. J. Med. 297:1197–1203, 1977.

Page, M. I., and King, E. O.: Infection due to *Actinobacillus actinomycetemcomitans* and *Haemophilus aphrophilus*, N. Engl. J. Med. 275:181–188, 1966.

Roughgarden, J. W.: Actinomicrobial therapy of rat-bite fever, Arch. Intern. Med. 116:39–54, 1965.

Schultz, M. G.: A history of bartonellosis (Carrión's disease), Am. J. Trop. Med. Hyg. 17:503–515, 1968.

Simerkoff, M. S., and Rahal, J. J.: Acute and subacute endocarditis due to *Erysipelothrix rhusiopathiae*, Am. J. Med. Sci. 266:53–57, 1973.

OTHER BACTERIA 435

Siverda, R., and Tan, S. H.: Pathogenicity of non-pigmented cultures of *Chromobacterium violaceum*, J. Clin. Microbiol. 5:514–516, 1977.

Weinman, D.: Genus *Bartonella*, in Buchanan, R. E., and Gibbons, N. E. (eds.): *Bergey's Manual of Determinative Bacteriology* (Baltimore: Williams & Wilkins Co., 1974).

24 / Chemotherapeutic Agents, Disinfectants and Sterilization

OVERVIEW

The development and use of antibiotics and other chemical agents for the control of microorganisms has minimized man's fear of many devastating diseases which in the past seriously affected his quality of life and survival. Unfortunately, introduction of these agents has created some new problems in regard to increased resistance of the microorganisms and production of altered host reactions (hypersensitivity and toxicity) to the chemotherapeutic agent.

One of the major infectious disease problems today is nosocomial infections caused by resistant bacteria. This problem resulted in part from a relaxation in attitudes toward infectious agents and disease — a concomitant of the development of antibiotics and their use in effective control of diseases of man. Paralleling the development and increased usage of modern chemotherapeutic agents, came many other important advances in the technology and science of medical practice. Drugs that affect host metabolism and resistance are used to treat diseases such as cancer. In addition, procedures that require use of intravenous and urinary catheters, prosthetic devices, and other instrumentation to maintain and prolong life became part of the armamentarium regularly used by the physicians. These procedures carry some risk of infection by introducing organisms into susceptible host tissue, by affecting host resistance, or both. Attempts to control these infections by use of antibiotics — in particular, indiscriminate use — compounded the problem by producing hypersensitivity to the antibiotics, drug toxicity, and selection of resistant forms. Thus the control of microorganisms in the hospital has become increasingly important and complicated in recent years.

To minimize these problems necessitates a return to basic concepts of disinfection and sterilization and requires knowledge of mechanisms of action and the pharmacology of the useful antibiotics. Most chemicals used to control and treat bacterial infections are relatively safe, provided one understands their properties and proper use. Chemotherapy is a multiedged sword, and rational use requires knowledge of toxicologic, pharmacologic and microbiologic properties.

INTRODUCTION

Definitions

The terminology used in describing the effects of physical and chemical agents on bacteria is confusing because of different meanings associated with these terms. Sterilization results in the complete absence of life, and this term should be used only when all viable forms (including viruses) are removed or killed. Often the term *sterilization* is applied to the use of antibiotics in preparation of the intestinal tract prior to surgery. This is incorrect usage because, at best, bacterial numbers may be decreased and some species eliminated by chemotherapy, but sterilization is not obtained.

Disinfectants in the classic sense are chemical agents that kill microbial cells and are used on inanimate objects such as table tops and certain instruments. Antiseptics are chemical agents that inhibit growth of pathogenic bacteria and are used on tissue in order to prevent sepsis or infection. In some cases a chemical can be used both as a disinfectant and as an antiseptic. Neither disinfectants nor antiseptics achieve sterilization.

In choosing a chemical agent for use as an antiseptic, disinfectant or chemotherapeutic agent, it is important to determine if the action is bacteriostatic or bactericidal. Bacteriostasis is the inhibition of growth; the organisms are viable and under conditions where the agent is removed or neutralizing compounds added, the organism will grow and reproduce. However, bactericidal agents result in death of the cell, an irreversible effect.

Characteristics

Many substances have been described which are effective inhibitors of microbial functions. Yet only a relatively small group of these compounds are effective in controlling bacterial growth and replication. The following discussion touches on some of the characteristics that determine usefulness of a substance as a disinfectant, antiseptic or chemotherapeutic agent.

Bacterial Factors

To affect the intact cell, the agent must reach a sensitive target site in the bacterial cell at a concentration sufficient to effect inhibition.

The cell surface is penetrated by passive diffusion, facilitated diffusion (carrier molecules), and active transport systems. Thus the chemical nature of the agent, i.e., partition coefficient, water solubility, degree of ionization and molecular size, as well as the properties of the bacterial cells, in particular, the selective properties of the cytoplasmic or inner membrane, determine whether the agent will reach a sensitive site. In addition to the cytoplasmic membrane, the outer membrane can also determine whether a cell will be sensitive or resistant. Mutants of gram-negative bacteria with changes in surface lipopolysaccharide, in either the lipid or carbohydrate portion, can have sensitivities that differ from those of the wild type of organism.

Some microorganisms can inactivate chemical agents. Enzymes such as B-lactamase (penicillinase), phosphorylases, adenylases and acetylases inactivate antibiotics by altering their structure and preventing them from reaching a sensitive site in a concentration level sufficient to inhibit the microorganism.

Host Factors

Several host factors are important in determining feasibility of a compound as a chemotherapeutic agent. First, it must be delivered to the site of infection, i.e., it must be adsorbed from the intestinal tract (if given orally) or be injectable, and it must reach concentrations at the site of infection sufficient to inhibit the microorganisms. The agent must be stable and not inactivated at the site of infection by pH or tissue fluids. Finally, for use as an antiseptic or chemotherapeutic, the agent must be selectively toxic for the microorganism. This means that at a concentration effective for inhibiting microbial growth in vivo it must not interfere in any major way with mammalian cell structure or function. Some chemotherapeutic agents are toxic for humans, but they are still valuable in treatment of disease. Use of these toxic agents requires monitoring the dose and observing closely the patient's response to the drug, e.g., neurologic functions, kidney and liver functions and hematologic parameters. In addition to primary toxicity for host cell function and structure, hypersensitivity can be produced and this may limit the agent's use.

CHEMOTHERAPEUTIC AGENTS

Chemotherapeutic agents are placed in two classes: (1) synthetic chemicals, such as the sulfonamides and isonicotinic acid hydrazide, and (2) antibiotics. Antibiotics are agents produced by other microorganisms. Many of the antibiotics in use today are now synthesized. Others, such as the penicillins, are semisynthetic in that the basal

TABLE 24-1.—MECHANISMS OF ANTIMICROBIAL ACTION

EFFECTS/ SITE OF ACTION	CHEMOTHERAPEUTIC AGENT	MODE OF ACTION
Cell wall	Bacitracin and vancomycin	Prevent polymerization of N-acetylmuramic acid and N-acetylglucosamine
	Cycloserine	Inhibits D-alanine racemase, D-alanyl-D-alanine synthetase, and consequently pentapeptide formation
	Penicillins and cephalosporins	Prevent transpeptidation and cross-linking of cell wall
Cell membrane: Nucleic acid synthesis and function:	Polymyxin B and colistin Rifampin	Act as cationic detergent Inhibits DNA-dependent RNA polymerase
	Nalidixic acid	Interferes with DNA template–DNA polymerase complex with cell membrane
Protein synthesis and structure:	Aminoglycosides (except spectinomycin) Spectinomycin Chloramphenicol and macrolides (erythromycin, clindamycin and lincomycin) Tetracycline Methenamine	Cause misreading of mRNA; interfere with initiation Prevents translocation Inhibit peptidyltransferase Inhibits binding of amino-acyl t-RNA Induces alkylation of proteins
Inhibitors of metabolism:	Sulfonamides, para-amino-salicylic acid, sulfones, diaminopyrimidines Isonicotinic acid hydrazide; ethambutol	Inhibit synthesis of folic acid Inhibit NAD synthesis; lipid synthesis

compound produced by the microorganism is used but it is altered chemically in order to produce an antimicrobial agent with different properties, i.e., better solubility, resistance to acid and inactivating enzymes.

Mode of Action

Chemotherapeutic agents affect microbial cells by (1) acting as an antimetabolite, (2) inhibiting cell wall formation, (3) damaging membranes, (4) inhibiting protein synthesis and (5) inhibiting RNA and DNA synthesis. Chemotherapeutic agents that act by inhibiting cell wall synthesis, cell membrane function, RNA synthesis or that interfere with protein synthesis by formation of nonsense proteins (aminoglycoside antibiotics) are bactericidal. The remainder are bacteriostatic. The mechanisms of antimicrobial actions are summarized in Table 24–1.

Synthetic Antimicrobial Agents

Inhibitors of Metabolism

Several synthetic chemicals function as inhibitors of essential metabolite production. Some of the important antibacterial drugs in this group are the sulfonamides, para-aminosalicyclic acid (PAS), sulfones, and a diaminopyrimidine (trimethoprim) (Fig. 24–1). These compounds all function by inhibiting the production of folic acid, which in its reduced form transfers one-carbon units required for synthesis of thymidine, the purines and several amino acids. Except for trimethoprim, these compounds inhibit the enzyme dihydropteroate synthase, which incorporates para-aminobenzoic acid (PABA) to form dihydropteroic acid and subsequently folic acid (Fig. 24–2). These chemotherapeutic compounds have a structure similar to PABA and compete for incorporation into folic acid. Folic acid is required by a number of microorganisms for synthesis of purines and pyrimidines, and growth of these stains is inhibited because the required compounds are not synthesized. Man requires exogenous folic acid and therefore selective toxicity is expressed. The action of these compounds is easily reversed by addition of PABA and tissue fluids.

Fig. 24–1.—Inhibitors of folic acid synthesis.

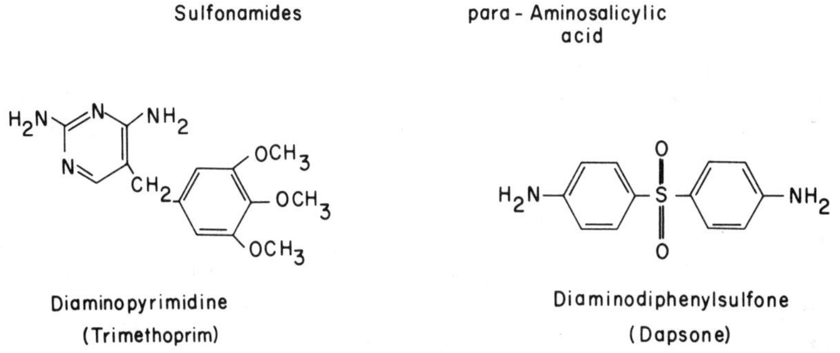

Sulfonamides

para - Aminosalicylic acid

Diaminopyrimidine (Trimethoprim)

Diaminodiphenylsulfone (Dapsone)

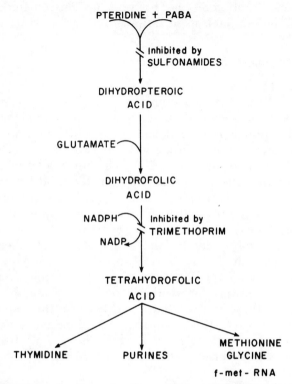

Fig. 24–2.—Sites of action of sulfonamides and trimethoprim in synthesis of tetrahydrofolate.

They are bacteriostatic agents. Some of the sulfonamides in use today are shown in Figure 24–3. The modification of the sulfonamide structure yields compounds that differ in solubility and are retained in vivo for shorter or longer periods of time. Some are used only topically.

Trimethoprim, a diaminopyrimidine, is a structural analogue of the pteridine part of dihydrofolic acid (see Fig. 24–1). It inhibits the enzyme dihydrofolic acid reductase (tetrahydrofolate dehydrogenase), which converts dihydrofolic acid to tetrahydrofolic acid. Trimethoprim is frequently used in combination with sulfamethoxazole. This combination is effective because two steps in the reaction sequence (see Fig. 24–2) leading to tetrahydrofolic acid are inhibited. This synergistic effect rapidly inhibits growth, and the effect may be bactericidal.

Isonicotinic acid hydrazide (INH) and ethionamide (Fig. 24–4), a

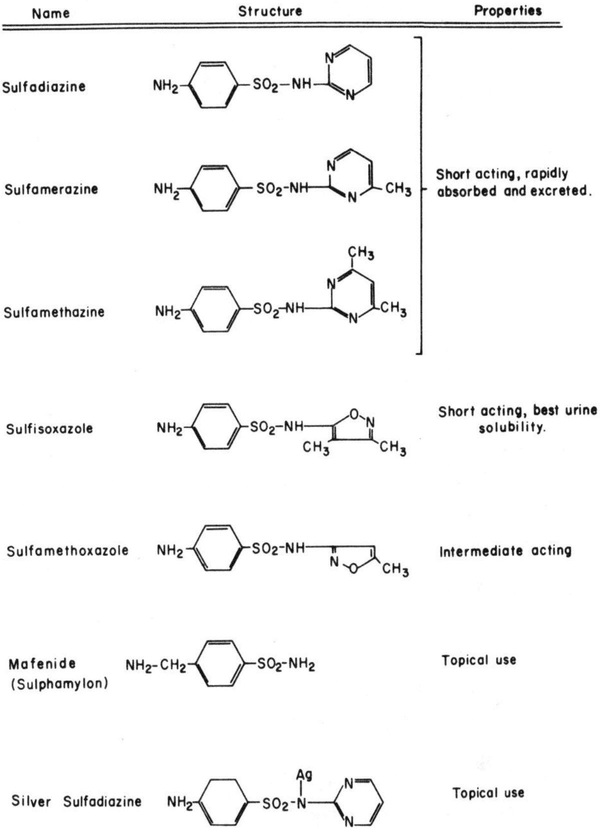

Name	Structure	Properties
Sulfadiazine		
Sulfamerazine		Short acting, rapidly absorbed and excreted.
Sulfamethazine		
Sulfisoxazole		Short acting, best urine solubility.
Sulfamethoxazole		Intermediate acting
Mafenide (Sulphamylon)		Topical use
Silver Sulfadiazine		Topical use

Fig. 24–3. — Sulfonamide derivatives: structure and properties.

Fig. 24–4. — Structures of isoniazid and ethionamide.

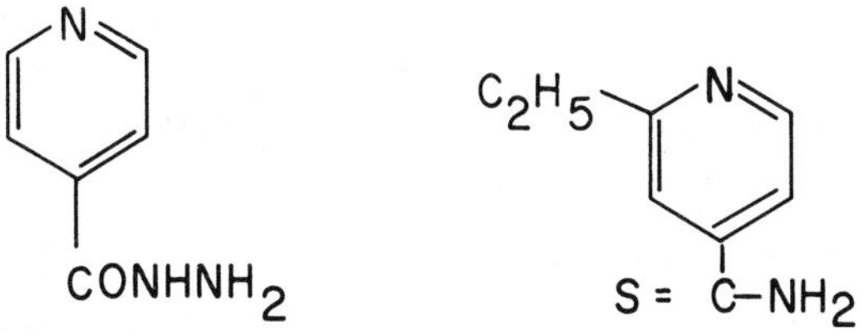

Isoniazid

Ethionamide

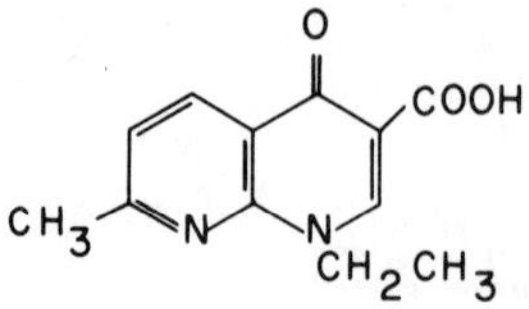

Nalidixic acid

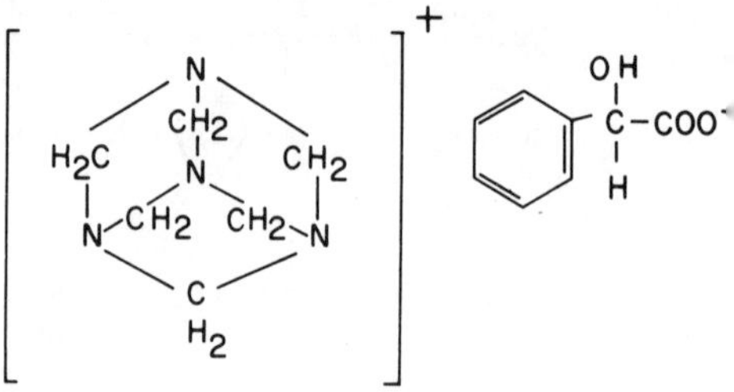

Methenamine mandelate

Fig. 24–5.—Structures of two chemotherapeutic agents used in treatment of urinary tract infections.

derivative of INH, are bactericidal drugs used in treatment of tuberculosis. Their mode of action is unclear, but they may be converted to isonicotinic acid, which is then incorporated into a nonfunctional analogue of NAD. INH also has been reported to interfere with lipid synthesis in *M. tuberculosis*.

Inhibitors of DNA Synthesis and Protein Function

Methenamine mandelate (Fig. 24–5) is a chemotherapeutic agent used as a urinary tract antiseptic. Methenamine itself does not inhibit bacteria, but as an acid pH it is hydrolyzed into ammonia and formaldehyde. The released formaldehyde alkylates proteins and is bactericidal. The functions of mandelic acid are to acidify urine, a requirement for hydrolysis of methenamine, and to maintain a low pH during hydrolysis and release of ammonia.

Nalidixic acid (see Fig. 24–5) is also used for urinary tract infections. It may inhibit DNA synthesis by interfering with an interaction between the DNA template–DNA polymerase complex and the cytoplasmic membrane.

Antibiotics

Two groups of microorganisms, the bacteria and fungi, produce antibiotics. Among the bacteria, the genera *Bacillus* and *Streptomyces* produce useful antibiotics; the fungal genera *Penicillium* and *Cephalosporium* are also important producers.

Inhibitors of Cell Wall Synthesis

Cell wall synthesis involves a series of biochemical events that are sensitive to a number of antibiotics. Because the protoplasmic osmotic pressure of the bacterial cytoplasm ranges from 5 atm in the gram-negative cell to 20 atm in the gram-positive cell, an alteration in the cell wall usually results in loss of cytoplasmic contents, a lethal or bactericidal effect.

One of the early steps in cell wall synthesis involves the addition of a pentapeptide to muramic acid. During this intracellular event L-alanine is first added to muramic acid. This is then followed by addition of the other amino acids with the final addition of D-alanyl-D-alanine. Cycoserine, a structural analogue of D-alanine (Fig. 24–6), inhibits (1) alanine racemase, which converts L-alanine to D-alanine, and (2) D-alanyl-D-alanine synthetase, which completes the terminal D-alanyl-D-alanine dipeptide. The pentapeptide is important because it is the point at which cross-linking of the peptidoglycan polymers takes place. The dipeptide of alanine is important because removal of the terminal D-alanine results in formation of energy required for cross-linking of the peptidoglycan, the final step in cell wall synthesis.

After synthesis of the linear peptide, a peptidoglycan polymer, consisting of muramic acid–pentapeptide and N-acetylglucosamine, is assembled to form a linear polymer. In this reaction a membrane phospholipid acts as a carrier for the disaccharide-pentapeptide to a cell wall acceptor (growing linear polymer). Vancomycin, a glycopeptide antibiotic, prevents transfer of the disaccharide-pentapeptide from the carrier to the cell wall acceptor and thereby prevents polymerization of the peptidoglycan polymer.

After transport to the cell wall acceptor and polymerization, the lipid pyrophosphate carrier must be hydrolyzed to lipid phosphate so that it can be available to again accept the muramic acid–N-acetylglucosamine pentapeptide and participate in further polymerization. Bacitracin, a polypeptide antibiotic, inhibits hydrolysis of the lipid pyrophosphate to lipid phosphate, thus preventing its reuse in mucopeptide synthesis.

Fig. 24–6.—Similarities in structure of D-cycloserine, an inhibitor of alanine incorporation during cell wall synthesis, and D-alanine.

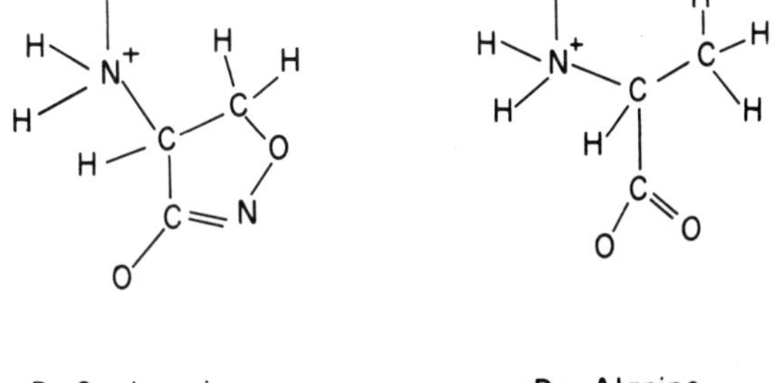

D-Cycloserine   D-Alanine

The final stage in synthesis of the cell wall is cross-linking of the linear peptidoglycan polymer to an adjacent polymer to give it rigidity. This reaction is a transpeptidation reaction and involves (1) cleavage of the terminal D-alanine to obtain energy for the reaction and (2) linkage via a pentaglycine bridge between the remaining D-alanine of one linear peptide and L-lysine on another linear peptide. The various penicillins and cephalosporins have a molecular configuration similar to D-alanyl-D-alanine, the two amino acids that make up the terminal end of the pentapeptide. Because of the similar structure, penicillin and the cephalosporins compete for the transpeptidase, thereby forming a complex with the enzyme. This results in inhibition of cross-link formation and an unstable cell wall. The structures of the penicillins and cephalosporins are similar (Fig. 24–7). The basic nucleus in the penicillin molecule is 6-amino-penicillanic acid and for cephalospor-

Fig. 24–7. — Structures of penicillin and cephalosporin.

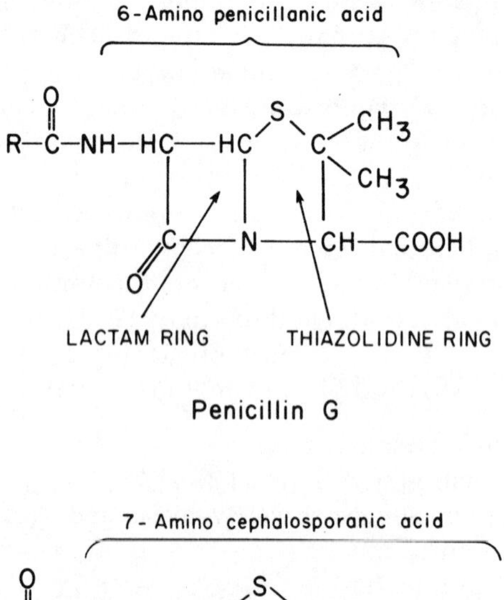

Penicillin G

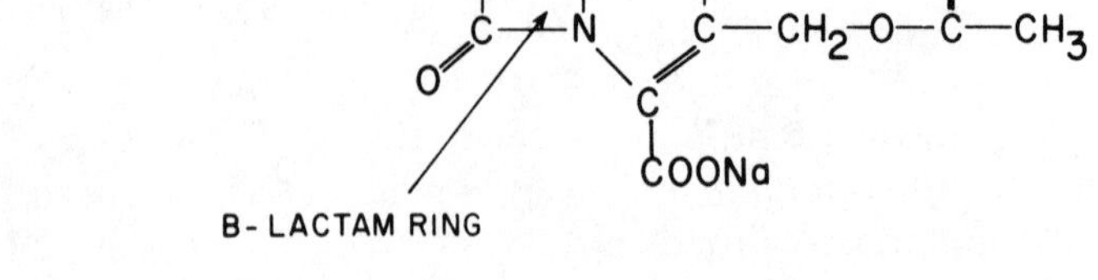

Cephalothin

	Side Chain	Stability in acid	Spectrum of action	β-lactamase Sensitivity (penicillinase)
Benzylpenicillin (Penicillin G)	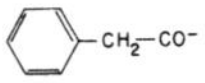 —CH₂—CO⁻	Unstable	Narrow	Sensitive
Phenoxymethyl penicillin (Pen V)	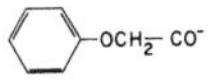 —OCH₂—CO⁻	Good	Narrow	Sensitive
Methicillin	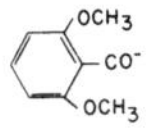 OCH₃ / CO⁻ / OCH₃	Unstable	Narrow	Resistant
Oxacillin	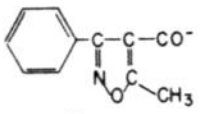 C—C—CO⁻ ... CH₃	Good	Narrow	Resistant
Dicloxacillin	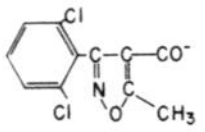 Cl ... C—C—CO⁻ ... CH₃	Good	Narrow	Resistant
Cloxacillin	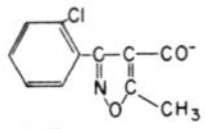 Cl ... C—C—CO⁻ ... CH₃	Good	Narrow	Resistant
Nafcillin	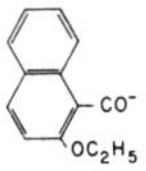 CO⁻ OC₂H₅	Poor	Narrow	Resistant
Ampicillin	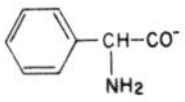 CH—CO⁻ NH₂	Fair	Broad	Sensitive
Amoxicillin	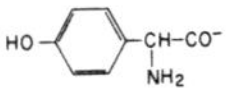 HO— CH—CO⁻ NH₂	Good	Broad	Sensitive
Carbenicillin	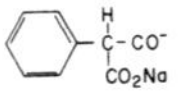 H ‖ C—CO⁻ CO₂Na	(not given orally)	Broad	Sensitive

Fig. 24–8.—Some characteristics of penicillin and semisynthetic derivatives.

in it is 7-amino-cephalosporonic acid. Both compounds contain a B-lactam ring, which is the determinant of antimicrobial activity. Splitting of this ring by acid or by a specific bacterial enzyme (B-lactamase) results in formation of an inactive compound. Modification of the side chains in both compounds results in a class of compounds with different chemical and biologic properties, i.e., resistance to acid, which permits oral administration, broad-spectrum activity and resistance to penicillinase (Fig. 24–8).

Agents Interfering with Cell Membrane Function

Two groups of antibiotics are in this group. One group, the polymyxins (polymyxin B and colistin), includes basic polypeptides produced by *Bacillus polymyxa*. The polymyxins bind to phosphate in the membrane phospholipids and act as cationic detergents. This results in disruption of the cell membrane and a bactericidal effect. The second group consists of the polyene antibiotics amphotericin B and

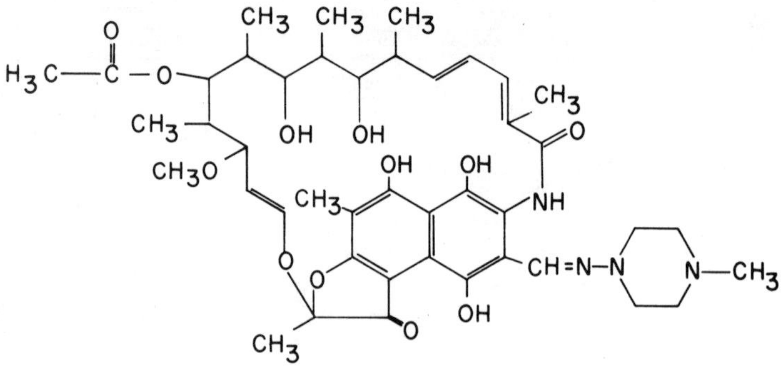

Rifampin

Fig. 24–9. — Structure of rifampin, an inhibitor of RNA synthesis.

nystatin, which are produced by actinomycetes. These compounds interact with eukaryotic membranes by binding to sterols. Except for the mycoplasma, bacteria do not contain sterols and are not susceptible to the polyene antibiotics. Polyenes are used in the treatment of fungal infection. Since the polyenes interact with eukaryotic membranes, they are toxic for humans.

Inhibitors of RNA Synthesis

Rifampin (Fig. 24–9) is an inhibitor of RNA synthesis which specifically affects the DNA-dependent RNA polymerase resulting in a bactericidal effect. The antibiotic does not affect the sigma factor, nor does it prevent binding of the polymerase to the DNA template. It apparently binds to the B subunit on the core enzyme and interferes with the initiation of RNA synthesis.

Inhibitors of Protein Synthesis

Protein synthesis is a complex chain of events with several major steps required for production of functional protein. These steps involve aminoacylation of transfer RNAs, messenger RNA readout in polysomes, and posttranslational modification of polypeptides. The major basis for the selective action of inhibitors of protein synthesis on microbes is the structural differences between bacterial and eukaryotic cell ribosomes. At the ribosome, the sequence of events for polypeptide synthesis is initiation, elongation and termination. Antibiotics that affect some of these steps are commonly used in chemotherapy. The effects of antibiotics on protein synthesis are somewhat variable, and this relates in part to concentration of antibiotic and the experimental system in which it is tested, and also to the difficulty in study-

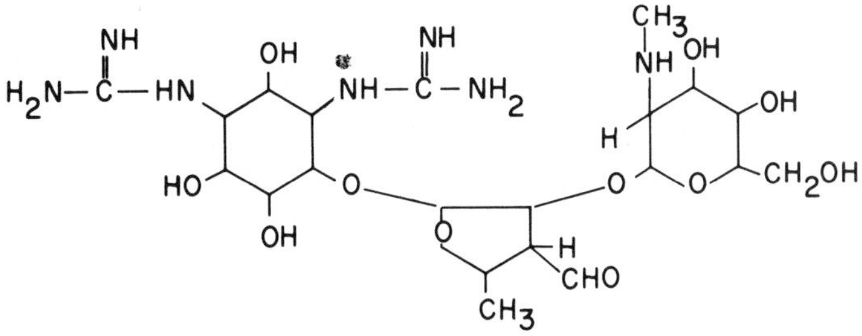

Streptomycin

Fig. 24–10. — Structure of streptomycin, an aminoglycoside antibiotic.

ing protein synthesis. Thus a given antibiotic may be shown to interfere at several steps. The major means by which commonly used antibiotics affect bacterial protein synthesis are described.

INITIATION. — The aminoglycoside antibiotics are large molecules that contain aminosugar residues connected by glycosidic bridges (Fig. 24 – 10). Included in this group are streptomycin, gentamicin, neomycin, kanamycin, tobramycin and amikacin. The modes of action are similar for each of the aminoglycosides. The aminoglycoside binds to a specific ribosomal protein and prevents an initiation complex with mRNA, an aminoacyl-tRNA and the initiation factors. Some work suggests that an initiation complex is formed but is "frozen in place," thereby preventing protein synthesis. The effect is on the 30S ribosomal subunit and is bactericidal.

MISREADING. — In addition to affecting initiation of protein synthesis, the aminoglycosides also affect elongation by causing a misreading of mRNA. This results in production of proteins with an incorrect amino acid sequence (nonsense proteins), which has a bactericidal effect.

ELONGATION. — After formation of the initiation complex, tRNAs carrying specific amino acids (aminoacyl-tRNA) attach to the decoding site on the 30S ribosome. The tetracyclines (Fig. 24 – 11) affect protein synthesis by inhibiting binding of aminoacyl-tRNA to the decoding site on the 30S ribosomal subunit. Tetracyclines also chelate with Mg^{2+}, but whether the binding with Mg^{2+} is related to the inhibition of aminoacyl-tRNA binding is unclear. The tetracyclines are bacteriostatic. Tetracyclines also inhibit protein synthesis in eukaryotic ribosomes but are more effective on prokaryotic cells.

Chloramphenicol, the macrolide antibiotic erythromycin, and both

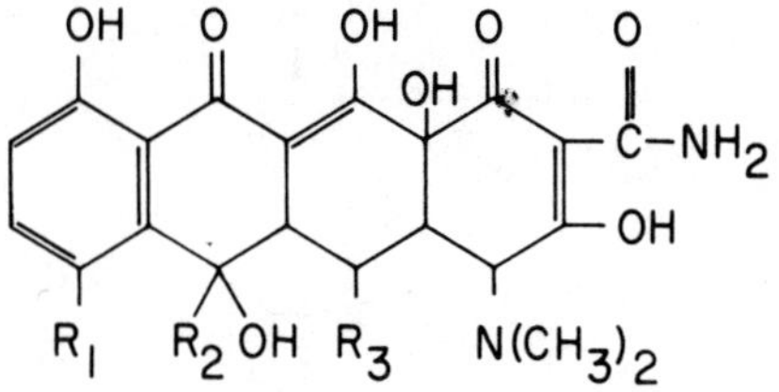
OH
O
OH
O
O
OH
C-NH2
OH
R1
R2 OH
R3
N(CH3)2

	R_1	R_2	R_3
Tetracycline	H	CH_3	H
Chlortetracycline	Cl	CH_3	H
Oxytetracycline	H	CH_3	OH
Demethylchlor-tetracycline	Cl	H	H

Fig. 24–11. – Structure of tetracycline group of antibiotics.

Fig. 24–12. – Inhibitors of peptide bond synthesis.

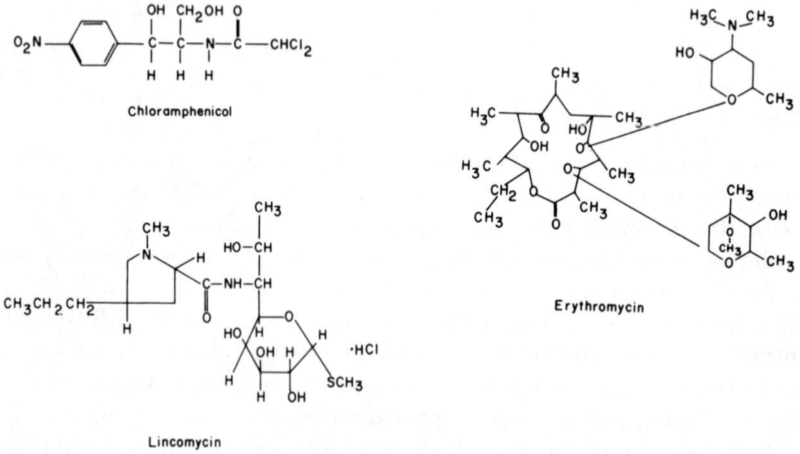
Chloramphenicol
Lincomycin
•HCl
Erythromycin

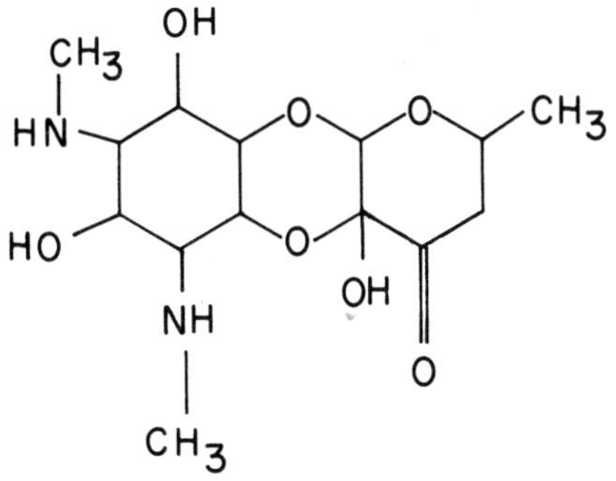

Fig. 24–13.—Structure of spectinomycin.

lincomycin and clindamycin (7-chloro-lincomycin) (Fig. 24–12) bind to the 50S subunit and inhibit peptide bond formation by inhibiting peptidyltransferase. The enzyme peptidyltransferase causes formation of a peptide bond between amino acids on the P and A sites and elongation.

Spectinomycin, an aminocyclitol, is classified as an aminoglycoside, but it is structurally and functionally different from other aminoglycosides (Fig. 24–13). Its bacteriostatic effect is exerted by inhibiting translocation, i.e., movement of the peptidyl-tRNA from the A site to the P site. This translocation is necessary for binding of an aminoacyl-tRNA at the A site and elongation of the peptide.

Resistance to Antibiotics

Resistance to antibiotics occurs either through adaptation, mutation or by transfer of genetic information from organisms of the same or different species. The major means of practical significance for development of resistance is through selection of mutants and by transfer of genetic information. Spontaneous mutation probably has little role in resistance because of the low frequency of mutation, but selection of resistant cells occurs through use of inadequate amounts of antibiotics. Under these conditions the resistant fraction of the bacterial population survives to fill the void. Plasmids with determinants for antibiotic resistance (R factor) are readily transferred from one species to another via transduction or conjugation. Transfer of resistance via plasmids is referred to as infectious drug resistance and can result in resistance to more than one type of antibiotic.

Resistance to antibiotics can be expressed in several ways (Table 24–2). Inactivation of a chemotherapeutic agent occurs by the action of specific enzymes coded for either by chromosomal genes or by plasmids. An enzyme, such as B-lactamase, inactivates penicillin by opening of the B-lactam ring. Acetyltransferases, phosphotransferases

TABLE 24-2.—PHENOTYPIC
EXPRESSION OF RESISTANCE

1. Inactivation of chemotherapeutic agent
2. Modification of sensitive site
3. Alteration of permeability
4. Increase in levels of inhibited pathway

or adenyltransferases inactivate antibiotics by enzymatically transferring a group (acetyl, phosphate and adenosine) to the antibiotic. In
some cases the sensitive binding site in the microbial cell may be
altered and result in resistance. This occurs in some organisms with
streptomycin resistance whereby the amino acids in a specific protein
in the 30S ribosomal subunit are altered. Binding of streptomycin
does not occur to the altered protein, and the antibiotic does not affect protein synthesis. Resistance to rifamycin is also expressed by
chromosomal mutation, which prevents binding of the antibiotic
to the DNA-dependent RNA polymerase.

Several mechanisms of resistance related to altered permeability to
the agent have been shown. Mutants of gram-negative rods with increased resistance to ampicillin have been reported in which resistance is associated with decreased permeability caused by changes in
the lipopolysaccharide in the outer membrane. Decreased permeability to the antibiotic may also be the result of an altered transport system. Mutants with decreased affinity of the condensing enzyme for
sulfonamide as well as mutants that produce large amounts of para-
aminobenzoate and folic acid have been isolated.

Examples of antibiotic resistance mediated by production of alternative metabolic routes or by development of a reduced requirement
for the product of the inhibited reaction have not been described for
the clinically useful chemotherapeutic compounds.

Cross-resistance to chemotherapeutic agents can exist between
antibiotics with both similar and different characteristics. In some
cases the chemical structures of the chemotherapeutic agents are similar and the mechanism responsible for resistance also affects these
similar structures. In other cases the binding sites or sites sensitive to
the chemotherapeutic agent are similar and resistance is expressed
between chemotherapeutic agents with different structures.

Considerations in Use of Chemotherapeutic Agents

Chemotherapeutic agents are probably the safest and best drugs
available to the physician for the treatment of infectious disease.

However, they are in many cases misused not only by the physician but also by the patient.

The sensitivity of the organisms (chap. 4) must be determined and used as a guide for selecting a chemotherapeutic agent in order to prevent use of an antibiotic to which the organism is resistant. The antibiotic should be chosen to specifically inhibit the isolated organism. Selection of an agent because it has broad-spectrum activity and unjustified use of antibiotic combinations only create additional problems such as resistant mutants or superinfection.

The use of low levels or inappropriate chemotherapeutic agents prior to obtaining a culture and a clinical diagnosis can impede diagnosis. In some cases aberrant forms (L-forms, large cocci, filaments) are induced, which complicates identification of the organism, and some of these aberrant forms are resistant to chemotherapy. For example, under appropriate conditions penicillin inhibits cell wall formation, but if the organism is in a part of the host where it can be protected against osmotic lysis, it can survive. Since it no longer has a cell wall it is not susceptible to inhibitors of cell wall synthesis. Further, the organisms will not be isolated by standard laboratory procedures, and the diagnosis can be confused.

Antibiotic combinations should be used only in selected circumstances, such as in treatment of infective endocarditis, anaerobic infections or tuberculosis. Penicillin and aminoglycoside combinations are proved effective for treatment of enterococcal endocarditis. Sulfonamides in combination with a diaminopyrimidine (sulfamethoxazole-trimethoprim) are effective particularly in treatment of some types of urinary tract infections. Combination therapy in tuberculosis is also used to prevent development of resistance. There is little evidence for use of other combinations of chemotherapeutic agents. Antibiotic combinations may be antagonistic, synergistic or additive in their effect on microorganisms; and, in the absence of prior clinical experience, these agents must be tested against the specific organism to prevent the use of antagonistic combinations. The axion to be remembered is "one drug—one bug."

In addition to determining sensitivity, the physician should determine the effect of the chemotherapeutic agent, that is, whether it is bacteriostatic or bactericidal. The latter drugs are important in serious infections such as infective endocarditis and diseases of the central nervous system and also in patients with a depressed immune system. Use of bacteriostatic agents requires participation of host factors to kill the microorganisms. In many patients, existing disease or treatment may reduce the efficiency of the immune system, resulting in poor patient response to a bacteriostatic agent.

The dose of antibiotic and the length of treatment are important. Inadequate doses serve to select resistant organisms from the population responsible for the infection or from the normal flora. Treatment for an inadequate length of time likewise selects resistant organisms and may result in relapse with the disease caused by a resistant microorganism. One of the problems associated with use of oral antibiotics is that patients often do not complete the therapy but stop the treatment when they feel better. Unfortunately, they may then self-prescribe the unused antibiotic at a later date.

Many chemotherapeutic agents are toxic and induce hypersensitivity. The levels of highly toxic drugs should be measured to minimize toxicity, and the appropriate tissue functions (kidney, liver, bone marrow) should be monitored to detect signs of toxicity. The patient's history should be obtained to determine if hypersensitivity exists or if the patient is likely to develop hypersensitivity. In some cases either testing for hypersensitivity should be done or the patient should be observed for symptoms of immediate hypersensitivity after administration and so treated. In patients with syphilis, leptospirosis, brucellosis and other diseases, treatment with antibiotics may result in a Jarisch-Herxheimer reaction. The mechanism is unknown, but it is related to release of microbial products and production of symptoms similar to those seen in endotoxin shock.

PHYSICAL AND CHEMICAL AGENTS

Physical agents commonly used to sterilize or reduce the number of bacteria in or on a substance (sanitize) include heat, filtration, radiation and high-frequency sound.

Microorganisms vary in their susceptibility to heat. Two parameters are used to describe these differences: thermal death point is the temperature at which killing occurs, whereas thermal death time is the period of time at a given temperature which is required for killing.

Dry Heat

Dry heat is used to sterilize objects whose structure or use would be affected by moisture, e.g., laboratory glassware. The temperature required for sterilization by dry heat (160 – 170 C) is higher than that necessary for sterilization with moist heat, and the time required (1 – 2 hours) is longer.

Moist Heat

Moist heat, generated in several ways, is the most common means of reducing bacterial numbers, or sterilization. The development and use of pasteurization have done more than any other technique to control many of the common diseases, such as tuberculosis, brucellosis, streptococcal and other infections, acquired by ingestion of contaminated milk or products made from such milk. There are two processes of pasteurization. The high temperature – short time method uses heating at 161 F (72.7C) for 15 seconds. The low temperature holding process requires heating at 145 F (62.8 C) for 30 minutes. Sterilization is not achieved by pasteurization because the process is directed primarily at killing pathogenic bacteria. Pasteurization is designed to use temperatures and time periods that do not affect the nutritional quality or the taste of the product.

Boiling is often used to sterilize instruments used in uncomplicated surgical procedures or to decontaminate materials. Although all vegetative bacteria are killed by boiling, spores of some organisms are resistant.

Fig. 24–14. – Cross section of an autoclave. (From Sokatch, J. R., and Ferretti, J. J.: *Basic Bacteriology and Genetics* [Chicago: Year Book Medical Publishers, Inc., 1976].)

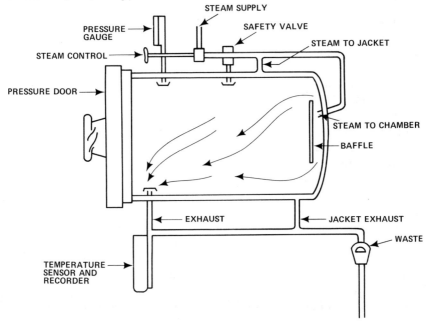

Steam under pressure is the most efficient method of sterilization. With an autoclave (Fig. 24–14), temperatures exceeding 100 C can be reached using saturated steam. The temperature obtained depends on the pressure. For example, at a pressure of 15 pounds per square inch (psi) a temperature of 121 C can be obtained. Autoclaving at 15 psi and 121 C for 15 to 20 minutes is sufficient for sterilization, provided that the objects to be sterilized reach 121 C for 15 to 20 minutes. Indicators such as strips or vials containing spores of *Bacillus stearothermophilus* should be placed in the center of the materials being sterilized to insure that all parts of the material reach the required temperature for the recommended period of time. After sterilization, the spores are placed in a culture medium, incubated, and observed for germination. If growth does not occur, then appropriate conditions were met and sterilization was accomplished.

Heat is commonly used to sterilize surgical drapes, dressings, instruments, bacteriologic media, and for decontamination of materials. Obviously, heat-sensitive materials, e.g., plastics, certain biologicals, cannot be sterilized by the use of heat at high temperatures. Gases and temperature-sensitive liquids are sterilized by filtration, radiation or gaseous sterilization.

Filtration

Thin filters (membrane filters) of cellulose esters manufactured with pore sizes that retain bacteria and fungi (0.22 and 0.45μm pore diameter) are commonly used to remove microorganisms from solutions or various gases (Fig. 24–15). Filters with small pore sizes that will retain viruses can be obtained but are used primarily for experimental or diagnostic purposes. Bacteria can be isolated and counted by using membrane filtration. For example, a known volume of liquid is filtered and the filters are removed and placed on an agar surface. Nutrients from the agar will diffuse into the filter, and the bacteria will grow on the filter surface. If the numbers of bacteria are sufficiently small, isolated colonies will form which can be counted and identified. The membrane filter is the filter type most commonly used today. One advantage is that it can be used to detect low numbers of organisms in large volumes of material.

Other types of filters made from asbestos, diatomaceous earth, porcelain or sintered glass are also in use. These filters retain bacteria in part by pore size but also because of electrical charge in the filter.

Filters referred to as high-efficiency particle accumulators (HEPA) retain more than 99% of microorganisms. These filters are available for sterilizing the air in biologic cabinets used in working with infec-

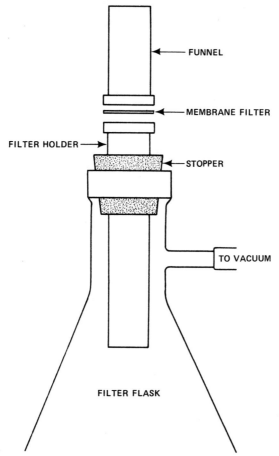

Fig. 24–15. – A membrane filter assembly. (From Sokatch, J. R., and Ferretti, J. J.: *Basic Bacteriology and Genetics* [Chicago: Year Book Medical Publishers, Inc., 1976].)

tious agents and for reducing the bacterial load in certain areas in some hospitals (surgical suites, burn wards, etc.). They are used in combination with monodirected air flowing at a constant rate which is termed laminar flow.

Radiation

Electromagnetic radiation generates rays that are lethal for microorganisms. Ultraviolet light in the range of 250 to 260 nm is used in research and hospital facilities to reduce the number of organisms in air and on surfaces. UV light has low energy and thus penetrates liquids only slightly and does not pass through physical barriers including glass. The lethal effect of UV light is due to formation of thymidine dimers between adjacent thymidine molecules in DNA thereby preventing replication of DNA. In addition to poor penetrability, a further limitation of UV radiation is that microbial cells can be reactivated by light (photoreactivation). Photoreactivation results in cleavage of the thymidine dimer by an enzyme active only in visible light. UV lights have limited lifetimes and should be monitored periodically to insure that the appropriate wavelength is being produced.

Ionizing radiation is also used to sterilize heat-sensitive products such as plastic items, catheters, gloves, and Petri dishes. Gamma rays are most commonly used because of excellent penetration. They have much higher energy than UV rays and cause ionization resulting in the formation of free radicals and the oxidation and reduction of essential molecules.

High-Frequency Sound

Ultrasonic waves at 30–100 kHz kill some microorganisms, but this method is not highly efficient. Organisms vary in sensitivity to ultrasonic sound, and ultrasonic waves are used primarily for cleaning of materials. Sound waves cause cavitation of gas in fluids, which disrupts the cell.

Desiccation and Dilution

Some bacteria do not survive if placed in areas of low humidity. One advantage in airing a room is that the rate of desiccation may be increased. In addition, the number of organisms is reduced by dilution.

Freezing

Some bacteria are killed by a freezing and thawing process but a significant number survive. Low temperatures are excellent ways to preserve bacteria, and lyophilization is used to preserve bacteria for long periods of time. In this process a suspension of organisms is frozen by dry ice and the water removed by evaporation from the frozen state. Microorganisms can be kept almost indefinitely in this state and, upon rehydration, will grow.

Sterilization by Gas

Ethylene oxide, B-propiolactone and formaldehyde (Fig. 24–16) kill bacteria by alkylation of proteins. Ethylene oxide is sporicidal and has good penetration. It is commonly used to sterilize heat-sensitive materials, such as plastics and some equipment, but the process is slow and requires 2–3 hours. Moreover, ethylene oxide is explosive, although it can be obtained premixed with Freon or carbon dioxide,

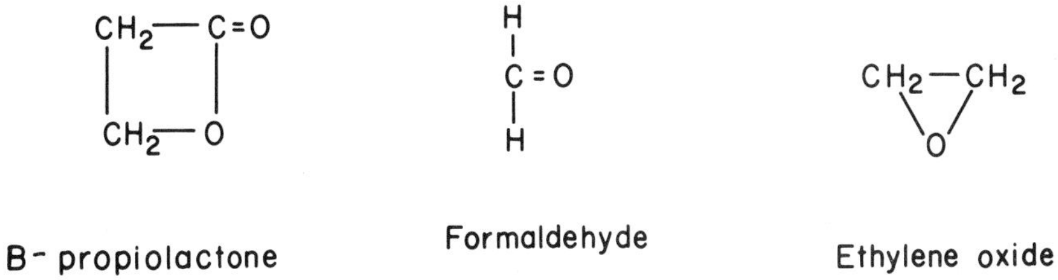

$$CH_2 \!-\! C\!=\!O$$
$$| \qquad |$$
$$CH_2 \!-\! O$$

B- propiolactone

$$H$$
$$|$$
$$C=O$$
$$|$$
$$H$$

Formaldehyde

$$CH_2 \!-\! CH_2$$
$$\diagdown \diagup$$
$$O$$

Ethylene oxide

Fig. 24–16. —Structures of B-propiolactone, formaldehyde and ethylene oxide, three agents used for gaseous sterilization.

thus minimizing the hazard. The gas is a vesicant for skin and mucous membranes, and the sterilized material must be aerated to remove residual gas. Commerical ethylene oxide sterilizers are available. Formaldehyde may also be used for sterilization. However, the gas is irritating to skin and mucous membranes. It polymerizes at room temperature and coats the material being sterilized. Thorough washings and aeration are required before use of the material. B-propiolactone is an effective sporicidal gas with rapid action. It dissipates readily but is toxic for man.

DISINFECTANTS AND ANTISEPTICS

General Principles

The effectiveness of a disinfectant or an antiseptic is governed by many factors, including the number and type of bacteria to be treated and the physical and chemical nature of the material to be treated. For example, liquid materials may require use of high concentrations because of dilution; semisolid or liquid materials require use of chemicals with penetrability. Organic material neutralizes the effect of chemicals such as heavy metals, and anionic agents such as soaps neutralize cationic agents. Many chemical agents do not inactivate spores, and some agents are less effective on organisms with high lipid content. Also, the stability of the agent at high or low pH and at high temperatures determines effectiveness. One must appreciate that antisepsis or disinfection is not accomplished by simply exposing tissue or inanimate objects to a chemical agent. Various interacting factors — environmental, host, bacterial, and the properties of the chemical agent — must be considered in attempting to reduce bacterial numbers to a safe level.

Chemicals used as antiseptics or disinfectants have three basic modes of action on microbial cells. They can interfere with structure and function of protein, alter cell membranes and permeability, or interact with nucleic acid. In many cases more than one mechanism may be involved. For example, the primary effect of phenol is on the cell membrane but phenol also denatures protein.

Protein Structure and Function

Effects on structure and function of proteins may occur via dehydration of proteins, alkylation or oxidation.

Ethanol (50–70%) and isopropanol (90–95%) are used as skin antiseptics. They are not effective against spores. In addition to their denaturing effect on proteins, they affect permeability through lipid solubility. Further, they dilipidate skin and in this way serve to clean skin by a mechanical means.

Other agents—the halogens, organic acids, permanganate, hydrogen peroxide and glutaraldehyde—oxidize proteins and cell membrane components. Chlorine and other chlorine-containing compounds are commonly used to disinfect water. Iodine solutions, alcoholic solutions of iodine (tinctures), and the iodophors are bactericidal agents with variable sporicidal activity. Iodophors are stabilized mixtures of iodine, such as polyvinyl pyrrolidone-iodine, that release iodine over a long period of time. Hydrogen peroxide is not a good antiseptic because it is rapidly decomposed by tissue catalase. Its best attribute may be that the bubbling action releases dirt and necrotic tissue from a wound.

Glutaraldehyde is effective as a disinfecting and sterilizing agent. It is bactericidal and viricidal at room temperature within 10 minutes, and its activity is affected only slightly by organic soil. The stabilized alkaline solution of 2% glutaraldehyde contains a surfactant to promote wetting and an anticorrosive agent. In the stabilized alkaline form, glutaraldehyde retains activity for 28 days.

Compounds that contain mercury and silver inactivate proteins by combining with sulfhydryl groups. These agents are bacteriostatic and they are readily inactivated by tissue fluids or compounds that contain sulfhydryl groups. Silver nitrate (Créde's solution) is used to prevent gonococcal infections of the eyes of newborn. Silver in combination with a sulfonamide is used for treatment of patients with *Pseudomonas*-infected burns.

Cell Membranes

Chemical agents with an effect on cell membranes include surfactants (anionic and cationic detergents), the phenols and chlorhexidine. Anionic detergents (soap and bile salts) are not bactericidal, whereas cationic agents such as the quaternary ammonium compounds and phenol are cidal. Some cationic agents that are good disinfectants are phenol and derivatives (orthophenylphenol, orthocresol and hexa-

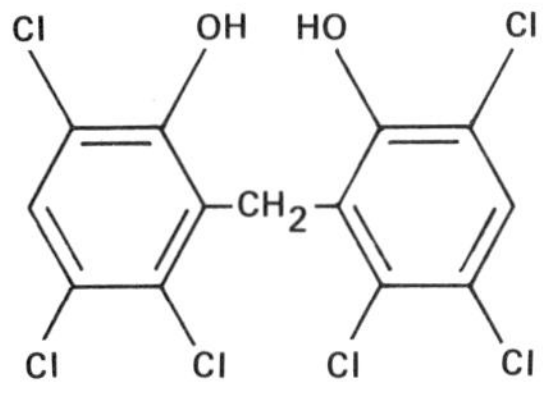

Hexachlorophene 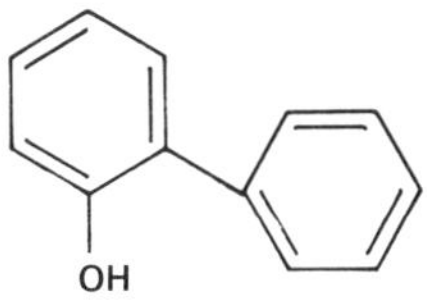   Orthophenylphenol

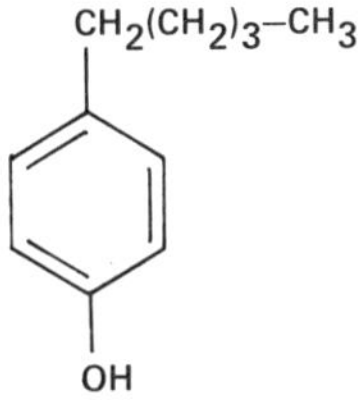

4–n–Amylphenol 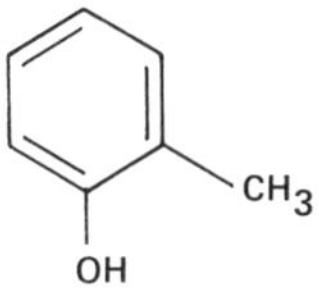   Orthocresol

Fig. 24–17.–Structure of phenolic compounds commonly used as anti-septics and disinfectants. (From Sokatch, J. R., and Ferretti, J. J.: *Basic Bacteriology and Genetics* [Chicago: Year Book Medical·Publishers, Inc., 1976].)

chlorophene) (Fig. 24–17). Hexachlorophene, the most widely used phenol compound, is a chlorinated biphenol and is effective as a dis-infectant and antiseptic. It was routinely used for bathing of newborns as a means of reducing staphylococcal organisms, but its use is now restricted because of the danger of neurotoxicity. Quaternary ammo-nium compounds (Fig. 24–18), such as benzalkonium chloride (Zephiran), cetylpyridinium chloride (Cepryn) and benzethonium chloride (Phemerol), are used as both disinfectants and antiseptics. They are bactericidal for vegetative cells but not for spores or the tu-bercle bacillus. *Pseudomonas* and other gram-negative organisms can survive in contaminated solutions of benzalkonium chloride and serve as a source for infection. These solutions must be routinely

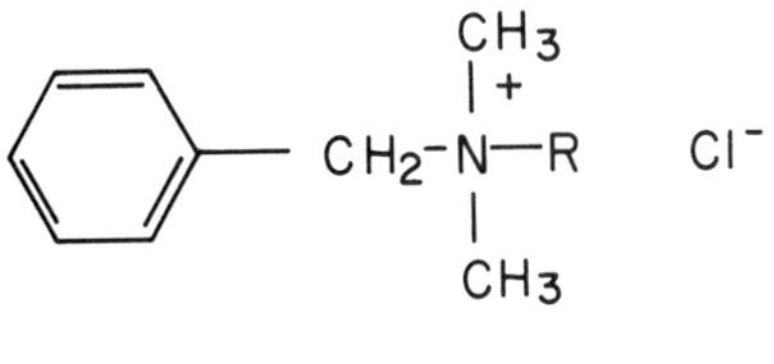

Fig. 24–18.–Benzalkonium chloride, a quaternary ammonium surfactant.

Benzalkonium chloride

changed and the containers adequately cleaned. Chlorhexidine is a biguanide that is not neutralized by soaps, body fluids or other organic compounds. It is used as a surgical scrub and for handwashing.

Nucleic Acid

Many of the dyes such as the triphenylmethane aniline compounds (gentian violet and malachite green), bind to acidic phosphate groups in nucleic acids as well as to proteins. The acridine dyes interfere with synthesis of DNA by intercalating between two successive bases in a DNA strand. Replication results in insertion of an extra base in the complementary strand.

Evaluation of Disinfectants

Disinfectants are usually evaluated by determining the phenol coefficient. Essentially, one determines the concentration of a disinfectant and the concentration of phenol that will kill selected microorganisms. The ratio of the reciprocal of the dilution of disinfectant being tested to phenol is the phenol coefficient (Table 24–3). This test has several drawbacks but does serve as a basis for comparison of disinfectants. However, tests that determine the dilutions which kill bacteria under conditions of use are more meaningful measures of effectiveness.

PROBLEM SOLVING AND REVIEW

GIVEN: When the patient was seen, he complained of diarrhea of 2 days' duration. He had a temperature of 37.8 C. Gram stain of the stool

TABLE 24–3.—PHENOL COEFFICIENT AS A
METHOD OF DETERMINING
EFFECTIVENESS OF CHEMICAL AGENTS

| | | Subculture tubes: 0 = no growth | | |
| | | + = growth | | |
	DILUTIONS	5 MIN	10 MIN	15 MIN
Brand X	1:100	0	0	0
(unknown)	1:125	+	0	0
	1:150	+	0	0
	1:175	+	+	0
	1:200	+	+	+
Phenol	1:90	+	0	0
	1:100	+	+	+

$$\text{Phenol coefficient of X} = \frac{150}{90} = 1.6$$

showed primarily gram-negative rods with a few pus cells. Stool was obtained and sent to the laboratory. *S. typhimurium* was isolated. The white blood cell count and red blood cell count were in the normal range. Chloramphenicol was prescribed, and 2 days after chemotherapy was started the patient developed a rash. Laboratory studies showed that the patient was leukopenic, anemic and had thrombocytopenia. Blood cultures were negative. The chloramphenicol was discontinued and an oral tetracycline was prescribed. The patient continued to have a diarrhea and began to complain of some soreness in the throat. The pharynx and tonsils were covered with a white exudate and were inflamed. Yeasts were found on gram stain of the exudate, and *Candida albicans* was reported on the culture.

PROBLEMS: — 1. What is the diagnosis? 2. Was the treatment appropriate? Why? 3. How do the rash, leukopenia, anemia and thrombocytopenia relate to the disease and/or treatment? 4. What was the rationale for treatment with tetracycline? 5. What caused the final episode of disease? (Ans. p. 463.)

SUPPLEMENTARY READING

Bryceson, A. D. M.: Clinical pathology of the Jarisch-Herxheimer reaction, J. Infect. Dis. 133:696–704, 1976.

Franklin, R. J., and Snow, G. A.: *Biochemistry of Antimicrobial Action* (2d ed.; New York: John Wiley & Sons, Inc., 1975).

Kagan, B. M. (ed.): *Antimicrobial Therapy* (2d ed.; Philadelphia, W. B. Saunders Co., 1974).

Pratt, W. B.: *Chemotherapy of Infection* (New York: Oxford University Press, 1977).

ANALYSIS

1. Gastroenteritis caused by *Salmonella typhimurium*. 2. Except in debilitated persons, chemotherapy is not recommended. It does not alter the course of this disease and it may prolong the carrier state. 3. Chloramphenicol is a toxic antibiotic. It is an inhibitor of protein synthesis and suppresses bone marrow function. 4. There is no rationale. Therapy should not have been continued. 5. Both the chloramphenicol and tetracycline therapy by inhibiting normal flora permitted overgrowth with *Candida* and consequent infection.

Index

465

Pox: rickettsial, 404
Prenatal congenital syphilis,
381–382
B-Propiolactone: structure of, 459
Proteases: *Staphylococcus*, 75
Protein
function
effect of disinfectants and
antiseptics on, 460
synthetic antimicrobial agents
as inhibitors of, 444
structure, effect of disinfectants
and antiseptics on, 460
synthesis, antibiotics as inhibitors
of, 448–451
Proteus, 283–285
antigens, 283–284
characteristics, 283
ecology, 283
infections, 284
laboratory procedures, 285, 286
pathogenicity, 284–285
species, 283
toxins, 283–284
treatment, 285
vulgaris, peritrichous flagella of,
32
Protoplasts, 35–36
Pseudomonas, 311–319
aeruginosa, 312–317
antigens, 313
cell wall, 312–313
enzymes, 313–314
genetics, 313
hemolysins, 313–314
immunity, 316
infections, 314–315
pathogenicity, 315–316
phages, 313
pyocins, 313
structures, 312–313
toxins, 313–314
treatment, 317–318
characteristics, 311
ecology, 312
laboratory procedures, 317–318
overview, 311
problem solving and review, 318
septicemia, skin necrosis in, 314
species, 311–312, 317

Puerperal sepsis: due to
Streptococcus pyogenes, 101
Pulmonary (*see* Lung)
Pus: laboratory procedures, 56
Pyelonephritis: kidney in, 276
Pyocins: *Pseudomonas aeruginosa*,
313

Q

Q fever, 404

R

Radiation, 457–458
Relapsing fever, 387–390
endemic, 389
epidemic, 389
laboratory diagnosis, 390
pathogenicity, 389
prevention, 390
problem solving and review, 395
treatment, 390
Renal (*see* Kidney)
Rheumatic fever: due to
Streptococcus pyogenes, 101
Rickettsia, 397–411
antigens, 400
characteristics, 397–398, 399
control, 408
ecology, 400
genera, 398–399
immunity, 407–408
infections, 401–405
infectivity of, 407
laboratory diagnosis, 408–409
overview, 397
pathogenesis, 405–406
prevention, 408
problem solving and review,
409–410
reservoirs for, 400
serologic tests, 407
species, 399
treatment, 408
vectors for, 400
Rickettsial pox, 404
Rifampin: structure of, 448
Risus sardonicus: in clinical tetanus,
176